MEDICAL
PARASITOLOGY

MEDICAL PARASITOLOGY

By JAMES T. CULBERTSON

ASSISTANT PROFESSOR OF BACTERIOLOGY
COLLEGE OF PHYSICIANS AND SURGEONS
COLUMBIA UNIVERSITY

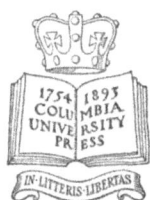

NEW YORK : MORNINGSIDE HEIGHTS

COLUMBIA UNIVERSITY PRESS

1942

PREFACE

THE HUMAN INFECTIONS caused by animal parasites are generally thought of as tropical diseases. Undoubtedly, as a group, they occur most commonly in the tropics, and some of the worst among them have existed there almost exclusively for centuries. But to consider the whole range of these infections as tropical is inaccurate and detracts unfairly from their importance. Many of the disorders for which animal parasites are responsible are serious public health problems the world over, and some have decidedly greater significance in the temperate zones than within the tropics.

Hitherto, comparatively little instruction upon the causes of these parasitic diseases has been offered in the medical schools of this country. But the changing circumstances of modern times require that these agents receive greater attention. It is now appreciated that in the past many cases of parasitic disease occurred among us but were overlooked because of our ignorance concerning them. What is even more important, all of these parasitic infections now seem likely to experience a new and widespread distribution to fresh areas as a consequence of the rise in business and travel which, in large part, air transport has made possible. Workers or travelers returning by airplane from areas long notorious as disease centers may not reveal symptoms of the infections they have contracted until after they have reached home. The chance of the spread of the disease to their relatives and other associates at home is thus enhanced. An added hazard is the transportation, unnoticed, aboard long-distance planes, of infected flies, mosquitoes, fleas, or other disease vectors which remain entirely capable of transmitting the diseases in the regions to which they are carried. Thus the parasitic diseases of the tropics, from which formerly we felt secure, now loom as a potential menace to the health of individuals everywhere. The greatest hope of protection against these dread maladies will come through a more adequate diffusion of knowledge of the agents which cause them.

The present volume offers a simple and brief description of the animal parasites and the diseases they cause. It is intended as a practical work and deals principally with the epidemiology, pathology, diagnosis, treatment, and prophylaxis of the infections for which the acknowledged human parasites are responsible. Details of the parasite morphology and taxonomy, which are of interest chiefly to zoölogists, have been restricted, although enough of these matters is offered, it is believed, to enable the student to identify and differentiate the organisms which are discussed. The book is in no sense designed for the accomplished specialist in the field of tropical medicine, and some information that the specialist might like to find is not included. Nor is the book intended as a research aid, for few references to the large literature are offered. It has been the author's purpose, rather, to supply a small book useful chiefly to medical students and medical practitioners, in which these persons will find a resumé of the significant information upon the animal parasites of medical importance.

The author acknowledges with pleasure the kindness of Professor J. G. Hopkins, Professor J. W. Jobling, Professor H. Smetana, and Mrs. C. R. Hulse of Columbia University, of Dr. J. Y. C. Watt of Cornell University, of Professor Laura Florence of New York Medical College, of Dr. H. Fox of Bellevue Hospital, and of Dr. E. R. Kellersberger of the American Mission to Lepers, in providing certain of the illustrative materials. He is particularly indebted to Mr. Martin Boldt and Mr. Julius Weber of Columbia University for their generous assistance in preparing the photographs. He wishes also to thank Miss Mildred Prinzing of the Columbia University Press, for carefully editing the manuscript, and Mr. J. Pearson Gould, of the Columbia University Press, for his skill in handling the technical problems of production. Finally, to his wife, Louise Barber Culbertson, he expresses his warm appreciation for her constant helpfulness and advice.

JAMES T. CULBERTSON

Columbia University
July 2, 1942

CONTENTS

viii CONTENTS

PLATES

ovale: macrogametocyte; M. Plasmodium falciparum: ring;
N. Plasmodium falciparum: microgametocyte; O. Plasmodium
falciparum: macrogametocyte

bothrium latum: egg; C. Diphyllobothrium mansoni: plerocercoid; D. Taenia solium: mature proglottid; E. Taenia
saginata: egg; F. Taenia solium: scolex; G. Taenia solium:
cysticercus in section of pork muscle; H. Taenia saginata:
gravid proglottid

FIGURES

TABLES

MEDICAL
PARASITOLOGY

Chapter I

INTRODUCTION

ALL ANIMALS are constantly competing with other animals for ultimate survival. This competition goes on not only among the numerous individuals within a single species but also between representatives of different species. Man hunts for certain game animals or even propagates some forms with the express purpose of utilizing their flesh as food for himself. At the same time he must- -in a broad biologic sense—be ever cautious that he himself be not devoured by other animals stronger or more numerous than he.

As a species, man has been eminently successful in overcoming all the animals of the field, forest, and jungle, as well as of the sea, and he no longer holds any of these forms seriously in dread. Certain other species of animal life exist, however, from which man has been much less successful in defending himself. These are the parasitic forms. Although the parasitic animals have no notable physical strength, they are, nevertheless, admirably adapted in one or another respect for survival, usually under the closest possible association with human beings. And, despite the fact that his parasites are feeding upon his own body substance, or upon the food he has ingested for himself, man may be wholly unaware of their presence within or near him. Sometimes, however, he is less fortunate, and suffers prolonged or perhaps eventually fatal torture from an insidious foe from which he cannot free himself.

It is with these parasitic animals that the present volume deals. The more significant forms are individually described, and the various manners by which they establish themselves upon human beings are pointed out. The precise ways in which man is injured by them are concisely stated, as are also the accepted methods of diagnosing the infections. Finally, the steps which man can take to prevent his infection with these parasites are described, together with procedures which have proved effective for eliminating the parasites from those persons already infected. The student is urged to familiarize himself with all these matters.

HISTORY OF INFECTION WITH ANIMAL PARASITES

The sequence of the discovery of animal parasites has reflected roughly the relative size of these forms, the larger ones being first observed and the smaller ones subsequently. With the larger species, human infection was perhaps first known, and only in comparatively recent years has the occurrence of the same or related forms in animals been appreciated. With the microscopic protozoan parasites the opposite situation often obtains. With these, the occurrence of a given type of parasite in animals was frequently first established, and only subsequently was man proved infected with similar forms.

HELMINTHS

Knowledge concerning the largest helminths—for example, *Ascaris lumbricoides* and the tapeworms—had begun to accumulate by the time of the first written records available today. In the Papyrus Ebers, of the sixteenth century B.C., a helminth is mentioned, along with a remedy for infection with it. Some of the teachings of Moses were directed toward protecting the Jews from the helminth parasites in scavenger animals. The "fiery serpent" mentioned in the Old Testament of the Bible is probably the Medina or guinea worm *Dracunculus medinensis,* which still parasitizes man in Egypt, the Near East, and other lands. Furthermore, Hippocrates, as well as other early medical men, recognized hydatid cysts and described methods for their removal, although the relationship of these cysts to tapeworms was not then suspected.

By comparatively recent times, A.D. 1000, beginnings had been made in the classification of the helminth parasites of man which were then known. The celebrated Arabian physician Avicenna recognized four groups: (1) long worms, probably the beef tapeworm *Taenia saginata;* (2) flat worms, probably single proglottids of *Taenia saginata;* (3) small worms, which were perhaps the pinworm *Enterobius vermicularis;* and (4) round worms, probably *Ascaris lumbricoides.* During the seventeenth century, the illustrious Italian, Redi, described practically all the larger helminths even now known to be common human parasites. Furthermore, he formulated the hypothesis that these parasitic forms were distinct species of animal life and were capable of reproducing themselves in a manner quite analogous to that of higher animals. But the task of finally classifying these helminth parasites in a system largely acceptable even to present-day taxonomists had to await the work of the Swedish parasitologist, Rudolphi, during the first years of the nineteenth century.

With the development of the microscope an entirely new world of parasites was opened to discovery, the limits of which have by no means been explored even to the present day. This instrument served not only to reveal the Protozoa, which will be discussed presently, but also the smaller stages of the helminths. Trematode cercariae, for example, were discovered by Müller in 1773, and eggs or other stages of many other parasites were soon found. Gradually, although slowly, the concept of life cycles for these helminths, involving two or even more hosts, was developed.

Trematodes.—The cercariae of trematode parasites were first believed to be protozoans, and only after careful observers pointed out striking homologies with the adult trematodes were the cercariae suspected of being parts of the life cycle of these organisms. A key to the problem was presented in 1818 when cercariae were found coming from certain comparatively shapeless structures (rediae) in snails. But progress was slow, and not until 1882 was the complete trematode life cycle known. The first cycle established was that of *Fasciola hepatica*, the sheep liver fluke, of which the adult had been known since 1379. Many other human trematodes were, meanwhile, discovered. Among the more important of these were: *Fasciolopsis buski*, which was first seen in 1843; *Heterophyes heterophyes* and *Schistosoma haematobium*, which were discovered in 1851; *Clonorchis sinensis*, which was found in 1874; and *Paragonimus westermani*, which was first observed in 1878. Knowledge of the complete life cycles of all these forms, however, awaited the twentieth century.

Cestodes.—The discovery of many of the cestodes dates from early history, as was previously pointed out. The unraveling of their life cycles, however, was a difficult problem requiring many centuries. In 1782 the "heads" from hydatid cyst membranes were shown to be similar structurally to the scolices of the adult taenioid worms. Furthermore, plerocercoids from fish were shown in 1790 to develop to adult tapeworms if fed to birds. The first very significant step toward completing a cestode life cycle, however, was taken in 1851, when cysticerci from a rabbit were fed experimentally to dogs, with the result that adult tapeworms were produced. In the next year, 1852, the hydatid cyst was proved experimentally to be a larval tapeworm, for adult forms developed in the intestine of dogs which were fed cattle hydatid membranes. Ten years later, in 1862, the adult *Taenia saginata* was proved experimentally to develop in man if the cysticercus from beef muscle was ingested. In 1883, man was shown to acquire his pseudophyllidean tapeworm, *Diphyllobothrium latum,* by ingesting a plerocercoid which occurs in the tissue of fresh-water fish. Finally, at the present time, the complete cycles of nearly all the human cestodes have been thoroughly established.

Nematodes.—Some of the larger human nematode parasites, such as *Ascaris lumbricoides* and *Dracunculus medinensis,* and even a few small forms, such as the pinworm *Enterobius vermicularis,* have, like most cestodes, been known since ancient times. Many others, however, are of comparatively recent discovery. *Trichuris trichiura,* for example, was probably discovered during the seventeenth century. *Loa loa* was seen in 1770. *Trichinella spiralis* was first found in human muscle in 1828 and in the muscle of the pig in 1846. The important human hookworm of the Old World, *Ancylostoma duodenale,* was not observed until 1843, and the New World hookworm, *Necator americanus,* was first described in 1902. The microfilariae of a filarial worm, *Wuchereria bancrofti,* were first observed in the blood of man in 1863, and the first adults of this species were found in 1876. *Strongyloides stercoralis* was also first seen in 1876.

Although the life cycle of *Trichinella* was established by 1859, that of most nematode forms was elucidated only very much later. The cycle of the filaria through its mosquito vector was determined by 1879, but its mode of returning to man was not worked out until 1900. The development of *Strongyloides stercoralis* was understood by 1902. The hookworm cycle was experimentally completed in 1897, and the full development of *Ascaris lumbricoides* was finally clarified in 1917.

PROTOZOA

The discovery of the protozoan parasites necessarily awaited the development of the microscope. Leeuwenhoek, the Dutch lens-grinder, probably was the first to discover a parasitic protozoan. In 1681, he observed and described what was probably *Giardia lamblia* in his own feces. Many years passed, however, before other protozoans were shown to be human parasites. A parasitic amoeba, *Endamoeba gingivalis*, was found in the human mouth in 1849. The largest human protozoan, *Balantidium coli*, was observed in a patient's feces in 1857. The very rare species, *Isospora hominis*, was seen in intestinal epithelial cells of man in 1860. But the first protozoan species to be discovered, which was seriously considered to cause disease in man, was *Endamoeba histolytica*. This form was seen in the stool of a patient with dysentery in 1875 and was experimentally introduced into the dog, in which symptoms also were caused. Stages of the human malarial parasites were first found in human blood in 1881, although deeply pigmented organs at autopsy had been for years considered diagnostic of malarial infection. Leishmania were seen in 1900, and a human trypanosome in 1901.

In contrast with the helminths, the life cycles of the protozoan parasites were completely known in most cases within a few years after the parasite was discovered, although the cycles of the leishmanias and some other forms have even now not been elucidated. The complex cycle for the important malarial organisms, however, was determined by 1898, and that of the human trypanosomes by 1909.

The problem of cultivation was an added one in the case of the protozoa. The development of the N.N.N. (Novy, Nicolle, and MacNeal) defibrinated rabbit blood agar medium in 1903 largely solved this problem for the leishmanias and some of the trypanosomes, but cultivation of the intestinal forms had to await the L.E.S. (Locke's solution, egg slant, serum) medium of Boeck and Drbohlav in 1925. This medium was found to serve for cultivating the important intestinal pathogen, *Endamoeba histolytica*, and for most of the other intestinal protozoans as well.

ARTHROPODS AS DISEASE AGENTS AND AS VECTORS

Infection of man by fly larvae has been known since ancient times, as has also the injury caused by stinging, biting, or skin-blistering insects. The first arachnid known to cause a specific human disease was the mite of scabies, *Sarcoptes scabiei*. The effects of this form were described as early as 1687 by Italian investigators, who were doubtless aided in their observations upon such comparatively small organisms by the microscopes which were then being newly developed. In the years since, many other arthropods have been proved capable of infecting man. Early in the twentieth century a paralysis which results from the introduction of venom during the bite of certain ticks was described.

The greater importance of arthropods in medicine lies not in the causation of disease but in the transmission of disease agents. Transmission, in a mechanical sense, by arthropods was long suspected in the case of many pathogens such as the bacteria of plague and the spirochete of yaws. But transmission of a quite different nature—namely, biological transmission—was first proved in 1869 in the case of the dog louse. The larvae of the double-pored tapeworm, *Dipylidium caninum*, were shown then to require development in this insect before the parasite could infect another dog or man. In the same year *Dracunculus medinensis*, the guinea worm, was shown to develop in the body cavity of the copepod, *Cyclops*, which thus served as an intermediate host and vector of the parasite. In 1879, the significance of the mosquito as a vector in filariasis was suggested by Manson, who traced the parasite development in the mosquito thoracic muscle. Subsequently, in 1900, the mode of transmission of this parasite back to man was determined. The female anopheline mosquito was proved the vector of human malaria in 1898. In 1900, a different species of mosquito (*Aëdes aegypti*) was shown to transmit yellow fever and in 1902 to carry dengue fever. The role of fleas in the spread of plague was established by 1908. In 1909 the tsetse fly *Glossina palpalis* was shown to transmit human sleeping sickness in Africa, and a cone-nosed bug, *Triatoma megista*, was found in the same year to transmit the South American trypanosome of Chagas's disease. Also in 1909, lice were proved to transmit typhus fever. In 1912, a tabanid fly, *Chrysops dimidiata*, was proved to be the vector of another filarial worm, *Loa loa*.

The importance of ticks and mites as vectors was first appreciated in 1893, when Theobald Smith proved that Texas cattle fever was spread by a tick. At the same time he showed that the cattle fever ticks transmitted the agent of the disease congenitally to their young. A larval mite was proved to spread tsutsugamushi fever in 1899, and a tick was shown in 1906 to carry the rickettsia of Rocky Mountain spotted fever. A spirochetal disease, relapsing fever, was found in 1904 to be spread by ticks in Africa, although later, in 1907, body lice also were proved capable of spreading this disease in other parts of the world.

CHEMOTHERAPY

When untreated, many parasitic infections endure for years, and some almost invariably end fatally. It is a most fortunate fact, therefore, that for most of these infections specific drugs are known which lead to cure. Sometimes the cures are dramatic and prompt, the parasite being eradicated at once and the symptoms being alleviated very soon.

The treatment of parasitic infection with drugs has a most extended history, with its beginnings in ancient times. An infusion of pomegranate bark was evidently the first substance employed successfully for removing tapeworms, its use being mentioned in the Papyrus Ebers about 1550 B.C. The principal material employed at the present time for eliminating tapeworms—*Aspidium filix-mas*—has also long been known. It was recommended about 300 B.C. by Theophrastus, a student of Aristotle. Many native plants, especially spices and plants rich in oil, were used by the early physicians to eliminate particularly the large intestinal helminths. The first protozoan disease for which a specific therapeutic became available was malaria. The crude bark of the cinchona tree was used for the purpose beginning about 1600, but this was superseded in 1820 by quinine, one of the alkaloid derivatives of the bark.

In recent times, great effort has been expended to perfect drugs which have a powerful action on the parasites but little or no effect on man. Many synthetic parasiticides are now available. For malaria, plasmochin was offered in 1926 and atebrin in 1933. In 1941, promin and sulfadiazine, two derivatives of the sulfonamide series, were also shown to have some antimalarial action. For amoebiasis, emetine was developed in 1912 and yatren in 1921; and for trypanosomiasis, germanin and tryparsamide were produced in 1920 and 1921, respectively. Tartar emetic was tried successfully in 1912 for leishmaniasis and in 1918 for schistosomiasis. The use of thymol for hookworm infection began in 1880, but oil of chenopodium was introduced in 1913, and this was followed by carbon tetrachloride in 1921 and by tetrachlorethylene in 1925. Gentian violet was employed for clonorchiasis in 1927, for strongyloidiasis in 1928, and for enterobiasis in 1938. Tetrachlorethylene was found effective in enterobiasis in 1937 and for tapeworm infection in 1938.

IMMUNITY

The fact that animals can acquire an immunity to a parasite with which they are infected was first proved by Smith and Kilbourne in 1893, in cattle infected with Texas fever. Man also has since been shown to acquire an immunity to amoebiasis and malaria. The immunity in man to these diseases is similar to that in cattle to Texas fever in that the immune state is coexistent with the persistence of the infection in latent form. Thus far, the most significant results of the application of principles of immunity to the parasitic infections of man have been in the diagnosis of disease. Various tests for antibody have been used with success in several important diseases, especially the helminthiases of the somatic tissues. Thus, both complement fixation and precipitin tests were devised in 1906 for hydatid disease, and a skin test was developed in 1911. Complement fixation tests, skin tests, and precipitin tests were developed for human schistosomiasis in 1910, 1927, and 1928, respectively. Precipitin and skin tests were devised for trichiniasis in 1928. Skin tests and fixation tests for filariasis were reported in 1930 and 1931, respectively. With the human protozoan infections, immunological tests have been less useful, although a complement fixation test for amoebiasis was presented in 1927, and agglutination and precipitation tests were devised for leishmaniasis as early as 1913. A promising complement fixation test for malaria was described in 1939.

Recently, investigation has been directed toward developing methods of immunizing man artificially against some human parasites. However, with the exception of work on Oriental sore, indicating that persons previously inoculated in a hidden part with *Leishmania tropica* will thereafter resist infection with this parasite in exposed areas such as the face, the studies on biologic prophylaxis have as yet yielded little. It is, nevertheless, not too much to hope that, when methods are developed for preparing suitable antigens of malaria parasites, of amoebae, and of other important forms, human beings will, through vaccination, be rendered at least relatively resistant to the effects of these organisms and possibly absolutely immune to infection by them.

DEFINITIONS

For adequate comprehension of the information presented in this book, certain terms commonly employed in discussing the parasitic diseases must be clearly defined at once and thoroughly understood by the student. Some of those which will be used most frequently in the text follow:

Parasite.—An organism which feeds in or on another organism, and at the expense of that organism.

Ectoparasite.—A parasite which lives on the skin, hairs, or other outside surface of another organism.

Endoparasite.—A parasite which lives within the body of another organism.

Temporary parasite.—An organism which has a parasitic existence during only part of its life.

Permanent parasite.—An organism which has a parasitic existence throughout its life.

Pathogenic parasite.—A parasite which injures its host to a greater or less degree, usually to an extent sufficient to cause clinical symptoms.

Sporadic or incidental parasite.—A parasite which develops in a species of animal in which it does not naturally dwell.

Host.—An organism which harbors a parasite.

Definitive host.—An organism harboring the sexual (adult) stages of the parasite.

Intermediate host.—An organism harboring the asexual (larval or immature) stages of the parasite. (Some parasites require more than one intermediate host. These hosts are then designated, in order of infection, "first intermediate," "second intermediate," etc.)

Reservoir.—A host, almost universally infected with a given parasite in nature, which is responsible for the endemicity of that parasite in any region.

Carrier.—A host which is responsible for the dissemination of a parasite but which itself manifests no symptoms of infection.

Vector.—An agent of transmission of parasites from one individual (or species) to another.

Mechanical vector.—An agent of transmission in which no development of the parasite occurs.

Biological vector.—An agent of transmission in which the parasite must first develop to a suitable stage which can infect the alternate host.

Infection.—The establishment of a parasite *within* a host, with or without the development of symptoms.

Infestation.—The presence of parasites *externally* upon a host or in the environment.

Prepatent period.—The time between invasion by a parasite and the recovery from the patient of some stage of the parasite development.

Patent period.—The time during which the parasite can be demonstrated in the patient.

Incubation period.—The time between invasion by a parasite and the appearance of clinical symptoms.

Convalescence.—The period from maximal symptoms till recovery.

Latency.—A period usually of considerable length and generally following convalescence when organisms are present but occur in too small number to cause symptoms.

Relapse.—The reappearance of symptoms following a period of latency.

Part One
GENERAL CONSIDERATIONS

Chapter II

INFECTION

SPECIES which observe a parasitic existence are found in all the phyla of the animal kingdom. However, those forms which parasitize man and which are important either as the cause of human disease or as transmitters of human disease agents occur in one of four phyla: Protozoa, Platyhelminthes, Nemathelminthes, and Arthropoda. Representatives of these several phyla may be quite easily identified and differentiated from each other by the following gross characteristics:

Protozoa.—Single-celled organisms.
Platyhelminthes.—Flatworms; alimentary canal, if present, not complete, an anus being absent; body cavity absent.
Nemathelminthes.—Roundworms; alimentary canal usually complete with anus; body cavity present; cilia absent from all stages.
Arthropoda.—Body and appendages encased in a chitinous exoskeleton; appendages jointed.

In each of these four phyla are numerous species of human parasites. Some of the most important ones in each phyla are mentioned in the following simple classification. The morphology of many forms is presented in the appropriate chapter in Part Two of this book.

PROTOZOA

The human protozoan parasites are found in four classes of the phylum Protozoa, which are distinguished by the adaptation of the cells for locomotion. The names of these classes, the means of locomotion, and the human representatives of each class which will be discussed in this book follow:

Class	Characteristics	Representatives
Rhizopoda	Pseudopodia for movement	Endamoeba histolytica Endamoeba coli Endamoeba gingivalis Endolimax nana Iodamoeba williamsi Dientamoeba fragilis
Mastigophora	Flagella for movement	Leishmania donovani Leishmania tropica Leishmania braziliensis Trypanosoma gambiense Trypanosoma rhodesiense Trypanosoma cruzi Giardia lamblia Chilomastix mesnili Trichomonas hominis Trichomonas buccalis Trichomonas vaginalis Embadomonas intestinalis Enteromonas hominis
Sporozoa	No locomotor organ	Plasmodium vivax Plasmodium malariae Plasmodium falciparum Plasmodium ovale Isospora hominis
Ciliata	Cilia for movement	Balantidium coli

PLATYHELMINTHES (FLATWORMS)

The phylum Platyhelminthes contains two classes in which human parasites are found: the class Trematoda (flukes) and the class Cestoda (tapeworms). The two classes are differentiated quite easily by the character of segmentation and by the presence or absence of a simple food tube. The trematodes are not segmented and have a simple food tube. The cestodes are segmented forms and lack even vestiges of such an alimentary tract. Some of the more important human trematodes and cestodes, which will later be described, follow:

Class	Characteristics	Representatives
Trematoda (flukes)	Simple food tube, ending blindly; body not segmented	Schistosoma haematobium Schistosoma mansoni Schistosoma japonicum Fasciolopsis buski Fasciola hepatica Clonorchis sinensis Paragonimus westermani Heterophyes heterophyes Metagonimus yokogawai Gastrodiscoides hominis
Cestoda (tapeworms)	No food tube; body segmented	Diphyllobothrium latum Diphyllobothrium mansoni Taenia solium Taenia saginata Echinococcus granulosus Hymenolepis nana Hymenolepis diminuta Dipylidium caninum

NEMATHELMINTHES (ROUNDWORMS)

The roundworms of the phylum Nemathelminthes comprise three classes: Nematoda (threadworms), Gordiacea (hairworms), and Acanthocephala (spiny-headed worms).[1] These classes, of which the species to be discussed later are named, may be differentiated by the following characteristics:

Class	Characteristics	Representatives
Nematoda	Intestine complete with anus in adult	Trichinella spiralis Trichuris trichiura Strongyloides stercoralis Necator americanus Ancylostoma duodenale Enterobius vermicularis Ascaris lumbricoides Dracunculus medinensis

[1] For many years the acanthocephalan parasites have been considered a class in the phylum Nemathelminthes. At present, many authorities feel these organisms are more closely related to the flatworms. There are some similarities to the cestodes in morphology and life cycle as well as in antigenic constitution.

Class	Characteristics	Representatives
Nematoda	Intestine complete with anus in adult	Wuchereria bancrofti Microfilaria malayi Loa loa Acanthocheilonema perstans Mansonella ozzardi Onchocerca volvulus
Gordiacea	Intestine incomplete or atrophied in adult	Gordius sp.
Acanthocephala	Intestine absent; protrusible organ for attachment armed with recurred spines	Macracanthorhynchus hirudinaceus Moniliformis moniliformis

ARTHROPODA

The phylum Arthropoda contains a very large number of human disease agents or vectors of such agents. These are found in four classes of the phylum: Hexapoda, Arachnida, Crustacea, and Myriapoda. Members of these classes are differentiated by the number of their legs and by several other characteristics, as stated below. A few representatives of each class are listed.

Class	Characteristics	Representatives
Hexapoda	Three pairs of legs; one pair of antennae; wings often present; respiration by trachea	Aëdes aegypti (yellow-fever mosquito) Anopheles quadrimaculatus (malaria mosquito) Culicoides austeni (gnat) Eusimulium damnosum (black fly) Chrysops dimidiata (horsefly) Glossina palpalis (tsetse fly) Musca domestica (housefly) Pediculus humanus (human louse) Xenopsylla cheopis (tropical rat flea)
Arachnida	Four pairs of legs; antennae absent; wings absent; res-	Sarcoptes scabiei (itch mite) Trombicula akamushi (harvest mite)

Class	Characteristics	Representatives
Arachnida	piration usually by trachea	Dermacentor andersoni (hard tick) Ornithodorus moubata (soft tick) Latrodectes mactans (black widow spider) Centruroides suffusus (scorpion)
Crustacea	Five pairs of legs; two pairs of antennae; wings absent; respiration by gills	Cyclops sp. (copepod) Astacus sp. (crayfish) Potamon sp. (crab)
Myriapoda	Many pairs of legs; one pair of antennae; wings absent; respiration by trachea	Scolopendra heros (centipede)

PORTALS OF ENTRY AND SITES OF FINAL RESIDENCE OF PARASITES IN MAN

Man becomes infected with animal parasites either by swallowing the infective stage or else by having the infective stage pass through his skin. Most intestinal infections result from swallowing the appropriate stage of the organism, usually along with food or drink. Sometimes the ingested parasite is not free but enclosed in the body of an alternate host such as an arthropod. When these alternate hosts are swallowed, man becomes infected with the parasites they carry.

The parasites of the blood are transmitted by bloodsucking arthropods. These vectors either inoculate the parasites they carry beneath the skin of man or else provide a skin wound through which the parasite may effect its own entrance. A few parasites can penetrate the intact human skin even without assistance from an arthropod vector.

Additional routes of infection are known. For example, mouth parasites may pass directly from mouth to mouth during kissing. Infection may pass congenitally from mother to young, at least when the placenta is in some way damaged. Some parasites are transmitted between male and female during sexual intercourse.

Parasites are occasionally found in strange or unexpected sites, but most species have a characteristic site—or type of site—in the hu-

TABLE 1

THE ROUTE OF INFECTION, FINAL SITE OF RESIDENCE, AND CHIEF EFFECTS OF THE PRESENCE OF IMPORTANT PARASITES IN MAN

Parasite	Infective Stage	Portal of Entry (via animal transmitter, if any)	Final Site of Residence	Effects in Man
Endamoeba histolytica	cyst	mouth	large intestine, liver, other tissues	dysentery, colitis, abscess
Giardia lamblia	cyst	mouth	small intestine, gall bladder	possibly local inflammation
Trypanosoma gambiense	trypanosome	skin (via tsetse fly)	blood, lymphatics, brain	lymphadenitis; encephalitis
Trypanosoma cruzi	trypanosome	skin (via cone-nosed bug)	blood, striated muscle, brain, other tissue	lymphadenitis; myositis
Leishmania donovani	leptomonas ?	skin (via sand fly)	spleen, liver, skin	reticulo-endotheliosis, fever
Leishmania tropica	leptomonas ?	skin (via sand fly)	skin	ulcers of skin
Leishmania braziliensis	leptomonas ?	skin (via sand fly)	skin, membranes of nose, mouth	ulcers of nose, mouth
Plasmodium vivax	sporozoite	skin (via anopheline mosquito)	erythrocytes, spleen, liver, brain	anemia, periodic fever (48-hr.)
Plasmodium malariae	sporozoite	skin (via anopheline mosquito)	erythrocytes, spleen, liver, brain	anemia, periodic fever (72-hr.)
Plasmodium falciparum	sporozoite	skin (via anopheline mosquito)	erythrocytes, spleen, liver, brain	anemia, periodic fever (48-hr.), blackwater
Balantidium coli	cyst	mouth	large intestine	colitis
Schistosoma haematobium	cercaria	skin	pelvic plexuses	cystitis

Parasite	Infective Stage	Portal of Entry (via animal transmitter, if any)	Final Site of Residence	Effects in Man
Schistosoma mansoni	cercaria	skin	mesenteric veins	cirrhosis; papillomata in intestine
Schistosoma japonicum	cercaria	skin	mesenteric veins	cirrhosis; papillomata in intestine
Fasciolopsis buski	metacercaria	mouth	small intestine	local inflammation
Clonorchis sinensis	metacercaria	mouth (via fish)	bile ducts, liver	cirrhosis; inflammation of bile ducts
Paragonimus westermani	metacercaria	mouth (via crab)	lung	cysts along bronchioles
Diphyllobothrium latum	plerocercoid	mouth (via fish)	small intestine	enteritis; anemia (?)
Taenia solium	cysticercus	mouth (via pig)	small intestine	enteritis; secondary cysticercosis
Taenia saginata	cysticercus	mouth (via cow)	small intestine	enteritis
Echinococcus granulosus	egg	mouth	somatic tissue	pressure; anaphylaxis if ruptured
Trichinella spiralis	larva	mouth (via pig)	small intestine, striated muscle	enteritis; myositis
Trichuris trichiura	egg	mouth	small intestine	enteritis
Enterobius vermicularis	egg	mouth	large and small intestine	enteritis; nervous upset; *pruritus ani*
Necator americanus	larva	skin	small intestine	"ground itch"; anemia; digestive upset
Ascaris lumbricoides	egg	mouth	small intestine	enteritis; duct obstruction
Strongyloides stercoralis	larva	skin	small intestine	enteritis
Wuchereria bancrofti	larva	skin (via *Culex* mosquito)	lymphatics	lymphangitis, elephantiasis
Loa loa	larva	skin (via tabanid fly)	subcutaneous tissue	calabar swellings
Onchocerca volvulus	larva	skin (via black fly)	subcutaneous tissue	fibrous modules in subcutaneous tissue
Dracunculus medinensis	larva	mouth (via copepod)	subcutaneous tissue	ulcers in skin

man body and are generally found in that location.[2] For example, adult tapeworms are restricted to the intestinal lumen and are not found in any of the somatic tissues. The malarial parasites, on the other hand, are blood forms which, so far as is known, never appear in the intestinal lumen. Nevertheless, some animal parasites seem able to develop in many locations. Thus, the hydatid cyst is usually found in the liver but may develop in the lung, spleen, kidney, brain, muscle, or bone and has been reported in the orbit. Likewise, the pathogenic amoebae are usually found in the intestinal wall, but lesions have been demonstrated in the liver, spleen, lung, kidney, brain, and skin. In Table 1, the typical portals of entry and final locations in man of the most important human parasites are given.

EFFECT OF PARASITES ON MAN

Some parasites cause essentially no damage to the human host. Certain forms—for example, trichomonads and amoebae—may reside in the mouth or the intestinal tract for years and elicit no symptoms at any time. Other species, however, cause the most profound effects, even death. For example, infection with the African trypanosomes leads invariably to death in untreated cases, and death is a common end of infection with the malignant malarial parasite *Plasmodium falciparum*. Between these extremes lie the majority of human parasites, some damage generally resulting from their presence and some symptoms generally developing.

The symptoms seen in a patient infected with an animal parasite depend largely on the kind of parasite involved and especially on the tissues or organs invaded. Dysentery may be seen following infection with *Endamoeba histolytica* or with other intestinal forms. Occasionally, intestinal parasites perforate the gut wall and peritonitis ensues. A myositis follows infection with *Trichinella spiralis,* which invades the skeletal muscle. A given parasite may be essentially harmless in one site but in another may cause extensive or serious damage. For example, the adult of *Taenia solium* in the intestinal lumen is of little concern, but if the larval forms of the same worm are carried to the brain, grave symptoms may be noted, which cannot easily, if at all,

---

[2] Parasites which dwell in the intestinal lumen are often called entozoic; those in the body cavity, celozoic; those of the blood, hematozoic; those of the cells, cytozoic; and those within nuclei, karyozoic.

be relieved. If a parasite blocks the duct of a gland, marked symptoms may result. Thus, a hydatid cyst may obstruct the bile duct and jaundice may result, or *Wuchereria bancrofti* may block lymph channels and elephantiasis of the part drained by the channel may develop. Appendicitis sometimes follows obstruction of the appendix by *Ascaris lumbricoides.*

Forms such as leishmanias and malarial parasites, which dwell in the blood-forming organs or the blood stream, cause severe anemia. Even the intestinal hookworms cause an anemia. These forms actually open the smaller vessels of the intestinal wall and blood escapes into the intestinal lumen.

In addition to these rather general forms of damage, certain parasites impair the function of specific organs. Thus the use of the eye is often lost in onchocerciasis or when cestode cysts develop in the eye. The nose and the soft palate are eroded away by the leishmanias in espundia. A "creeping eruption" of the skin follows infection with larval *Ancylostoma braziliense* or with the maggots of *Dermatobia hominis.*

ADAPTATIONS OF PARASITES FOR INFECTING THEIR HOSTS

Every human parasite is adapted in some manner for survival in man, else its prolonged residence in him would be impossible. With some, the adaptation is apparently passive, involving chiefly the capacity of the parasite to resist the digestive enzymes of the host or the antagonistic action of its blood and defensive cells. Other parasites, however, have adaptations for infection of a more active order. For example, *Endamoeba histolytica* can invade the colon wall because it elaborates a lysin which digests away the intestinal epithelium. Likewise, the schistosome cercariae can penetrate the skin because they possess cephalic glands whose secretion lyses a path into that tissue.

The larger intestinal worms generally have hold-fast organs by which they remain attached. Thus the flukes have a pair of muscular suckers, and the tapeworms have either sucking grooves or suckers and often hooklets as well on their scolex. Even the embryos of the tapeworms are equipped with spines which enable them to catch on to and penetrate the intestinal wall after escaping from the ingested egg. The intestinal nematodes are less obviously equipped with organs of attachment to maintain their position in the intestinal lumen. The hookworms, however, have a buccal capsule armed with teeth or plates by which they fix themselves to the tissue of the wall.

Some forms are adapted not so much by structure as by their tropisms to infect their hosts. Thus, hookworm larvae in the soil generally rise to the top of the soil (negative geotropism) where they will be more likely to contact human skin. Furthermore, these same larvae, as well as those of other helminths and also of insects (*Dermatobia hominis*), are attracted to the warm human skin (positive thermotropism). One of the nicest adaptations of parasites is seen with two species of filarial worms, *Wuchereria bancrofti* and *Loa loa*, which are, respectively, transmitted biologically by two insects, *Culex fatigans*, which is a night-biting mosquito, and *Chrysops dimidiata*, which is a day-biting fly. The parasite adaptation lies in its appearing in the peripheral blood of the human only during those parts of the twenty-four-hour day during which its potential arthropod vector bites man.

Chapter III

EPIDEMIOLOGY

THE INCIDENCE of infection with any human parasite in a given community depends on the availability of susceptible hosts, a satisfactory means of transmission, and an environment favorable to those stages of the parasite which must exist or develop outside the host body. These environmental factors are largely responsible for the geographic distribution of many species of parasites. When the several factors which govern the transmission of parasites are so correlated that the parasite is able constantly to maintain itself in the community yet is restrained from making unusual inroads upon the population at large, the infection may be said to be endemic in that region. If conditions are altered so that the parasite gains the ascendency and large numbers of people suddenly become infected and suffer from its effects, then the infection is said to be epidemic in that community.

SUSCEPTIBLE HOSTS

Susceptibility to infection with animal parasites depends on many factors. Some of these are intrinsic in the host, such as its genetic constitution and age (natural resistance) and its previous exposure to the same infectious agent (acquired immunity). Further factors, such as living conditions, occupation, clothing, education, and customs, also contribute toward probable infection or freedom from infection with a given parasite. In some cases, animals are present which can substitute for man as the vertebrate reservoir in the parasite life cycle. The parasite can, then, propagate itself through the animal when susceptible humans are not available.

NATURAL RESISTANCE

As is indicated in Chapter IV below, man is absolutely resistant to many parasites of lower animals. Likewise, some human parasites are unable to infect any vertebrate besides man. A few forms, such as malarial parasites and the hookworms, develop better in persons of the white race than in Negroes, and some parasites are able to infect only younger individuals of any race. When persons of susceptible race and age are absent from a community, the chance for the transmission of that parasite in that area is severely reduced.

ACQUIRED IMMUNITY

Often as a result of infection with a given parasite, persons acquire an immunity which protects them from subsequent infection with the same organism. When essentially the entire population has been thus immunized, the parasite encounters difficulty in maintaining itself in that community. On the other hand, if a parasite is introduced into a community where it has not occurred previously, the entire population may be particularly susceptible and for a time thereafter the parasite may occur epidemically among the inhabitants. Such epidemics are often seen when a new strain of malarial organism is freshly introduced into a community.

CARRIERS

Persons who have recovered from parasitic infection frequently remain carriers of the causal organism. Such individuals may themselves show no symptoms whatsoever, but they are able, through transmitting appropriate stages of the parasite, ultimately to lead to active infection in other persons. The percentage of carriers of an organism represents the level of endemicity of that parasite in any given community. Carriers exist for all parasites. Human carriers are important in the transmission of amoebiasis, malaria, filariasis, enterobiasis, and hookworm disease. Occasionally the carrier experiences a relapse of the infection that he harbors.

Not only human beings but also many other vertebrates serve as carriers of some human parasites.[1] The human leishmanias may be

---

[1] A distinction is drawn between an animal carrier and an animal alternate host in this connection. The carrier is one which substitutes for man. The alternate host is one which harbors stages of the parasite different from those found in man.

carried by dogs, and the human pathogenic amoeba is sometimes found in the *Macacus* monkey, although this animal is probably only rarely the source of human infection. The African trypanosomes of man dwell in antelopes and domesticated animals, as well as in the human, and the trypanosome of Chagas's disease usually lives in the armadillo or opossum rather than in man. *Balantidium coli* generally dwells in the pig. The sheep and many other forms serve as animal carriers of *Echinococcus granulosus* in place of man, and the dog carries *Dipylidium caninum*, which, indeed, man only occasionally harbors. Many fish-eating mammals besides human beings carry *Diphyllobothrium latum* as well as the trematode *Clonorchis sinensis*. Another trematode, *Paragonimus westermani*, occurs in several animals besides man which eat crayfish or crabs. The human nematode *Trichinella spiralis* is normally carried by rats or pigs.

OTHER FACTORS

Even when individuals are susceptible to infection with a given parasite, they may not harbor it. The possible reasons for their freedom from the infection are many. Sometimes the parasite does not occur in the geographic area where the person dwells. The employment of the individual may not be of a kind to expose him to the parasite. For example, rice-field workers in endemic areas of the Orient are almost certain to have schistosomiasis, whereas persons who work in urban centers in the Orient probably will not contract this disease. *Balantidium coli* occurs chiefly among pig-raisers. Sometimes the wearing of clothing prevents infection. For example, hookworm disease is often prevented by the wearing of shoes. Certain foods transmit parasites. Those persons who consume raw fish or raw meat, for example, are especially likely to harbor such parasites as *Diphyllobothrium latum*, *Taenia saginata*, or *Trichinella spiralis*, which these foods transmit. Some religious practices expose persons unduly. For example, bathing in sacred pools in India may lead to schistosomiasis, hookworm disease, amoebiasis, or infection with other parasites spread through water contaminated with feces. Other religious teachings, on the other hand, may essentially prevent the spread of certain parasites. For example, Mohammedans and Jews are instructed to avoid eating pork, through which *Taenia solium* and *Trichinella spiralis* are conveyed. Hindus, who hold the cow sacred, seldom harbor *Taenia saginata*. The heavy infection with schistosomiasis among Egyptians along the Nile valley is explained by the habit of many of these people of entering water for purposes of defecation or micturition.

Perhaps more than any other factor, the educational level of a community determines the parasite burden, for improved education is usually accompanied by greater cleanliness and a general improvement in living conditions. More than anything else, from a public health point of view, education implies instruction in the proper disposition of human body wastes, through which many parasites are disseminated. Indeed, if the water and the food of man can be protected from fecal contamination, the incidence of infection with intestinal protozoans particularly, and of some other parasites as well, will be sharply reduced.

MEANS OF TRANSMISSION

Parasites are spread from one person to another (1) directly, (2) indirectly, or (3) through an animate vector. Vectors may have merely a mechanical role, possibly through transporting the parasite to a location where infection of man is more likely to occur. In some cases, however, the vector plays a biological role, and the parasite must experience development in the body of the vector before it can cause infection in the next individual.

DIRECT TRANSMISSION

A few parasites are transmitted directly from one person to another. The amoeba (*Endamoeba gingivalis*) and the trichomonad (*Trichomonas buccalis*) of the human mouth are spread in this manner. It is possible that the leishmanias of Oriental sore or espundia also are directly passed through contact. *Trypanosoma gambiense* and *Trichomonas vaginalis* are said to be transmitted directly in sexual intercourse. One of the few helminth parasites transmitted directly from one person to another is the pinworm *Enterobius vermicularis*.

INDIRECT TRANSMISSION

Many parasites, in passing from one person to another, dwell for an interval of indefinite length outside the host body. This is seen especially among intestinal parasites. These forms are generally adapted for their residence outside the body through their capacity to produce stages resistant to the outside environment. The intestinal protozoa usually form encysted stages. The helminths form eggs enclosed in shells. When these cysts or eggs are later ingested along with food or drink by another person, the organisms resume their parasitic life and lead to the infection of that individual. Such transmission is seen with all the intestinal protozoa (except *Dientamoeba fragilis* and *Trichomonas hominis*), as well as with such nematodes as *Enterobius vermicularis*, *Ascaris lumbricoides*, and *Trichuris trichiura*. Usually with the helminths, some development must first go on outside the body before the organism can produce infection. With some species, following such development, infection can occur either by mouth or percutaneously, as with the hookworms.

BIOLOGIC TRANSMISSION BY ANIMATE VECTORS

A large number of parasites are transmitted biologically by animate vectors. These are often blood and fixed-tissue parasites, but many intestinal forms which require an alternate host may also properly be said to employ this host as a biologic vector.

Malarial organisms are probably the best-known parasites which require a vector. They are transmitted in anopheline mosquitoes. The human trypanosomes of Africa develop in tsetse flies, and the South American trypanosome is spread by a cone-nosed bug. Trematodes require development in a mollusk, snails being used by the trematodes of man. Some species of trematode, such as *Clonorchis sinensis* and *Paragonimus westermani*, must, subsequently to their development in the snail, become encysted on fish, crayfish, or other animals, which thus act as second intermediate hosts. Cestodes often require development in an alternate mammal. For example, *Taenia saginata* develops as a cysticercus in cattle, *Taenia solium* as a cysticercus in pigs, and *Echinococcus granulosus* reaches its adult stage not in man but in the dog. Some tapeworms (e.g., *Dipylidium caninum*) develop in insects which must later be swallowed. One species, *Diphyllobothrium latum*, requires two intermediate hosts—the crustacean *Cyclops* and fresh-water fish. Certain nematode parasites likewise require alternate hosts for transmission. For example, *Wuchereria bancrofti* is spread by *Culex* mosquitoes, *Loa loa* by tabanid flies, and *Onchocerca volvulus* by black flies. The guinea worm, *Dracunculus medi-*

nensis, is spread through the crustacean *Cyclops.* The rare acantho-cephalan parasites of man usually dwell as larvae in the grubs of beetles, and human infection occurs when the infected grub is accidentally swallowed.

MECHANICAL TRANSMISSION BY ANIMATE VECTORS

As indicated earlier in this section, many vectors act merely as mechanical transmitters of parasites. Thus, flies which visit human fecal deposits may transport on their feet or body protozoal cysts or helminth eggs which eventually are deposited on human food stores or on food about to be consumed by man. Sometimes these cysts or eggs even survive passage through the fly intestine.

Bloodsucking arthropods may, under unusual circumstances, also act as mechanical transmitters of blood protozoa which normally experience biological transmission. If a mosquito or tsetse fly is interrupted while feeding on an infected person, it will usually try to complete its blood meal at once on the next available individual. If viable organisms remain on the mouth parts of the mosquito or fly, these may be introduced when it bites the second person, and infection will then ensue without development of the parasite in the body of the insect.

THE GEOGRAPHICAL DISTRIBUTION OF PARASITES (ENVIRONMENTAL FACTORS)

Unless an individual comes in contact with an infective stage of a parasite, he cannot contract infection with that form. The distribution of some parasites is, however, essentially cosmopolitan, and adequate contact for potential infection is assured at some time in the life of nearly everyone. Other forms, however, are so sharply restricted in distribution and by the circumstances of their transmission that little possibility of infection exists unless the individual visits the precise areas where the parasite is endemic.

The reasons for the restriction in distribution of parasites are various. Often temperature or climate is an important factor. Hookworms, for example, require warm moist soil for their development to the infective larval stage. Very often, however, the presence of a suitable vector appears to be the most serious limiting factor. The human trypanosomes of Africa occur only in that continent probably because the tsetse flies are restricted to that part of the world. Likewise, the human trematodes of the Orient have never come to the Western world evidently because suitable snail hosts for these parasites are not found in this area. But, even given adequate environmental conditions and suitable vectors, some parasites are nevertheless absent from certain localities. This can often be explained by the fact that the parasite itself has not been introduced or, if introduced, has died out. This circumstance is known to be responsible for the absence of even so common an affliction as malaria from some of the smaller South Sea islands.

In Table 2 the geographic distribution of most of the important parasites is indicated. In the chapters of Part Two of this book the distribution of each form is more precisely stated.

TABLE 2

THE GEOGRAPHICAL DISTRIBUTION OF IMPORTANT HUMAN PARASITES [a]

Parasite	North America			West Indies	Central America	South America				Europe						Africa					Asia					Japan	Philippine Islands	East Indies	Australia
	CANADA	UNITED STATES	MEXICO	West Indies	Central America	VENEZUELA	BRAZIL	ARGENTINA	PERU	SCANDINAVIA	RUSSIA	GERMANY	BALKANS	ITALY	IBERIAN PENINSULA	NORTH COAST	EGYPT	NIGERIA	CONGO	RHODESIA	SIBERIA	NEAR EAST	INDIA	CHINA	SOUTHEAST ASIA	JAPAN	PHILIPPINE ISLANDS	EAST INDIES	AUSTRALIA
Leishmania donovani											+		+	+	+	+	+	+			+	+	+	+					
Leishmania tropica			+								+					+		+	+			+	+		+				+
Leishmania braziliensis				+	+	+	+	+	+																				
Trypanosoma gambiense																		+	+										
Trypanosoma rhodesiense																				+									
Trypanosoma cruzi		+	+		+	+	+																						
Plasmodium ovale													+		+			+	+			+					+		
Schistosoma haematobium																+	+	+	+	+		+					+		
Schistosoma mansoni				+		+	+										+	+	+										
Schistosoma japonicum																								+		+	+	+	
Paragonimus westermani																							+	+	+	+	+		

Species												
Fasciolopsis buski	+					+	+	+		+		+
Clonorchis sinensis							+	+	+	+	+	
Heterophyes heterophyes				+			+	+	+	+	+	+
Metagonimus yokogawai			+		+		+	+	+			
Gastrodiscoides hominis							+	+	+			
Diphyllobothrium latum	+		+	+		+	+	+	+		+	
Diphyllobothrium mansoni	+						+	+	+	+	+	+
Echinococcus granulosus	+	+	++	++	+	+	+	+	+	+	+	+
Necator americanus	+	+	++		+	+	+	+	+	+	+	+
Ancylostoma duodenale	+	++	++		+	+	+	+	+	+	+	+
Wuchereria bancrofti	+	++	+	+	+	+	+	+	+	+	+	+
Loa loa		+	+	+								
Acanthocheilonema perstans	+	++	+	+	+						+	
Onchocerca volvulus	+	+	++	+								
Dracunculus medinensis		+	+	+	+	+	+	+	+	+		+

a Species having essentially cosmopolitan distribution: intestinal amoebae, intestinal flagellates, *Plasmodium vivax*, *Plasmodium malariae*, *Plasmodium falciparum*, *Balantidium coli*, *Fasciola hepatica*, *Taenia solium*, *Taenia saginata*, *Hymenolepis nana*, *Dipylidium caninum*, *Trichinella spiralis*, *Trichuris trichiura*, *Strongyloides stercoralis*, *Enterobius vermicularis*, and *Ascaris lumbricoides*. Some of these forms (e.g., *Plasmodium falciparum*) are largely confined to the tropics and warmer parts of the temperate zones.

Chapter IV

NATURAL RESISTANCE AND ACQUIRED IMMUNITY

THE MODES of resistance to infection of which an individual is capable represent forces which parasites must overcome before they can establish themselves in that person. Against most forms of parasitic life (e.g., those parasites which occur exclusively in lower animals) human beings are by nature entirely resistant. Often, however, this natural resistance is only slowly developed as the person matures, and it may be lacking in the young child. To other parasites (e.g., those which are primarily human parasites) man never becomes naturally resistant but throughout life remains susceptible to infection on initial exposure. In some of these cases, the infected person acquires, as a direct result of his first infection, a specific immunity which protects him against a subsequent infection with the same species of parasite. The factors which govern the natural resistance and the acquired immunity of man against animal parasites are discussed in the present chapter.[1]

NATURAL RESISTANCE

Although all persons are naturally exposed to a broad variety of parasites, actual infection is experienced with but few species. The failure of some parasites to establish themselves in man has been shown to be due to the antagonistic effects of special defensive mechanisms—a few of which are mentioned later in this chapter—which man brings naturally to bear upon these parasites. Sometimes, however,

[1] Information upon natural resistance and acquired immunity in infections of both man and other animals is summarized in W. H. Taliaferro, *The Immunology of Parasitic Infections*, New York, Century Co., 1929, and in J. T. Culbertson, *Immunity against Animal Parasites*, New York, Columbia University Press, 1941.

merely the body temperature, the age or diet, or other aspects of human physiology seem to account for insusceptibility. When no unfavorable factor exists, man is usually susceptible to infection since he then supplies an adequate physiological environment for the parasite development.

HOST-PARASITE RELATIONSHIPS

Many parasites cause little or no damage to the persons they invade and are able to propagate themselves and eventually reach new hosts with ease so that the parasite species will be indefinitely perpetuated. Such a host-parasite relationship represents a quite satisfactory condition of balance. It is seen particularly among human infections with the intestinal flagellates, the group of nonpathogenic amoebae, and even with some of the larger intestinal worms, such as *Taenia saginata*.

Very commonly, however, such perfect balance is not attained, and either the host or the parasite survives to the serious detriment of the other. If *Trypanosoma equiperdum,* which causes dourine of the horse, be injected in man, for example, no infection whatsoever results, for man is completely resistant to this parasite. The same organism inoculated to the rat, however, will kill the rat in about five days with no opportunity for transmission to new hosts. In neither man nor the rat, then, could this parasite possibly perpetuate itself. In the horse, however, in which the parasite occurs normally, the organism causes an infection which, although eventually fatal, is so prolonged that the natural transmission of the parasite to new hosts is generally assured.

Some parasites experience abnormal or incomplete development in strange hosts. If the infective larvae of the hookworms of dogs enter the skin of man, for example, they do not invade the deeper tissues or eventually reach maturity in the intestinal lumen as they would in the dog, but they remain undeveloped and are confined to the skin sometimes for years, where they cause a form of "creeping eruption."

Usually, parasites which cause severe or fatal infections in man may be considered poorly adjusted or even abnormal parasites for the human host. Often, as with *Trypanosoma rhodesiense,* they are known to have been acquired only recently—in an evolutionary sense—by the human species. Forms which have been known as human parasites since ancient times, on the other hand, generally cause little damage to man. As a result of their long association with man, these older forms seem either to have lost their pathogenicity for him, or else man, possibly by a process of elimination of the more susceptible individuals, has as a species become better able to cope with the invading parasite.

RANGE OF HOST SUSCEPTIBILITY

Some parasites characteristically infect a variety of taxonomically widely dispersed species of host. Others are confined to a few closely related hosts or even to a single host species. Usually, where both man and lower animals are infected by the same parasite, the course of the infection is essentially similar in all hosts. The experimental study of the infection is then greatly facilitated. When no experimental animal is known for a given human parasite, knowledge of the infection caused by that parasite is generally greatly limited.

Parasites with narrow host range.—The human parasites with narrowest host range are found, among the Protozoa, in the class Sporozoa, and, among the helminths, in the classes Cestoda and Nematoda. Among the sporozoans, all of the human malarial parasites are naturally restricted to man alone, and in no other animal does any species cause an infection equivalent to that in man. Furthermore, man is quite resistant to the malarial organisms of other animals, except for several species found in certain apes. The human intestinal sporozoan, *Isospora hominis*, is also probably exclusively a human parasite, although as yet relatively little is known about this form. One species of intestinal flagellate, *Giardia lamblia,* is also evidently a parasite chiefly, if not exclusively, of man.

Among cestodes, the most marked restriction in host range is seen with adult worms of the genus *Taenia. Taenia saginata* and *Taenia solium* occur as adults almost exclusively in man, and the cysticercus of each is confined to but a few herbivorous hosts. The adult worm of *Echinococcus granulosus* occurs only in a few canine animals, but the larval form (the hydatid cyst) invades a rather wide range of species including man. In the class Nematoda, the pinworm (*Enterobius vermicularis*), the filarias, and *Strongyloides stercoralis* have the most extreme host restriction, being found only in man or in a few closely related species.

Parasites with broad host range.—A broad variety of animals can be infected with *Endamoeba histolytica*, the human trypanosomes, the leishmanias, and most of the intestinal flagellates. *Endamoeba histolytica* can establish itself in the dog, cat, rat, pig, and *Macacus* monkey, besides man. The human trypanosomes can infect representatives of essentially all orders of mammals. The human leishmanias can invade the dog, cat, and many rodents. *Trichomonas hominis* from man can infect the rat and mouse, the kitten, the chick, and probably others. *Balantidium coli* will establish itself fairly well in the monkey and the pig besides man.

The trematodes as a group have a rather broad host range. *Schistosoma japonicum*, for example, will infect man, the laboratory monkey, cat, cow, horse, rat, and mouse. *Clonorchis sinensis* is found naturally in man, dog, cat, hog, and guinea pig, among others. Tapeworms outside the family Taeniidae generally invade as adults several kinds of hosts. Thus *Hymenolepis nana* occurs in man and various rodents, and *Dipylidium caninum* occurs in man and in the dog, cat, and other carnivores. *Diphyllobothrium latum* is found in man, hog, dog, and cat, among others. Among nematodes, probably *Trichinella spiralis* has the broadest host range, being infective for man, carnivores, rodents, and ungulates, as well as for mammals of other orders. Even some birds are susceptible to *Trichinella*. The guinea worm, *Dracunculus medinensis*, also has a broad host range, and even the New World human hookworm, *Necator americanus*, can develop at least occasionally in such species as dog, rat, pig, horse, and pangolin.

FACTORS INFLUENCING NATURAL RESISTANCE

Genetic constitution.—Persons of different races often differ sharply in their natural resistance to infection with certain parasites, perhaps chiefly as a result of unlike genetic constitution. Negroes, for example, are as a race much more resistant to most kinds of malarial parasites than are white persons, and only the more virulent forms of these organisms are able to elicit symptoms in Negroes. Similarly, the Negro is more resistant to hookworm disease, as well as to the cestode *Hymenolepis nana*, than are white individuals. It seems quite possible that still other parasites—especially tropical forms—will also eventually be found to have greater infectivity for white persons than for Negroes.

Age.—Older persons are often more resistant to infection with a given parasite than are young individuals, even when the older persons have not been previously exposed to it. This so-called age resistance is manifested by man against malarial parasites, *Trypanosoma cruzi,* and *Giardia lamblia,* among the protozoans, and, among the helminths, against *Hymenolepis nana* and probably against *Ascaris lumbricoides* and the hookworms.

The explanations of age resistance are still obscure. Some authorities feel that, as the individual ages, his tissues become less favorable physiologically as a medium for the parasite development. Others consider that the difference with age is related chiefly to the greater capacity of older individuals to make an effective specific immune response—that is, that older individuals are more effective as antibody formers.

Sex and reproduction.—Persons of the two sexes are probably about equally susceptible to most parasites, although generally if any greater resistance of one sex is apparent, it is shown by the female. Women are, particularly, more resistant than men to amoebiasis and seldom suffer from amoebic abscess of the liver. In leishmanial infections such as kala azar, women also appear more resistant than men. The strain of reproduction is known to have a marked depressing influence upon the resistance of animals, and in man, too, this effect is sometimes suggested. Malaria frequently flares up in pregnant women, for example, or even after parturition.

Intercurrent infection.—Little is known of the effect of intercurrent infection upon the natural resistance of man to parasites. When malaria is superimposed on tuberculosis, the tuberculous lesion is said often to light up or extend, even in those about to recover. Conversely, malaria is reported to be stimulated to relapse by an injection of tuberculin. When *Plasmodium vivax* and *Plasmodium malariae* are introduced simultaneously into man, the *vivax* organism is decidedly the dominant one, the infection with *Plasmodium malariae* often being completely inhibited. The *vivax* parasite is also dominant over *Plasmodium falciparum.*

Diet.—In animals, the diet exerts a profound influence particularly on the parasitic infections of the alimentary canal. Somewhat less is known experimentally of the role of the diet in human parasitic disease, although a well-balanced diet of ample quantity is known to favor resistance in amoebiasis. In malaria, a diet rich in sugar is believed to favor relapse. In general, from the studies in animal infections with parasites, diets high in protein favor resistance to infections, whereas those rich in carbohydrates seem to depress resistance.

Little on the role of diet in resistance is yet established in the human helminthiases, but in hookworm disease a poor diet is believed to lower the resistance.

Special organs.—In studies performed in animals, effects which interfere with the function of the reticulo-endothelial system are generally found to depress resistance. Exposure to X ray or extirpation of the spleen will quite often reduce the resistance drastically in animals, and similar effects should apparently develop in man after the same treatment. As yet, however, little is established so far as man is concerned as to the function of specific tissues in resistance to the animal parasites. Malarial parasites, nevertheless, are usually lodged in the reticulo-endothelial tissues, especially that in the liver and spleen, evidently because of the marked activity of the phagocytic cells of this system.

SPECIAL DEFENSIVE MECHANISMS OF THE HOST

The mechanisms by which infected persons defend themselves from animal parasites stem from the function of the cells of the host. This function may be largely that of phagocytosis but may involve the elaboration of secretions which attack the parasites. The digestive juice, for example, is destructive of certain parasites. When free hydrochloric acid is plentiful in the stomach, infection with *Endamoeba histolytica* is less likely to occur, for the cysts will be killed by the acid while passing through the stomach. Likewise, the intestinal juice will digest the larval stage of some tapeworms which are infective only for lower animals.

The normal serum of man is lytic for the natural trypanosomes of game animals in Africa, and the resistance of man to these parasites is believed to stem from this capacity of human serum. The resistance of man to certain trematode parasites, likewise, may be related to a similar lytic function of human serum upon the cercarial stage of the parasite.

ACQUIRED IMMUNITY

As stated in the introduction to this chapter, man can be readily infected with some species of parasites on first exposure to them, but often, as a direct result of such initial infection, he assumes a new and specific capacity of resistance which may largely or even perfectly protect him thereafter against these forms. Such individuals are said to have acquired an immunity to these parasites. The immune state depends on the development of specific antagonistic substances. called antibodies, for a given parasite as a result of previous infection with that parasite or previous vaccination with its constituent antigens. These antibodies persist for long periods in the immune individual, since their production goes on continuously. Even if the production lags or ceases, it can be initiated anew by an appropriate stimulation, should an occasion requiring the antagonistic substances arise.

Immunity can also be passively acquired. In passive immunity, antibodies which are developed in one individual are transferred with blood or serum to another in which they act. There is no production of antibody in the passively immunized person, and the level of the antibody concentration drops continuously from the time the serum containing the antibody is introduced. Usually, within from four to six weeks, all traces of the transferred antibody are lost.

IMMUNITY ACQUIRED BY INFECTION

Man is known to acquire a specific immunity through infection with several parasites, primarily the protozoans. Most important among these are *Endamoeba histolytica*, *Leishmania tropica*, and the malarial parasites. Probably the most convincing example is seen with *Leishmania tropica*, which causes Oriental sore. From quite early times, mothers in endemic areas have safeguarded the facial beauty of their daughters from disfiguration by deliberately inducing a sore in some hidden area. Following recovery from this initial lesion, the inoculated person is immune to reinfection. Evidently nothing short of living, fully virulent organisms capable of developing a primary cutaneous lesion will serve for immunizing human beings; vaccines prepared of killed organisms are ineffectual for the purpose.

The immunity developed in amoebiasis and malaria are similar in that, with each, the causal organism must remain in the body of the individual and must propagate itself continuously at a low level. This conditional immunity is known as *premunition*. When the organisms are ultimately eradicated, either spontaneously or by the administration of therapeutic drugs, man loses his acquired immunity and resumes his normal susceptibility to the infection.

Very little immunity is acquired by man against most of the important helminths. If all but the scolex of a tapeworm be dislodged during treatment, for example, the form promptly regenerates itself, with no immune effect of the previous infection being notable. Likewise, when *Ascaris lumbricoides* or hookworms are eliminated by drugs from natives in the tropics, reinfection occurs with discouraging promptness and regularity. Yet since the patients develop a substantial sensitivity, especially to the roundworms, reinfection although possible after treatment, is probably less intensive than it otherwise would be and less likely to cause symptoms.

IMMUNITY ACQUIRED BY VACCINATION

As yet, with no parasitic infection has the vaccination of man been tried significantly. In malaria, the few attempts which have been reported have been rather discouraging. The problem of preparing a vaccine of the malarial organisms is, as yet, no simple one. Experimental vaccination against malaria in monkeys has also resulted unfavorably, although some success has been reported in the case of the experimental bird malarias.

IMMUNITY ACQUIRED PASSIVELY BY THE INJECTION OF IMMUNE SERUM

Malaria is the only protozoan disease of man in which immune serum therapy has been tried as a means of treatment. In the hands of a few investigators, favorable results have been obtained, but even in these the results of such treatment have not been strikingly successful.

Among the helminth infections, serum therapy has been tried in trichiniasis, and some authorities feel that, as a result of administering the immune serum, the symptoms of the disease are allayed.

Immune serum has never attained general use for treating trichiniasis, however, or any other helminthic disease.

MECHANISM OF SPECIFIC IMMUNITY

The mechanism of immunity has not been revealed in the case of any parasitic infection of man. Probably, however, in man as well as in several animal infections which have been thoroughly studied, the immunity depends on the specific antagonistic action of the host's cells and especially on the antibodies produced by these cells. These antibodies have the remarkable capacity of uniting either chemically or physically with the constituent antigens of the parasites. In the case of the smaller forms, such as the protozoans, the parasites may be directly killed or lysed by the antibody. With the larger forms, such as the helminths, the antibody may form a precipitate by uniting with the parasite antigens. The precipitate thus formed sometimes so completely occludes vital passages of the worm or otherwise interferes so profoundly with the normal function and physiology of the worm that the parasite dies.

The phagocytic cells function in acquired immunity primarily as scavengers of the parasites which occur in the somatic tissue. They are seldom able to approach the fully virulent parasite, but if the parasite be first exposed to antibody, and thus opsonized, the cells will then respond. In the case of the protozoa, these cells engulf the parasites and digest them. In the case of the large helminths, many cells act in concert, first forming nodules about the parasites and then clearing away those worms which are killed in such nodules. The death of the parasites in the nodules is probably an effect of the antibody rather than of phagocytosis.

Chapter V

DIAGNOSIS

THE ACCURATE DIAGNOSIS of parasitic infections is of prime importance to the medical man, for often, if the infecting agent can be correctly identified, a specific therapeutic material can be employed to eradicate or check the invader. In most parasitic infections, clinical symptoms are not adequate for accurate diagnosis, and observations performed in the laboratory upon blood, feces, tissue substance, or other material from the patient assume critical importance in establishing the etiology of the disease. The methods used in diagnosing parasitic infections have as their purpose: (1) the direct observation of the parasite, (2) the indirect demonstration of the parasite, or (3) the setting forth of presumptive evidence for the presence of the parasite. These will be discussed individually, but are summarized in Table 3. The technical procedures involved in some of these methods are described in the Appendix.

DIAGNOSIS BY THE DIRECT OBSERVATION OF THE PARASITE

Stages which are distinctive for certain parasites can be observed directly in feces, urine, sputum, lachrymal secretion, blood, or tissue substance of infected individuals. Usually, special staining procedures are helpful in revealing their presence and in finally identifying them, and often, special procedures for concentrating them must be resorted to.

PARASITES IN FECES

Essentially all of the intestinal parasites, whether found in the lumen of the intestine, in the intestinal wall, or in ducts or organs

TABLE 3

PROCEDURES EMPLOYED FOR DIAGNOSING INFECTIONS WITH ANIMAL PARASITES

Parasite	Microscopic Observation						Cultivation			Animal Inoculation			Antibody Test			Other Procedures			
	FECES	URINE	SPUTUM	TISSUE	BLOOD	SPINAL FLUID	BOECK'S MEDIUM	N.N.N. MEDIUM	OTHER SPECIAL MEDIUM	RAT	HAMSTER	KITTEN	PRECIPITIN	COMPLEMENT FIXATION	SKIN TEST	MONOCYTOSIS	EOSINOPHILIA	SPLENIC EN-LARGEMENT	X RAY
Endamoeba histolytica	+						+					±		+					
Endamoeba coli	+																		
Leishmania donovani				+				+			+			+				+	
Leishmania tropica				+				+											
Trypanosoma gambiense					+	+		±		+						+			
Trypanosoma cruzi					+			+		+				+					
Giardia lamblia	+																		
Trichomonas hominis	+						+												
Plasmodium falciparum					+											+		+	
Plasmodium vivax					+											+		+	
Isospora hominis	+								±										

Balantidium coli

Clonorchis sinensis

Fasciolopsis buski

Schistosoma haematobium

Schistosoma mansoni

Paragonimus westermani

Diphyllobothrium latum

Taenia saginata

Echinococcus granulosus

Hymenolepis nana

Trichinella spiralis

Trichuris trichiura

Enterobius vermicularis

Strongyloides stercoralis

Necator americanus

Ascaris lumbricoides

Wuchereria bancrofti

Onchocerca volvulus

Dracunculus medinensis

[a] Proglottids seen macroscopically.
[b] Embryos in fluid from skin ulcer.

which drain into the intestine, can be diagnosed through careful observation of the feces of the patient.

Protozoa.—Among the protozoan infections, all those caused by the amoebae (excepting the mouth form, *Endamoeba gingivalis*), the intestinal flagellates, the human coccidian, and the ciliate *Balantidium coli* can be identified by observing either cysts or trophozoites in the feces. Cysts of most of these forms characteristically occur in the feces, although in severe infections or during periods of diarrhea, whether these are caused by the parasite or otherwise, the trophozoites may appear in the stool. One of the flagellates, *Trichomonas hominis*, and an amoeba, *Dientamoeba fragilis*, are unique among intestinal protozoans in that they never produce cysts. The trophozoites of these forms are found in the feces.

Helminths.—Among the trematodiases, infections with *Fasciolopsis buski, Heterophyes heterophyes*, and *Metagonimus yokogawai*, as well as some others which dwell in the intestinal lumen, and *Clonorchis sinensis* and *Fasciola hepatica*, which dwell in the bile ducts or liver, all can be diagnosed by finding eggs in the feces. Even the eggs of the lung trematode, *Paragonimus westermani*, may be found in feces if the sputum which contains them is swallowed by the patient. Likewise, eggs of the schistosome trematodes, particularly those of *Schistosoma mansoni* and *Schistosoma japonicum*, of which the adults dwell in the mesenteric venules, but occasionally those of *Schistosoma haematobium* also, occur in the feces.

Infections with most human cestodes can be diagnosed by finding eggs in the feces. With such forms as *Dipylidium caninum, Hymenolepis nana, Hymenolepis diminuta*, and *Diphyllobothrium latum* the egg specifically identifies the form. The eggs of *Taenia saginata* and *Taenia solium*, however, are identical and the differentiation of these species is possible only when—as usually occurs—gravid proglottids are recovered in the feces and carefully examined as to the number of branches in the uterus. Rarely, when the hydatid cyst ruptures into the bile duct, scolices of *Echinococcus granulosus* appear in the feces of man.

Among the nematodiases, essentially all but those caused by the filarioid worms and by *Dracunculus medinensis* and *Trichinella spiralis*, can be identified by finding the characteristic egg in the feces. This includes infections with the hookworms, *Ascaris lumbricoides*, and *Trichuris trichiura*. In *Strongyloides stercoralis* infection, the rhabditiform larva generally is found in the feces, the egg usually having hatched before leaving the intestine. In trichiniasis, the adult parasites occur in the feces, the male worms alone during the first days after infection and the females subsequently. The adult worms usually, and the eggs sometimes, of *Enterobius vermicularis* likewise occur in the feces, especially after the patient has received an enema.

PARASITES IN URINE

The presence of parasites in the kidney or the bladder, or in any other part which drains into the urinary tract, can often be established by finding some stage of the parasite in the urine. In amoebic abscesses of the kidney, for example, *Endamoeba histolytica* occurs in the urine. *Trichomonas vaginalis* may be found in the urine of both men and women who harbor this parasite. Eggs of the schistosomes, particularly *Schistosoma haematobium*, are found in the urine, as are also those of the rare kidney worm *Dioctophyma renale*.[1] Microfilariae of *Wuchereria bancrofti* appear in chylous urine.

PARASITES IN SPUTUM AND SALIVA

Comparatively few infections with parasites can be diagnosed by examining the sputum, or saliva. Eggs of the lung fluke *Paragonimus westermani* are seen in sputum, and rarely the migrating larvae of *Ascaris*, hookworm, or *Strongyloides* are found. Scolices or "sand" (hooklets) from ruptured hydatid cysts of the lung also may be found in the sputum. In saliva or material from between the teeth, the mouth amoeba *Endamoeba gingivalis* or the flagellate *Trichomonas buccalis* often is seen, particularly if the teeth are carious.

PARASITES IN THE EYE, THE CONJUNCTIVA, OR THE LACHRYMAL SECRETION

Only very few parasites cause infection of the eye or the conjunctival tissue. Nevertheless, on rare occasions, *Endamoeba histolytica* and leishmanias have been reported in the conjunctival sac, and the nematode *Thelazia callipaeda* has been found in the lachrymal canals and glands. The adult of *Loa loa* and the microfilariae of several species of filarioid worms have been found in or near the eye. Larvae

[1] A nematode, found usually in dogs, which is somewhat closely related to *Trichinella spiralis* and *Trichuris trichiura*.

of *Trichinella spiralis* have been demonstrated in the muscles which move the eye. In the eyeball itself, cysticerci of *Taenia solium* are occasionally reported, as are hydatids of *Echinococcus granulosus*. In the Orient, plerocercoids of *Diphyllobothrium mansoni* are sometimes recovered from the conjunctival tissue of natives.

PARASITES IN BLOOD

Many protozoans as well as many helminths occur in the blood and can be identified by examining the blood. Usually, these forms are those transmitted by insects, although some other parasites also occur in the blood stream.

Protozoa.—Trypanosomes, malarial parasites, and, rarely, leishmanias can all be identified in blood films, and the infections which they cause thus diagnosed. Usually, in surveys of the general population, thick blood films are used, although where details of the parasite structure must be seen, thin films are advised. (See Appendix, for preparation of thick and thin blood films.)

Helminths.—Examination of the blood is used to diagnose all the human filarial infections except that with *Onchocerca volvulus*. Thick films stained with hematoxylin or, quite advantageously, fresh preparations are examined to detect the microfilariae of the parasites. With considerable difficulty, trichiniasis also can be diagnosed by examining the centrifugated lysed blood, the embryos of *Trichinella spiralis* sometimes thus being detected.

PARASITES IN TISSUE SUBSTANCE

Tissue of the living patient can often be removed and parasites seen in it directly or after sectioning and staining. In some cases, however, tissue can be obtained only at autopsy but on examination then will readily reveal the parasite or evidence of pathologic change which has diagnostic significance.

Protozoa.—Fluid withdrawn from an amoebic cyst of the liver will often reveal the moving trophozoites, and sections of the intestine or other organs containing lesions will also present the organism. Likewise, stained films from skin lesions in Oriental sore or stained smears of fresh spleen or liver substance in kala azar will show *Leishmania tropica* or *Leishmania donovani*, respectively. Tissue sections of these organs also will reveal the parasites. Tissue of the brain from fatal cases of trypanosomiasis will present a characteristic perivascular leucocytic infiltration helpful in the diagnosis of African sleeping sickness, although usually the living trypanosome itself can be seen earlier in juice from the cervical lymph nodes or from the spinal fluid. Sections of the heart muscle reveal the leishmanial stage of *Trypanosoma cruzi* and thus serve to identify Chagas's disease at autopsy. The tissue of nearly all organs of patients dead of malaria shows deep pigmentation as well as the presence of many parasites either within phagocytic cells or else free in capillaries. Sections of the intestinal wall reveal the schizogonous stages of coccidia as well as lesions containing trophozoites of *Balantidium coli*.

Helminths.—Biopsy of striated muscle is quite frequently used in the diagnosis of trichiniasis. The living parasite can be seen if the muscle is teased apart or pressed between glass plates. Stained sections also reveal the coiled larval organisms. The microfilariae of *Onchocerca* occur in fluid aspirated from a cutaneous nodule harboring the parasite and are also sometimes demonstrable in tissue fluid other than that from nodules and in fluid from the eyeball. Stained sections of the surgically removed cutaneous nodule in onchocerciasis reveal the adult worms. Sections of infected lymph nodes show the intercoiled adults of *Wuchereria bancrofti*. Fluid from the cutaneous ulcers caused by the guinea worm, *Dracunculus medinensis*, can be examined directly with the microscope, and the worm embryos may be seen. Cysticerci of *Taenia solium* or of hydatid cysts occur particularly in the liver but also in many other sites, such as the brain, and are shown by sections. Sections of the liver may reveal *Schistosoma mansoni* or its eggs, which are generally in pseudotubercles. The eggs of *Schistosoma haematobium* are often seen in lung sections. Lung sections also reveal the lung fluke *Paragonimus westermani*.

DIAGNOSIS BY INDIRECT DEMONSTRATION OF PARASITES

In several procedures highly useful in diagnosis, the parasite is not directly found in the specimen from the patient but can be observed after this material has been especially handled. For example, the parasite may be cultivated from the blood, feces, or other source, or the parasite may appear in laboratory animals inoculated with the specimen from man. Finally, a procedure called "xenodiagnosis" may in unusual circumstances be resorted to; in this an arthropod vector is permitted to feed on man, and the parasite is later demonstrated in the arthropod.

CULTIVATION

Protozoa.—Several of the protozoan parasites found in the intestine can be grown in culture. *Endamoeba histolytica,* the other intestinal amoebae, and *Endamoeba gingivalis, Trichomonas hominis, Chilomastix mesnili,* and *Balantidium coli* all can be grown in Boeck's and Drbohlav's medium or in modifications of it. The nonpathogenic amoebae generally die out in a few generations although *Endamoeba histolytica* survives indefinitely if frequently transferred. The leishmanias and *Trypanosoma cruzi* grow well in N.N.N. medium. The African trypanosomes always grow poorly, although about as well in N.N.N. medium as in any other, subcultures seldom being obtained. Malaria parasites survive for a considerable time in defibrinated blood and may rarely experience two or three schizogonous cycles. *Giardia lamblia* and *Isospora hominis* cannot be cultivated.

Helminths.—The free-living stages of a number of helminths can be cultivated in artificial medium. Feces containing hookworm eggs, if incubated for a few days, sometimes advantageously mixed with charcoal, will show the third-stage infective filariform larvae. The nematode infection for which cultivation is usually employed in diagnosis is *Strongyloides stercoralis.* This form can be propagated in vitro for an indefinite period, since the form is a facultative parasite and free-living propagative stages develop in culture.

ANIMAL INOCULATION

Many of the human parasites can infect lower animals, and experimental infections in such animals sometimes are resorted to as a laboratory diagnostic procedure. This is done especially when the experimental animal is decidedly more susceptible to the infectious agent than is man. Feces containing amoebae cysts from man if inoculated into the kitten or puppy frequently leads to an acute disease which ends fatally. Likewise, trypanosomiasis can be diagnosed by transferring blood from an infected patient to the rat or mouse. Animal inoculation is seldom used for diagnosing helminth infections, although tissue containing cysts or *Trichinella spiralis* promptly leads to infection in the mouse or rat.

XENODIAGNOSIS

A few parasitic infections can be diagnosed by permitting blood-sucking insects to bite man, although usually other simpler procedures are available. Nevertheless, *Trypanosoma cruzi* does develop in the cone-nosed bug (*Triatoma megista*), as well as in many other blood-suckers, and the African trypanosomes of man develop in tsetse flies (*Glossina* spp.) which are fed on infected patients. Xenodiagnosis is, however, largely of academic interest and has had little use as a method of diagnosing parasitic infection.

PRESUMPTIVE DIAGNOSIS OF PARASITIC INFECTION

The presumptive methods for diagnosing parasitic infection do not reveal the parasite itself but supply evidence for present or past infection with the parasite. The presumptive methods involve the demonstration by in vitro procedures of the antigens of the parasite or of the antibody which the infected patient has developed against these antigens. The reaction which occurs in the skin of some persons after a specific antigen is injected also is presumptive evidence of their infection with the homologous parasite. Some other special procedures, such as determining variations in the blood picture, or the enlargement of the spleen, or the use of the X ray, are also invoked for eliciting presumptive evidence of the presence of certain parasites.

TESTS FOR ANTIGEN

Although the test for antigen is a particularly favorable procedure for diagnosis because it would, presumably, be positive very early in the course of an infection, it has not yet been used for human parasitic diseases. In such parasitic infections of animals as trichiniasis, malaria, and trypanosomiasis, it has been employed experimentally, although even in these it has had but small trial. Possibly future years will find greater exploitation of the test for antigen of the human parasites.

IN VITRO TESTS FOR ANTIBODY

Two types of in virto tests for antibody have been used in diagnosing human parasitic infection: precipitin tests and complement fixation tests.

Precipitin tests.—Although precipitin tests for amoebiasis, trypanosomiasis, and malaria have been described, in none of these diseases has the test received general use. Among certain of the somatic tissue helminth infections, however, fairly widespread use has been attained, particularly in schistosomiasis, cysticercosis, echinococcus disease, filariasis, and trichiniasis. Often the test remains positive for many years.

Complement fixation tests.—The complement fixation test is probably the most delicate of all tests for antibody. Because of the difficulty of the technique, however, results obtained with it by any except an experienced worker generally are unreliable. It has been quite widely tried with success in amoebiasis and is probably useful in kala azar, trypanosomiasis, and malaria. It has proved of great value in diagnosing schistosomiasis, echinococcus disease, and human filariasis.

SKIN TESTS

Skin tests are particularly useful diagnostic aids because they can be performed simply. They have not proved useful as yet in protozoan diseases, but among the helminthiases they have become in many cases the diagnostic procedure of choice. They are used for schistosomiasis, echinococcus disease, trichiniasis, and filariasis. Immediate reactions of the wheal and erythema type are generally noted in man, although often a delayed reaction of the Arthus type also occurs.

OTHER PROCEDURES

Three other procedures useful in diagnosing human parasitic infection will be mentioned: variations in the leucocyte picture, enlargement of the spleen, and X-ray photography.

Variations in the leucocyte picture.—In several infections with the blood protozoans, a drop in the total leucocyte count and a relative increase in the number of monocytic cells are noted. These changes are seen in malaria, beginning a few days after infection. A relative monocytosis occurs also in trypanosomiasis and in leishmaniasis.

A most striking change in the leucocyte picture is seen in the helminthiases as a group, especially when somatic tissue is invaded. This change is the rise in the relative number of eosinophilic leucocytes. Whereas these cells normally constitute about one percent of the total leucocyte count, during intensive helminth infection their proportion may rise to fifty percent or more. The rise begins during the second week, and the high level is usually maintained for several weeks or months thereafter. An eosinophilia has been reported in practically all the helminth infections but is especially useful in identifying cases of schistosomiasis, cysticercosis, echinococcus disease, filariasis, and trichiniasis.

Enlargement of the spleen.—Many parasitic infections lead to splenic enlargement, but the most important in this respect is malaria. A usual preliminary procedure in estimating the incidence of malarial infection in a community is to determine the percentage of enlarged spleens. Kala azar also leads to marked enlargement of the spleen, and in those comparatively restricted regions where kala azar occurs, the splenic index is not satisfactory as an estimate of the level of malarial infection. The spleen also becomes greatly enlarged in schistosomiasis.

X-ray photography.—X-ray photography is employed widely as an aid in diagnosing hydatid disease, particularly when the cyst is lodged in the lung or the liver. When cysts become calcified, their outline is sharply shown. X-ray photographs also reveal calcified cysticerci of *Taenia solium* and the calcified adult of *Wuchereria bancrofti*.

Chapter VI

SPECIFIC THERAPY

M ANY SUBSTANCES, both natural and synthetic, are employed in the therapy of parasitic infections. Some of these are useful upon but one or two kinds of parasites; others manifest their destructive action upon several varieties. The mode of action of some drugs is fairly well appreciated, but that of others is quite obscure despite, often, a very marked excellence in effect.

Most substances used in treating parasitic infection can be put in one of three groups: (1) natural plant products and their alkaloids, (2) synthetic organic chemicals, and (3) inorganic chemicals. The most important chemotherapeutic materials of each of these groups will be briefly discussed. Some of the substances are also mentioned in Table 4.

NATURAL PLANT PRODUCTS

A number of plant species are the source of chemotherapeutic substances which are used for eliminating animal parasites. Some of these can be employed in their natural form; others must be highly refined. In some cases, specific derivatives, such as enzymes or alkaloids, are known to be responsible for their action.

ARECA CATECHU (ARECOLINE)

Derivatives of seeds of an Oriental plant, *Areca catechu* (betel nuts), have been extensively used for eliminating tapeworms for centuries. The active principle is the alkaloid derivative *arecoline*. The drug is administered in the morning on an empty stomach, and, unlike most vermifuges, requires no cathartic subsequently.

TABLE 4

DRUGS USED FOR TREATING INFECTIONS WITH ANIMAL PARASITES

Drug	Route Administered	Susceptible Infections
Alkaloids		
Arecoline	oral	intestinal cestodiases
Ascaridol	oral	ascariasis; hookworm disease
Emetine	subcutaneous	amoebiasis; fascioliasis
Ficin	oral	trichuriasis
Filicin	oral	intestinal cestodiases
Papain	oral	trichuriasis
Pelletierin	oral	taeniasis
Quinine	oral	malaria
Aliphatic chlorides		
Carbon tetrachloride	oral	hookworm disease; intestinal cestodiases
Tetrachlorethylene	oral	hookworm disease; enterobiasis
Phenolic derivatives		
Hexylresorcinol	oral	ascariasis; intestinal cestodiases; fasciolopsiasis
Thymol	oral	hookworm disease
Beta-naphthol	oral	hookworm disease; fasciolopsiasis
Para-aminobenzene derivatives		
Sulphur compounds		
Promin	oral	malaria
Sulfadiazine	oral	malaria
Arsenic compounds		
Tryparsamide	intramuscular; intravenous	African sleeping sickness
Antimony compounds		
Stibosan	intravenous	kala azar
Neostibosan	intravenous	kala azar; Oriental sore
Simple organic compounds of metals (antimony)		
Tartar emetic	intramuscular; intravenous	kala azar; clonorchiasis; schistosomiasis
Fuadin (neoantimosan)	intramuscular; intravenous	schistosomiases
Quinoline derivatives		
Plasmochin	intramuscular; intravenous	malaria
Yatren	oral; retention enema	amoebiasis
Acridine derivative		
Atebrin	oral	malaria
Aniline derivative		
Gentian violet	oral	clonorchiasis; strongyloidiasis; enterobiasis
Urea-aminonaphthalene sulfonic acid derivative		
Germanin	intravenous	African sleeping sickness

ARTEMISIA SP. (SANTONINE)

The Levant wormseed (*Artemisia cina*) and other related species of *Artemisia* have been used as anthelmintics since the time of the early Greek physicians. Originally the crude material was employed, but finally an alkaloid derivative, santonine, was developed. Formerly this derivative was the drug most widely used for eliminating *Ascaris lumbricoides*. In recent years its use has been largely abandoned since it affects principally female worms and since it seldom leads to complete cure. It has little toxicity but is readily absorbed. Some patients develop nervous symptoms, such as headache, drowsiness, hallucinations, and even coma following its use.

ASPIDIUM FILIX-MAS (FILICIN)

The substance most widely used for eliminating tapeworms is obtained from the male fern *Aspidium filix-mas*. Either the oleoresin or the extract may be employed, this being administered by duodenal tube to the patient on an empty stomach. The drug apparently acts directly on the worm. The active principle of the fern plant is *filicin*, which comprises about one fourth of the oleoresin. Derivatives of the fern plant have been used for eliminating tapeworm since before the dawn of the Christian era.

CARICA PAPAYA (PAPAIN)

The fruit of the papaya plant, *Carica papaya*, is said to be an active anthelmintic, effective especially upon *Trichuris trichiura*. It owes its action to an enzyme of the fruit juice, *papain*.

CHENOPODIUM AMBROSIOIDES (ASCARIDOL)

The oil of American wormseed, *Chenopodium ambrosioides* var. *anthelminthicum*, is an effective drug for eliminating the large nematode *Ascaris lumbricoides*, as well as hookworms. The active ingredient of the oil is *ascaridol*, which constitutes about seventy-five percent of the crude substance. The drug is given on an empty stomach and intestine, a purgative having been previously administered. It is a highly toxic substance especially irritating to the mucous membranes and must be administered with great caution.

CINCHONA SPP. (QUININE)

The bark of trees of the genus *Cinchona* has been used for treating malaria since 1600. In 1820, the alkaloid derivative *quinine* was shown to be the active principle of the bark. The precise mode of action of the drug is not known, although since the parasites in blood films from patients who have received quinine stain peculiarly, some authorities believe the action of the drug is direct. Others, however, feel that phagocytosis is stimulated by the drug. Quinine bisulphate is given in gelatin capsules by mouth; quinine dihydrochloride is administered intravenously or intramuscularly.

FICUS SP. (FICIN)

The sap (*leche de higueron*) of certain fig trees, particularly *Ficus glabrata,* is an efficient anthelmintic, acting especially on *Trichuris trichiura.* The active principle is an enzyme, *ficin.* The native sap is best used fresh, although if preserved by adding sodium benzoate, a considerable activity is retained on storage. The drug is administered by mouth some hours after a purgative has been given.

IPECACUANHA (EMETINE)

Ipecac root has long been known to be of benefit in chronic diarrheas, and in recent years it has come to be considered a specific for amoebic dysentery. It is also useful in amoebic abscess of the liver or lung. A highly toxic alkaloid derivative, *emetine,* has largely superseded the natural ipecac root in treating amoebic infections. This material is injected subcutaneously or intramuscularly. Since the drug has marked in vitro action, it may act directly upon the parasite in the patient, likewise. The drug has also been used in fascioliasis and paragonimiasis.

PUNICA GRANATUM (PELLETIERIN)

Derivatives of the pomegranate, *Punica granatum,* have been used for eliminating *Taenia saginata* since early Egyptian times (1550 B.C.) and are still employed. The alkaloid *pelletierin* is the active principle.

SYNTHETIC ORGANIC COMPOUNDS

Many organic compounds have been synthesized in an effort to find substances which will manifest powerful action upon the parasites and yet have little or no harmful effect upon man. Often, these synthetic materials depend for their action upon essentially the same organic radical or base that occurs in certain of the natural plant substances previously mentioned. Thus, there is a fundamental chemical similarity between quinine and the synthesized plasmochin, between emetine and synthesized yatren, and between santonine and betanaphthol. The advantages of the synthesized drugs are several: they are usually more powerful in action so that smaller doses are required; furthermore, inert components of the crude materials are absent from the synthetic material and the toxicity of the synthetic drug is thus proportionately reduced.[1]

ALIPHATIC CHLORIDE COMPOUNDS

Carbon tetrachloride (CCl_4).—Carbon tetrachloride has, since 1921, been used widely for the treatment of hookworm disease and has been tried in late years also in tapeworm infections (*Taenia solium, Taenia saginata,* and *Diphyllobothrium latum*). Although effective on the parasites, the drug is highly toxic, and many deaths have been reported following its administration. It is given by mouth, diluted in milk, on an empty stomach. A saline purgative should be administered both the night prior to and several hours subsequent to the drug treatment.

Tetrachlorethylene (C_2Cl_4).—Tetrachlorethylene has been, since 1925, the drug of choice for the elimination of hookworms. It is relatively low in toxicity and is almost as effective in removing the worms as carbon tetrachloride. It has also been tried in pinworm infection. It is given by mouth.

PHENOLIC DERIVATIVES

Hexylresorcinol (*a dihydric phenol*).—Under the name caprokol, crystoids of the dihydric phenol, hexylresorcinol, are given by mouth

---

[1] The author wishes to thank Dr. Charles L. Fox, Jr., for his advice upon the interrelationships of the synthetic organic compounds. The compounds are presented in a sequence suggested by him.

for treating several helminth infections. The drug is the one of choice, because of its low toxicity, for eliminating *Ascaris lumbricoides*. It has also been used in hookworm and pinworm infections and in infections with *Hymenolepis nana*, *Taenia saginata*, and *Fasciolopsis buski*.

Thymol (methyl-isopropyl-phenol).—Thymol is one of the oldest drugs used for eradicating hookworms, being employed for this purpose since 1880. It is quite effective but has marked toxicity. Its use has been largely superseded by that of tetrachlorethylene.

Beta-naphthol (beta-hydroxynaphthalene).—During the first two decades of the twentieth century, beta-naphthol was widely used for eliminating hookworms, largely replacing thymol for this purpose because of its lower toxicity. The drug is not atoxic, however, and its use has largely been discontinued because of its irritating effect upon the mucous membranes. Furthermore, it seems to be less effective than thymol or some other drugs upon hookworms. At the present time it is used little except for treating *Fasciolopsis buski* infections.

PARA-AMINOBENZENE DERIVATIVES

Many compounds which contain antimony, arsenic, or sulphur have been employed as chemotherapeutic materials. They usually resemble each other fundamentally in that one or another of these elements is found in the para-amino position of the benzene ring.

Derivatives containing sulphur (sulfanilamide derivatives).—Two derivatives of sulfanilamide, promin (sodium P, P^1-diamino-phenyl-sulfone N, N^1-didextrosulfonate) and sulfadiazine (2-sulfanilamido-pyrimidine) have been shown to have a therapeutic effect in human malaria. The action of these substances, however, is probably less powerful than that of quinine or certain quinoline derivatives. Thus far, comparatively little trial of the drugs has been possible.

Derivatives containing arsenic.—The most important benzene derivative containing arsenic is tryparsamide (sodium salt of N-phenyl-glycineamide-p-arsonic acid). It is the most satisfactory arsenic compound for treating African sleeping sickness. It is particularly useful in infections that have gone on for some time, since it benefits even those cases in which the central nervous system has become involved. The drug is given either intramuscularly or intravenously. Although it has relatively low toxicity, some peculiarly sensitive persons manifest serious effects following its administration. Optic neuritis is a somewhat frequent effect, and blindness may ensue.

Derivatives containing antimony.—One of the most successful para-aminobenzene derivatives containing antimony is stibosan (meta-chlor-para-acetylaminophenyl-stibiate of sodium). It is a relatively atoxic substance in which the antimony is pentavalent. It is used for kala azar, the drug being given intravenously. A related pentavalent antimonial, neostibosan (amino salt of para-aminophenyl stibinic acid), which contains forty percent of metallic antimony, is also used in kala azar, as well as for Oriental sore.

SIMPLE ORGANIC COMPOUNDS OF METALS

Several relatively simple compounds of trivalent antimony are useful in chemotherapy. One of these, tartar emetic (potassium antimonyl tartrate), has been used since 1912 in the treatment of kala azar and cutaneous leishmaniasis and since 1918 for schistosomiasis. The drug is also said to have an effect in infections with *Clonorchis sinensis*. It has comparatively low toxicity and is generally given intravenously. The sodium salt (sodium antimonyl tartrate) is also used, especially for treating schistosomiasis. Neoantimosan or fuadin (antimony pyrocatechin disulphonate of sodium) is another compound of trivalent antimony used particularly in schistosomiasis. It is relatively atoxic and is injected intramuscularly. Soon after these compounds are given, eggs of the schistosomes will cease to appear in the feces, although treatment is usually continued for at least two weeks.

QUINOLINE DERIVATIVES

Plasmochin(N-diethylamino-isopentyl-9-amino-6-methoxyquinoline).—Plasmochin was introduced in 1926 for the treatment of malaria. Although it was at first believed to act upon all stages of the malarial parasites, its use has since been largely abandoned except for eliminating the gametocytes of *Plasmodium falciparum*. Plasmochin is the only drug which is known to act on these forms of the malignant parasite. The drug is administered both intramuscularly and intravenously.

Yatren (sodium iodoxyquinoline sulphonate).—Yatren (chiniofon, anayodin) is used particularly in amoebic infections. It is administered not only by mouth but also by retention enema. The drug is evidently the one of choice for completely curing infections with *Endamoeba histolytica,* although preliminary treatment with the related but much more toxic substance emetine is often advised in order first to bring the infection, if severe, under control.

ACRIDINE DERIVATIVE

Atebrin.—The most important acridine derivative used in chemotherapy is atebrin (2-chloro-7-methoxy-5a-diethylamino-8-pentyl-amino-acridine), which was developed in 1933. The substance is similar to plasmochin, but presents an acridine base in lieu of the quinoline base of plasmochin. The drug has a most powerful therapeutic action in malaria. Evidently some prophylactic effect, at least for brief periods, follows its use. Atebrin acts on all stages of all species of malarial parasites, excepting the gametocytes of *Plasmodium falciparum.* The drug also has a remarkably efficient therapeutic effect in giardiasis. It is usually administered by mouth, two or three tablets, of one-tenth gram each, being given daily for five days.

ANILINE DERIVATIVE

Gentian violet.—Gentian violet is a complex aniline dye which has proved useful in treating infections with *Clonorchis sinensis, Strongyloides stercoralis,* and *Enterobius vermicularis.* It is usually administered by mouth in enteric-coated tablets or, rarely, by duodenal tube. In the case of *Strongyloides stercoralis,* the drug seems to act directly upon the protoplasm of the female worm in the intestinal wall.

UREA-AMINONAPHTHALENE-SULFONIC ACID DERIVATIVE

Germanin (Bayer 205).—The unusually complex drug known as germanin or Bayer 205 (urea of acid dimeta-aminobenzoyl-meta-amino-para-methylbenzoyl-1-naphthylamino-4-6-8-trisulfonate of soda), which was first prepared in 1920, has a most extraordinarily powerful action upon the trypanosomes of African sleeping sickness. The best effect is obtained early in the infection before the parasites invade the central nervous system. Germanin has comparatively low toxicity and is usually given intravenously. The action is prompt, the trypanosomes being eliminated from the peripheral blood within twelve hours or so after the drug is given. Since the drug seems to manifest comparatively little action on the parasites in vitro, some authorities feel it produces its effect in the patient chiefly by stimulating phagocytosis. The drug has quite remarkable powers to combine with the tissue proteins and, probably because of this, serves in the chemoprophylaxis of trypanosomiasis. After receiving one gram of drug, human beings appear to resist infection with the African trypanosomes of man for about three months. The drug has no action upon *Trypanosoma cruzi.*

INORGANIC CHEMICALS

Several inorganic chemicals are useful in the chemotherapy of parasitic infections. Many of these, such as magnesium sulphate (Epsom salts) are themselves not active against the parasites but are employed as purgatives in conjunction with some of the substances mentioned earlier in this chapter. The purgative flushes from the bowel the parasites which have been loosened from the wall by the essential therapeutic agent. The purgative is also employed prior to the administration of the specific drug, in order to remove all food from the intestinal tract and thus better expose the parasites to the drug subsequently administered.

Iron compounds are quite frequently given as adjuvants to the specific therapeutic agent. In hookworm disease, for example, the elimination of the worms is not enough to cure the patient, for the hookworm anemia persists after all worms are eradicated. The anemia can be improved only by administering iron. Indeed, the iron is generally given even before the patient is treated for his worms, since if his hemoglobin level and erythrocyte count can be elevated, the patient will be fortified against the disease.

A few inorganic chemicals, however, are directly effective in parasitic diseases. One of these is carbon dioxide snow. This material applied directly to the skin over the tunnels of the larvae of *Ancylostoma braziliense, Ancylostoma caninum,* or the larvae of *Gasterophilus* flies in creeping eruption will kill the offending parasite. The treatment is also recommended in scabies.

Chapter VII

PROPHYLAXIS

EVERY LARGE CITY at the present time employs in its public health department trained experts whose responsibility it is to protect the general population from infection with animal parasites. Meat inspectors, sanitary engineers, and persons who strive to keep down the mosquito nuisance, for example, all contribute, as does the physician, to the community effort to avoid parasitic infection. Generally, the prophylactic measures utilized are directed either (1) toward destroying the parasite or lessening the possibility of its invading human beings or else (2) toward raising the level of resistance of individuals to the parasite. In addition, the education of the general population in the principles of personal hygiene and in the significance to health of infection with animal parasites does much to prevent infection by these forms.

MEASURES TO DESTROY THE PARASITE

Measures designed to destroy an animal parasite are generally directed at what is considered the most vulnerable point or points of its life cycle. These may involve the stages found in man himself, and the treatment of infected persons is then advised. Sometimes, however, the stages of the parasite found in human waste products are more easily killed or diverted than those in the body of man. Often the most expeditious procedures involve eliminating potential arthropod vectors, such as mosquitoes and flies or ticks. Some parasites must be specifically searched for in foods, and any foodstuff found to contain them must be condemned, usually for the use of animals as well as man.

Particularly with the protozoan infections, treatment of every infected individual is generally practiced. This is true especially in amoebiasis, for one individual may often more or less directly lead to infection in other human beings. Those who prepare or handle food, for example, may seed the cysts of *Endamoeba histolytica* into the food and thus infect all those who later ingest it. Likewise, the potential arthropod vectors of malaria (mosquito) or of African sleeping sickness (tsetse fly) will not become transmitters if they bite persons whose infections have been cured.

In some helminth infections, likewise, community prophylaxis involves primarily the treatment of each human case in turn. Pinworm infection is an outstanding example among these, for in it the transmission occurs directly from person to person. The elimination from infected persons of such other forms as hookworms, *Ascaris lumbricoides,* and *Trichuris trichiura,* and of tapeworms is also advised so as to avoid the pollution of soil, food, or drink with the eggs or larvae of these species.

SAFE DISPOSAL OF HUMAN WASTES

Intestinal parasites, or forms of which the transmitting stage is passed in urine or feces, can often be controlled by proper disposal of such human wastes. The waste may be treated with disinfectant or heated, or even stored for a protracted period until the parasite dies. In any event, the greatest care must be taken to prevent the contamination of human food or drink with the wastes containing the parasite. Infected feces must not be used as fertilizer, since cysts of amoebae or embryonated eggs of *Ascaris,* for example, may persist on vegetables such as fresh celery for weeks and infect persons when the vegetables are swallowed without cooking. If feces containing hookworm eggs reaches moist soil, infective larvae develop and remain for some time in such soil, ever a potential source of infection if human skin be exposed to them. Sometimes, as in schistosomiasis, the stage of the parasites found in the urine or feces must first infect a water snail before passing to another human being. If infection of the snail can be prevented by properly disinfecting the urine or feces before its disposal, or by first storing the waste for some time if it must be used as fertilizer, man will at the same time be protected from the parasite. The same is true, particularly in the Orient, with the feces of persons harboring *Fasciolopsis buski* and *Clonorchis sinensis*.

INSPECTION OF FOOD AND WATER

Many kinds of food must be examined carefully for the presence of certain specific parasites, and if these are found, the use of such food by man must be prohibited. The meat of cattle, pigs, and other domesticated animals used as food is, in the larger commercial slaughtering houses, examined especially for such helminths as the cysticerci of cestodes. In some countries, especially in Central Europe, the muscle tissue of the pig is examined microscopically for the presence of *Trichinella spiralis*. Usually the organisms themselves are searched for in each case, although skin tests or antibody tests with the serum from the animal also are useful in revealing presumptively the presence of the parasite. Generally, meats which have been refrigerated for a long period are safer for use than is that from recently slaughtered animals.

Vegetables may carry the cysts or eggs of many human parasites. Before they are eaten, vegetables should be peeled or hulled, if possible, or else washed or cooked. Infection with amoebae, *Ascaris, Trichuris*, and many other intestinal forms can thus be avoided.

Water as it comes from the faucet in a city with a well-guarded water supply will usually be devoid of animal parasites. It is well to remember, however, that chlorination, as generally carried out, does not kill the cysts of *Endamoeba histolytica*, although usually such cysts are removed by sand filtration or by sedimentation. Water from natural sources, on the other hand, may harbor a number of parasites, especially in the tropics. These include all the intestinal forms and those species, such as some pseudophyllid tapeworms and *Dracunculus medinensis*, which spend their larval stage in the microscopic copepod, *Cyclops,* or its relatives.

DESTRUCTION OF POTENTIAL RESERVOIRS

Man is the natural reservoir of most human parasites, but a number of animals are also potential reservoirs of some species. Game animals (antelopes) are potential or actual reservoirs of the human trypanosomes in Africa. The armadillo and opossum are natural reservoirs of *Trypanosoma cruzi* in South America. *Schistosoma japonicum* of the Orient can develop in several domesticated animals. *Diphyllobothrium latum* and *Clonorchis sinensis* occur in many fish-eating animals, and *Paragonimus westermani* in those species which eat crabs. *Trichinella spiralis* is found in rats and pigs. *Dracunculus medinensis* occurs in a broad variety of reservoirs. Generally, however, the protection afforded to man by eliminating these animal reservoirs from any given community is small or insignificant and temporary.

DESTRUCTION OF POTENTIAL VECTORS

Many diseases—some caused by animal parasites and some by agents of other nature—are best controlled by controlling the arthopod vector. Areas where malaria, yellow fever, and dengue fever occur can be rendered inhabitable by controlling the mosquito population. This is an enormous task, even for small communities. But since many kinds of disease-carrying mosquitoes are primarily house-dwellers or dooryard dwellers and do not characteristically fly more than a few hundred feet from their birthplace, their control is not beyond human capacity. Large-scale measures also are profitable. Swamps can be drained or ditched. Waters which cannot be channeled can be oiled, or sprayed with Paris green or other larvicide. The waters can also be stocked with fish (*Gambusia* sp.) which feed on mosquito larvae or with plants such as *Chara* sp. which presumably are repellant to egg-laying adult mosquitoes. Some of the world's greatest engineering accomplishments, such as the construction of the Panama Canal and the erection of the naval base at Singapore, were possible only after the mosquito problem of the given area was solved.

The control of African sleeping sickness is in some communities possible by killing the slow-breeding tsetse fly. Usually, the larva or pupa is searched for in underbrush, or else the underbrush itself in which the adults breed is cleared away. Because each female tsetse fly produces but few young each year, and because relatively few flies at most become infected with the trypanosome, the disease in man will be largely checked by an active anti-fly campaign.

The control of black flies, tabanid flies, and houseflies is a very great problem. Black flies live as larvae in splashing or turbulent water, such as in mountain brooks, and tabanid flies experience their larval development rather inaccessibly in the bottoms of pools, lakes, or streams. The housefly, however, lives in manure piles or garbage cans as a larva, and if these be kept covered, the number of flies will be reduced.

Lice and ticks, which carry especially rickettsial and spirochetal diseases, are also quite difficult to control. Louse-ridden individuals must be treated individually, the clothing and the body of each person being deloused. Prophylaxis for ticks also involves removal of each form found on the person and the wearing of special protective clothing when in tick-infested communities.

The control of schistosomiasis and of other trematode infections is sometimes possible through attack upon the snail vector. If copper sulphate be added to open beds of water, snails are often killed. The draining of irrigation canals in which snails usually breed checks their propagation, and if copper sulphate treatment be combined with such drainage and the whole procedure be carried out periodically, the number of snails will be so much reduced that the trematode infection will decline as a public health problem.

MEASURES TO RAISE INDIVIDUAL LEVEL OF RESISTANCE

Individual prophylaxis involves especially the administration of drugs which act protectively. In a few cases, individuals can be rendered immune by vaccination or by recovery from prior infection.

CHEMOPROPHYLAXIS

Persons can be protected against two protozoan diseases by the administration prior to infection of a drug specific for the disease. In malaria, the administration of quinine and, perhaps even more favorably, of atebrin is known to confer a temporary resistance against the symptoms of disease, although usually when the administration of the drug is stopped, the disease develops and symptoms appear. Similarly, the administration of germanin (Bayer 205) will confer temporary resistance on man against the African trypanosomes. One gram of drug injected in an adult will usually protect for about three months against trypanosomiasis.

IMMUNOLOGICAL PROCEDURES

The only parasitic infection in which the vaccination of man is routinely practiced is Oriental sore. In endemic areas, where a large percentage of the population is infected, lesions in hidden sites in children are deliberately induced by inoculating material from a sore in the hope thus of developing in the child an immunity which will prevent disfiguring natural lesions on the face or other exposed site. The fully virulent living parasite must be used in this vaccination.

In the case of several parasitic infections, immunity is acquired through prior infection (see Chapter IV). This is true in infection with *Endamoeba histolytica* and with malarial parasites, although evidently, in each case, low-grade or latent infection must continue if the immune state is to be preserved. With no helminth has an absolute immunity to reinfection been demonstrated in man, although some degree of immunity seems likely to result from an initial infection with the somatic tissue helminths. Vaccination or deliberate infection is, however, not practiced as a prophylactic measure against any helminth disease.

EDUCATION

Even in an endemic center, informed persons generally can devise means of protecting themselves from a given parasite. Often comparatively small changes from the routine of the natives suffice to afford the informed person perfect protection from the parasite in question. If drinking water be boiled, for example, infection by parasites spread through water can often be avoided. If meat be cooked thoroughly, it likewise will be safe to use. If even thin-soled shoes be worn, hookworm larvae will not be able to invade the skin of the foot. And considerable protection from tropical insects and the infectious agents they transmit will follow the screening of houses or sleeping beneath mosquito nets.

Custom is strong, however, especially when fortified by religious teachings, and native peoples are particularly loath to change their ways, despite the perfect logic of educational programs. But however slow the progress, education is probably in the end the most effective method of prophylaxis, for without appreciation of both the danger

of infection and also the advantages of freedom from it, the layman
—in the temperate zone as well as in the tropics—will be slow to en-
deavor either to protect himself from animal parasites or to coöper-
ate in affording protection to his fellow man.

Part Two

INFECTIONS CAUSED BY
ANIMAL PARASITES

Chapter VIII

THE AMOEBIASES

AMOEBAE are one-celled protozoans (class Rhizopoda) which can be identified chiefly by their possessing, in the "vegetative" or growing stage, pseudopodia which enable the organisms to move. Many amoebae are free-living forms, but some characteristically live as parasites in the bodies of other animals. A few species are parasitic upon man.

Altogether, six distinct species of amoeba can infect man. Only one of these forms, however—namely, *Endamoeba histolytica*—is known to invade tissue and thus to cause disease; the others—*Endamoeba coli, Endamoeba gingivalis, Endolimax nana, Iodamoeba williamsi,* and *Dientamoeba fragilis*—are harmless commensals. All of the human amoebae are found in the large intestine excepting *Endamoeba gingivalis,* which occurs in the mouth. The various species are differentiated by the characters mentioned in the following key:

A. Nucleus with peripheral chromatin, small karyosome
  I. Intestinal form; trophozoite actively motile, often with phagocyted erythrocytes, nucleus with central karyosome; cysts quadrinucleate —*Endamoeba histolytica*
  II. Mouth form; trophozoite actively motile, often with phagocyted erythrocytes, nucleus with central karyosome; no cysts—*Endamoeba gingivalis*
  III. Intestinal form; trophozoites somewhat sluggish, never (seldom) with phagocyted erythrocytes; nucleus with eccentric karyosome; cysts with eight nuclei—*Endamoeba coli*
B. Nucleus without peripheral chromatin, large karyosome
  I. Intestinal form; trophozoite sluggish; cysts quadrinucleate—*Endolimax nana*
  II. Intestinal form; trophozoite sluggish; cysts with single nucleus and one or more glycogen masses—*Iodamoeba williamsi*

C. Nucleus without peripheral chromatin; nuclear chromatin divided to four or five masses around a central dot; two nuclei usually present; cysts unknown—*Dientamoeba fragilis*

ENDAMOEBA HISTOLYTICA AND AMOEBIC INFECTION

Endamoeba histolytica [1] was first described in 1875 by Lösch, who had observed the parasite in the dysenteric stool of a Russian boy in St. Petersburg. Although he succeeded in transferring the amoebic infection to a dog by injecting the animal rectally with some of the patient's feces, Lösch did not consider the amoebae the cause of the patient's disease. Support was accorded *Endamoeba histolytica* as a possible pathogen, however, when Robert Koch in Egypt in 1883 observed the parasite deep in the tissues of the intestinal wall of dysenteric cases. Kartulis later observed the parasite in abscesses of the liver (1887) and of the brain (1904). Two objections were raised, however, against accepting amoebae as the etiological agent in dysentery: (1) amoebae were often present without dysentery, and (2) cases of dysentery were known in which no amoebae occurred. The first of the objections was met by the work of Quincke and Roos in the United States, who showed that other species of amoebae besides the pathogenic form occur in man. Their work was later confirmed by other observers, and in 1903 Schaudinn named the pathogenic species *Endamoeba histolytica*. Meanwhile, the second objection was set aside by the discovery, in 1898, by Shiga, that some forms of dysentery are caused by bacteria.

The question of the pathogenicity of amoebae was not finally settled until 1913 when Walker and Sellards performed a classical experiment upon sixty inmates of a prison in Manila, Philippine Islands. The men were divided into three equal groups. To the first, cysts of free-living amoebae were fed. The second group received cysts of the obligate intestinal parasite, *Endamoeba coli*. The third group were fed cysts of *Endamoeba histolytica*. Although amoebic cysts appeared in the feces of some of the men in each group, it was only among those of the third group, which had received cysts of *Endamoeba histolytica*, that symptoms were observed. In this group of twenty men, seventeen became infected with the parasite within a few days, and four of these developed acute cases of dysentery.

[1] Common synonyms: *Entamoeba histolytica; Entamoeba dysenteriae.*

Endamoeba histolytica has world-wide distribution, with its greatest incidence in warmer regions. It is common in China, Indo-China, the Philippine Islands, India, the Near East, countries bordering the Mediterranean Sea, the West Indies, Central and South America, and southern United States.

MORPHOLOGY AND LIFE CYCLE

Endamoeba histolytica occurs as a trophozoite in the large intestine or in tissue and as a cyst in the feces (Figure 1A). The trophozoite, when viewed in fresh preparations, is an actively motile form. Usually it measures about twenty-five microns in diameter, although forms as small as fifteen microns or as great as seventy-five microns in diameter sometimes are encountered. The cell is made up of both ectoplasm and endoplasm. The fingerlike or bladelike pseudopodia, by which the organism moves, consist of ectoplasm. The endoplasm, which contains the nucleus and food vacuoles, flows into the ectoplasmic pseudopodia as these are developed. When the organism is stained by the iron-alum-hematoxylin technique, the detailed morphology of the nucleus becomes visible. There is a thin, nuclear membrane with small black granules or dots evenly spaced over its inner surface. In the exact center of the nucleus is the small black-staining karyosome, which is connected with the nuclear membrane by fibrils forming a linin network.

The cysts of *Endamoeba histolytica* are spherical bodies five to twenty microns in diameter. After being stained by the iron-alum-hematoxylin technique, four nuclei can usually be seen. These, although smaller, are morphologically like the nucleus of the trophozoite. Food vacuoles are absent from the cyst, but a deeply staining chromatoidal mass, which is absent from the trophozoites, characteristically is found in the cyst. The cyst wall is not stained by the usual methods, and remains as a clear hyaline border of the cell.

The quadrinucleate cysts of *Endamoeba histolytica*, after being swallowed by man, are carried to the posterior small intestine or the anterior large intestine before excystment takes place. Here the amoebae, after one more nuclear division, finally divide to eight small forms, representing young trophozoites. These soon multiply many

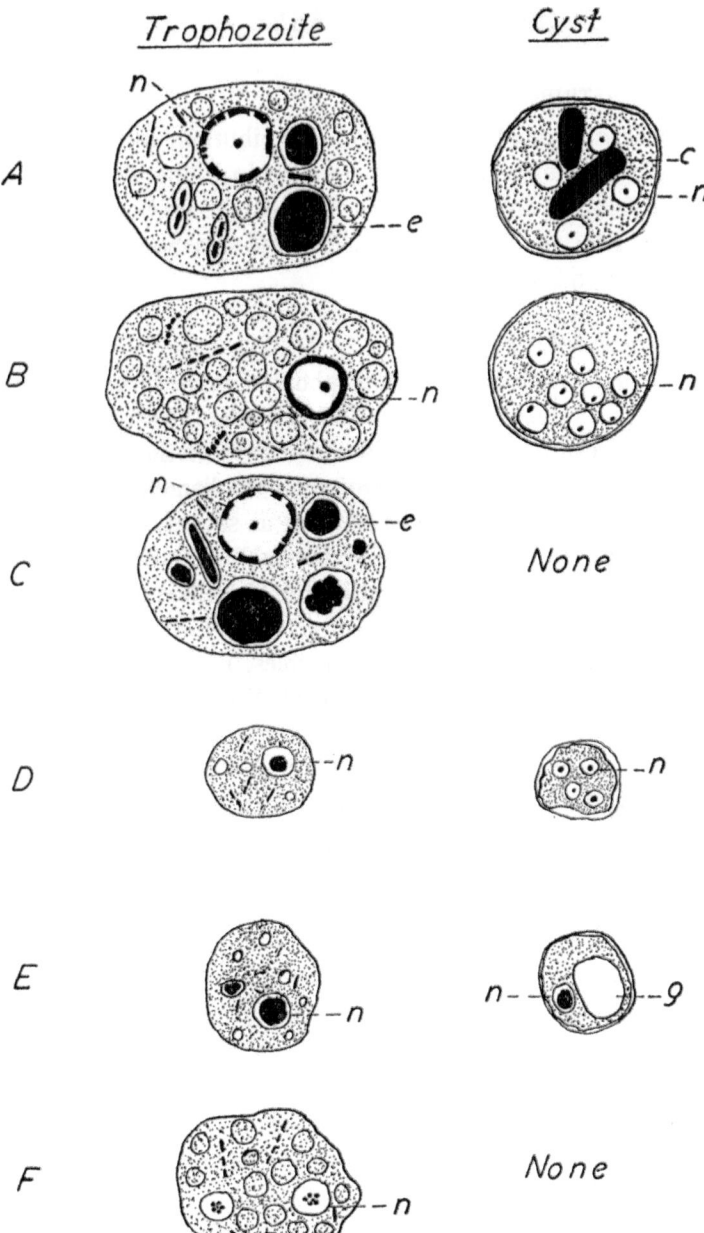

Figure 1. The amoebae of man: A, *Endamoeba histolytica*; B, *Endamoeba coli*; C, *Endamoeba gingivalis*; D, *Endolimax nana*; E, *Iodamoeba williamsi*; F, *Dientamoeba fragilis*. c = chromidial bar; e = erythrocyte in food vacuole; g = glycogen mass; n = nucleus.

times by fission. They promptly penetrate the tissues of the large intestinal wall, lysing their course beneath the epithelium by secreting a cytolysin. Those forms which do not invade tissue may become encysted, and these cysts are passed out with the feces. The cysts are rather resistant bodies which may survive for weeks in water or another favorable medium until they are ingested by another individual. They pass through the stomach unchanged, because of their resistance to the gastric juice, but they excyst in the intestine, since trypsin digests the cyst wall.

CULTIVATION

Endamoeba histolytica was first cultivated in 1925 by Boeck and Drbohlav in L.E.S. medium (see Appendix, p. 261). Cultures in this medium must be transferred every forty-eight hours or so but can be maintained indefinitely. Both trophozoites and cysts are formed in cultures. If the culture is left at room temperature for several hours, cysts with more than four nuclei often develop. Another medium which has been devised by Tsuchiya (see Appendix, p. 261) is said to require less frequent transplantation of the organism. The parasite generally maintains its virulence despite continued cultivation for several years.

Bacteria-free cultures of *Endamoeba histolytica* have been obtained by the inoculation of sterile media with the bacteria-free pus of an amoebic liver abscess, as well as by other procedures. Thus far, however, the organism has survived for only a few days in such cultures.

EPIDEMIOLOGY

The incidence of infection with *Endamoeba histolytica* varies much in different parts of the world, although generally it is higher in warmer regions. In Iraq from thirty to forty percent of the general population are infected, and in Egypt at least fifteen percent harbor the parasite. In southern United States, the incidence is generally said to be approximately ten percent. Northern Europe has a peculiarly low incidence, according to most reports, the incidence there being about 5 percent.

With respect to amoebiasis in the Western Hemisphere, Faust has stated, "there is substantial evidence that amoebiasis exists in an appreciable portion of the Western Hemisphere from Central West

Canada (52°30′ N. latitude) to the Strait of Magellan (52° S. latitude); that it is much more intensely endemic in the American tropics than in the temperate zones; and that in areas like the United States the incidence figure may possibly average as high as 20 percent, or double that of previously accepted estimates." [2]

Infection with *Endamoeba histolytica* is maintained in any community by carriers of the parasite—that is, by persons who often are unaware of their infection. These persons constantly eliminate cysts of the parasite in their feces. If these cysts reach the food, especially fresh vegetables and fruits, or the drink of other individuals, such persons are then exposed to infection. Quite often, food handlers or those who prepare foods are carriers of the organism and unwittingly lead to the infection of those who ingest the food which they prepare or handle.

Amoebic Dysentery, Report of Epidemic.—An epidemic of amoebic dysentery developed among visitors to Chicago, Illinois, during the summer of 1933, the first year of the Chicago World's Fair, "Century of Progress." Between June 1, 1933, and June 30, 1934, 1,409 cases with 98 deaths were reported among such persons, this number undoubtedly representing but a part of the total of those infected. Essentially all of the cases were among the guests of two large hotels in Chicago. Investigation finally revealed that the infections resulted from faulty plumbing in these hotels, there having been installed cross-connections between the sewerage system and the water conduits. The epidemic was, then, water borne, infection resulting from drinking polluted water. A careful survey of the regular employees of the hotels showed more than thirty-five percent were infected with *Endamoeba histolytica*.[3]

Active cases of amoebic dysentery are not responsible for the spread of the infection, for such cases pass in their feces only trophozoites which soon die when outside the body. Even if these trophozoites while still alive are swallowed by a susceptible individual, infection is unlikely, since the trophozoite will be digested. Only the cyst stage is able to resist the stomach acid while passing to the intestine.

Lower animals are not significant, probably, as vectors of *Endamoeba histolytica*. In dogs and cats only trophozoites are produced. The *Macacus* monkey acts as a natural host of the parasite, but little chance exists of widespread human infection from the monkey. The

[2] E. C. Faust, *American Journal of Tropical Medicine*, 22: 93 (1942).
[3] H. Bundesen, National Institute of Health, *Bulletin*, 1936.

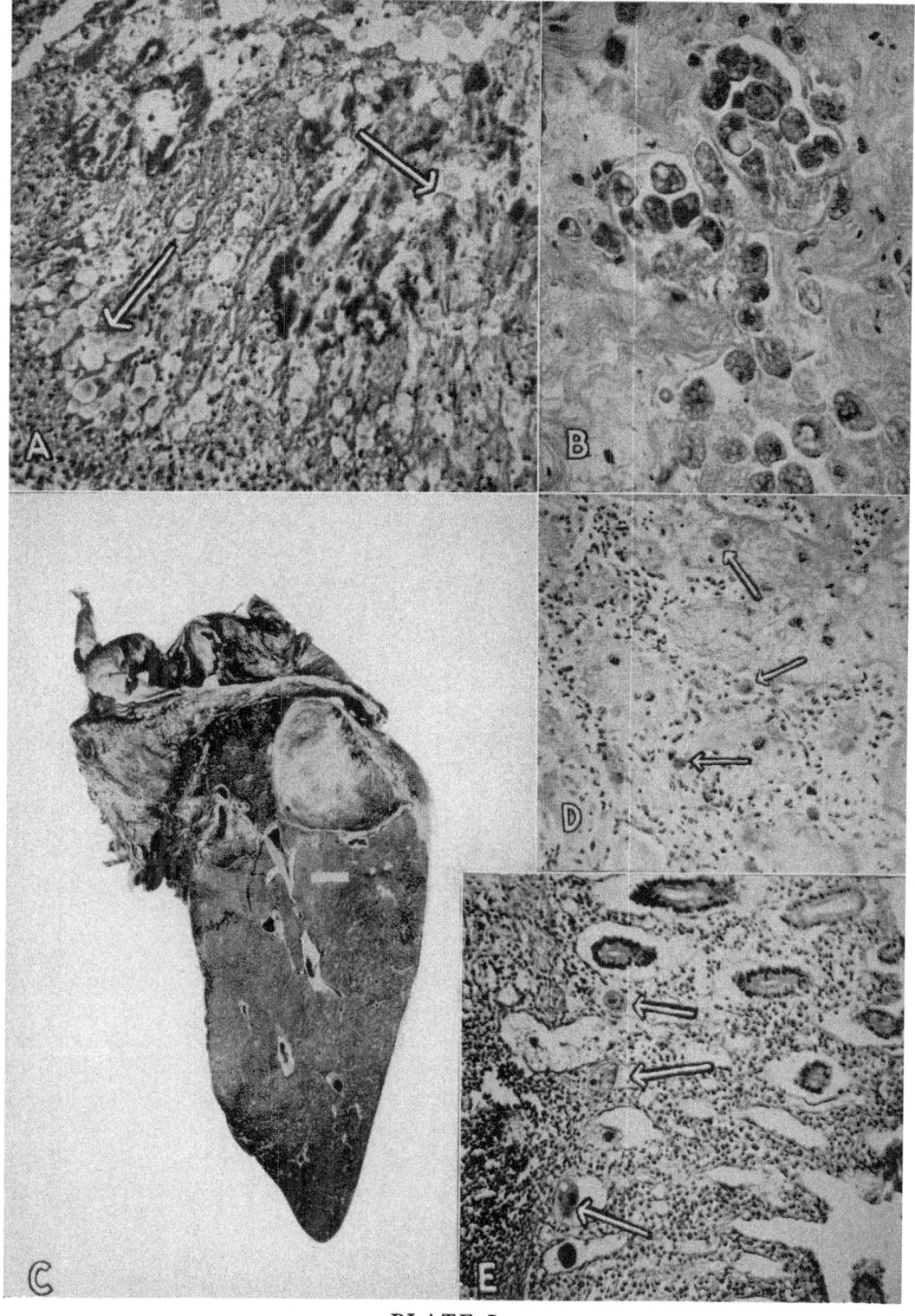

PLATE I

A. *Endamoeba histolytica* in intestinal lesion. Arrows indicate areas where many amoebae can be seen. (x100)   B. Nest of *Endamoeba histolytica* in section of intestinal mucosa. (x200) C. Amoebic abscess in liver. Gross section.   D. *Endamoeba histolytica* in lung abscess. Arrows indicate some of the amoebae. (x100)   E. Balantidiasis: lesion of large intestine showing *Balantidium coli*. (x100)

rat is the only lower animal which may prove to be a significant vector. Cysts are sometimes formed in this host, and the animal's habit of visiting human food stores provides opportunity for contaminating these foods with cysts of the parasite. Houseflies and some other insects may often act as mechanical vectors of the parasite cysts.

PATHOGENICITY

Most infections with *Endamoeba histolytica* are confined to the intestinal wall, where the organism causes the disease amoebic dysentery, or primary amoebiasis. With some frequency, however, metastatic lesions develop in other organs, chiefly in the liver. These are cases of secondary amoebiasis.

Primary (intestinal) infection.—Infection with *Endamoeba histolytica* generally takes the form of a chronic disease. The lesions which occur in the intestinal infection are generally confined to the colon. Any part of the colon length may present lesions, although they usually occur just behind the ileocaecal valve or else in the sigmoid flexure. Often the lesion is limited to the mucosal or submucosal layers of the wall, but sometimes muscle layers also are involved, and occasionally perforation of the intestinal wall occurs, with consequent peritonitis. Because of the tendency of the parasite to undermine the superficial mucosal tissue, the young ulcers are generally flask-shaped —with comparatively small openings from the intestinal lumen but extensive damage beneath the surface. Later, interconnecting serpiginous channels are formed deep in the tissue. Tissues surrounding uncomplicated lesions characteristically are not infiltrated by polymorphonuclear leucocytes or other cells from the blood. There is evidence that the parasite produces a histolysin, since the invaded tissue is eroded and finally completely digested. The lysin probably is secreted and passed into tissue in advance of the parasite, for the tissue is certainly killed prior to invasion by the amoebae. Indeed, this lysin may also make possible the initial penetration of the intestinal epithelium. (See Plate I, A and B, facing page 78.)

As a result of the erosion to the intestinal wall, blood vessels are opened and blood is found in the stools of infected persons. When the damage is extensive, a true dysentery develops with frequent copious bloody stools. In the carrier, often no symptoms are evident. The majority of patients finally check the progress of the parasite, even without treatment. In some, however, the injury spreads until use of the colon is lost. Sacculation of the colon, or obstruction through adhesions and strictures, commonly occurs. Colostomy may be necessary. Death from complicating factors is the frequent end.

Secondary amoebiasis.—In a considerable percentage of patients with intestinal amoebiasis, amoebic abscesses develop in other sites, probably largely as the result of the parasite lysing its way into small venules of the colon wall and being transported in the blood to the other organs. Most such abscesses occur in the liver, because this organ is most directly exposed to the amoebae entering venules of the portal system. In one large survey of 3,680 amoebic dysentery cases which came to autopsy, twenty-one percent showed abscesses of the liver. Oddly, liver abscess seldom occurs in women or children. It is rare also among natives—both male and female—in the tropics, despite a high incidence of intestinal amoebiasis among the native population. Other blood filters also may harbor abscesses. They have been described in the brain, spleen, lung, kidney, bones, and, indeed, practically all sites, including the orbit. Lesions of the skin are also known, occurring most frequently in the perianal region, but in other sites as well, such as about the sinus of a draining liver abscess. These infections result probably exogenously from local contamination. (See Plate I, C and D, facing page 78.)

The liver, and other organs also, may be largely incapacitated by destruction and lysis of tissue. Often a liter or more of fluid will be drawn from a liver abscess. Amoebae usually are few in this fluid, but are many in the unlysed but dead tissue bordering the abscess cavity. Cysts are seldom produced in the abscesses. Not infrequently the intestinal infection will be held in essentially complete abeyance or will even be eliminated spontaneously while extensive damage is going on in the liver or other organs.

IMMUNITY

Amoebiasis is generally an infection of adult persons, cases being comparatively rare among children. Most adults are probably relatively resistant to *Endamoeba histolytica.* Among those who contract infection, few manifest severe symptoms. The so-called "healthy carriers" of the parasite normally maintain a fair balance between repair of old lesions and the development of new ones and seldom become aware of their infection. Occasionally, this relative resistance will be lost, however, especially by persons who imbibe large amounts of alcohol.

An acquired immunity to *Endamoeba histolytica* evidently depends on premunition—that is, on the persistence of a latent infection with the parasite. When an infection is cured, either spontaneously or by drug treatment, the patient becomes once more susceptible to the infection. All infected individuals, including carriers and experimentally infected animals (dogs, cats, monkeys) develop antibodies against the organism, and these are detectable in the patient's or animal's serum by the complement fixation test.

DIAGNOSIS

Amoebic infection can be diagnosed (1) by observing the parasite directly in the feces with the microscope, (2) by cultivating the parasite, and (3) by detecting antibodies in the patient's serum.

Microscopic observation.—The diagnosis of intestinal amoebiasis is usually carried out by direct microscopic examination of the feces. Trophozoites are found only in those persons with acute dysenteric symptoms. Cysts occur in the feces of healthy carriers of the parasite. For best results, the patient is given a saline laxative and the stool is passed in the laboratory. It should be examined immediately after it is passed, since motile trophozoites will then probably be seen. An effort should be made to keep the stool warm until the examination is completed, and a warm-stage microscope is recommended for the examination. Generally a number of examinations of stools obtained on six or seven successive days must be found negative before the individual can safely be declared uninfected, for sometimes parasites are few and appear only at intervals. The parasites in the fresh stool can often be stained sufficiently for specific recognition by mixing a portion of the stool with iodine prior to examination, although saline or aqueous smears also are satisfactory. The iron-alum-hematoxylin technique is undoubtedly the finest staining procedure, but because of its difficulty it is not often resorted to. Simpler, more rapid staining methods are also available (see Appendix, p. 260). Usually the presence of erythrocytes in the motile trophozoite is sufficient to establish its identification.

The presence of Charcot-Leyden crystals (five to twenty-five microns in length) in the feces are regarded by some individuals as presumptive evidence of infection with amoebae. Such crystals also occur in coccidiosis (*Isospora hominis*), and various helminth infections, as well as in malignancy of the rectum and mucous colitis. They do not occur in bacillary dysentery.

Culture.—The diagnosis of amoebiasis is also possible by cultivating the stool in an appropriate medium. Usually some modification of Boeck's L.E.S. medium proves satisfactory (see Appendix, p. 261). The parasite can be found in such cultures after from twenty-four to forty-eight hours.

Complement fixation test.—In recent years the complement fixation test has been applied successfully for diagnosing amoebiasis. It is particularly useful in identifying abscess of the liver or of other organs when the parasite may not appear in the feces. The test is positive also in carriers of the parasite. When patients or carriers are cured of their infection, the complement fixation test becomes negative, but it is once more positive in cases which relapse. The antigen for the fixation test is prepared either from cultures of the parasite or from scrapings of colonic lesions in young puppies.

Sigmoidoscope examination.—When other methods for diagnosis fail, the sigmoidoscope may be used to identify intestinal infection with *Endamoeba histolytica*. Small, yellow ulcers are seen in the wall of the rectal canal, and if these are scraped with a probe passed through the sigmoidoscope, motile amoebae may be demonstrated microscopically in the scrapings. In old cases or in carriers, the lesions may be so small as to require a sigmoidoscope with a magnifying eyepiece for detection. Most authorities feel that the use of the sigmoidoscope seldom reveals cases that cannot be identified by the simpler procedures described above.

SPECIFIC THERAPY

Three drugs have been widely used for the treatment of amoebic infection: emetine, yatren (chiniofon or anayodin), and carbarsone. Emetine, an alkaloid of ipecacuanha, has probably received more extensive employment than the others, although recently authorities have largely agreed that this drug seldom or never wholly eradicates the parasite. It is still used very generally, however, for bringing a fulminating infection under control. It is very toxic, and must be given subcutaneously or intramuscularly. Emetine bismuth iodide, an insoluble powder, is especially useful for chronic carriers. It is given by mouth in gelatin capsules.

The drug of choice for amoebiasis at the present time is yatren, an iodine compound which seems to eliminate *Endamoeba histolytica* from lesions not only in the intestine but also in the liver and other sites. It can be given by mouth or by enema. By some authorities yatren is employed in conjunction with emetine-bismuth-iodide, the two drugs being given at the same time.

The third drug, carbarsone, has been less extensively employed than the others, but, in the hands of a few, has given satisfactory results. Its use is not advised for hepatic infections.

PROPHYLAXIS

Protection against amoebic infection generally is afforded by safeguarding food and drink from fecal contamination. Not only must stored food be protected from such contamination, but also food which is being prepared or served. Chefs, waiters, and others who handle the food immediately before its consumption may contaminate it with cysts carried on the hands or beneath finger nails. A mother cooking for her family may be responsible for the infection of that family. Food handlers should be inspected at regular intervals, and those found infected should be treated until cured, or else encouraged to find other occupation.

THE NONPATHOGENIC AMOEBAE

The nonpathogenic amoebae have a cosmopolitan distribution, with their greatest incidence in the warmer parts of the world. All the forms inhabit the human intestine except *Endamoeba gingivalis*, which occurs in the mouth. Most of the intestinal species—*Endamoeba coli, Endolimax nana,* and *Iodamoeba williamsi*—are transmitted when in the cyst stage, generally by the contamination of food or drink with feces from an infected carrier. *Dientamoeba fragilis* evidently forms no cysts but is passed as a trophozoite. *Endamoeba gingivalis*, which also forms no cysts, is probably spread directly from mouth to mouth. Although none of these parasites is pathogenic, the intestinal forms often increase in number during periods of diarrhea.

The diagnosis of these infections is usually established by observing the parasites in the feces, but all of the forms can be cultivated for at least a few generations in Boeck's L.E.S. medium. No drugs are available and none is needed for the eradication of these organisms. Persons can be protected from infection with the intestinal forms by safeguarding food or water from fecal contamination.

ENDAMOEBA COLI

Endamoeba coli (Figure 1, B) has been known as a parasite of man since 1870, when it was first described by Lewis. It is an especially common parasite, occurring in about fifty percent of the general population in the United States. It does not invade tissue and will not even ingest erythrocytes so long as other food is present. Its trophozoites are like those of *Endamoeba histolytica* in size and superficially resemble them in general structure. The organism moves, however, very sluggishly, and its endoplasm contains rather large vacuoles. The single nucleus when stained has a rather conspicuous eccentric karyosome and the peripheral chromatin is disposed in rather larger particles than in *Endamoeba histolytica*. The stained cyst characteristically reveals eight nuclei like that of the trophozoite. A chromatoidal mass is often present, its shape being less regular than that of the mass in cysts of *Endamoeba histolytica*.

ENDAMOEBA GINGIVALIS

Endamoeba gingivalis (Figure 1, C) is the only amoebae found in the human mouth. It occurs in about twenty-five percent of the general population. Its trophozoite stage is essentially identical in all respects with the trophozoites of *Endamoeba histolytica*. Even erythrocytes generally can be observed within it. Unlike *Endamoeba histolytica*, however, no cyst stage is known for *Endamoeba gingivalis*. Evidently, its transmission occurs directly from mouth to mouth, as during kissing. The parasite is commonly found about the teeth, especially if these are carious or if the gums have pyorrheal pus pockets. It is not deemed to be the cause of such conditions, however, and probably when in these sites is merely performing a scavenger function.

ENDOLIMAX NANA

Endolimax nana (Figure 1, D), commonly called the dwarf amoeba because of its small size, was first seen by Wenyon in 1912. It occurs in about twenty-five percent of the population. The very sluggish trophozoite measures up to twelve microns in diameter and has a nucleus with a very prominent karyosome but no peripheral chromatin. The cysts measure up to ten microns in diameter and are quadrinucleate. The cyst nuclei are smaller than, but otherwise similar to, those of the trophozoites.

IODAMOEBA WILLIAMSI

Iodamoeba williamsi [4] (Figure 1, E) was discovered by Wenyon in 1915. It is a fairly common form, occurring in about ten percent of the population. The trophozoite measures up to fourteen microns in diameter and is characteristically sluggish in its movements. Its nucleus has a large central karyosome, but no peripheral chromatin. The cysts are spherical, generally about ten microns in diameter, and—in distinction from all other parasitic amoebae of man—have a single nucleus in which the karyosome is eccentric. One or two conspicuous glycogen masses are characteristically present in the cyst.

DIENTAMOEBA FRAGILIS

Dientamoeba fragilis (Figure 1, F) is a rare parasite, whose trophozoites measure up to twelve microns. Characteristically, two nuclei are present, each with a central karyosome divided into several units. Little evidence is yet available for the occurrence of cysts. Some authorities believe this form responsible for disease symptoms.

[4] Common synonym: *Iodamoeba bütschlii*.

Chapter IX

THE LEISHMANIASES

THE ORGANISMS of the genus *Leishmania* are those protozoans which possess a single flagellum (order Protomonadina, class Mastigophora) and which have in their development only two stages: a leishmania and a leptomonas. The leishmania stage occurs principally in the vertebrate host and the leptomonas principally in an invertebrate. Three species of *Leishmania* infect man: *Leishmania donovani,* which causes the visceral infection kala azar, and *Leishmania tropica* and *Leishmania braziliensis,* which cause cutaneous (Oriental sore) or mucocutaneous (espundia) infections, respectively. The parasites responsible for these several disease entities are indistinguishable in morphology, but the diseases are easily differentiated.

LEISHMANIA DONOVANI AND VISCERAL LEISHMANIASIS (KALA AZAR)

Leishmania donovani [1] was first observed in 1900 by Leishman in the spleen of a soldier dead in India of kala azar or dumdum fever. Later, in 1903, the organisms were found by Donovan in biopsy material from the spleen of a patient with the disease.

Geographical distribution.—*Leishmania donovani* occurs in China, India, Mesopotamia, southern Russia, all the countries bordering the Mediterranean Sea, Ethiopia, the Sudan, and Nigeria. The parasite probably also occurs in Brazil and Argentina of South America. The infection in the countries of the Mediterranean area is generally confined to children of six years of age or less.

Morphology and life cycle.—*Leishmania donovani* is a small oval parasite, as seen in human tissue, measuring only about three microns in its greatest dimension. It contains a comparatively large, somewhat

---

[1] Common synonym: *Leishmania infantum.*

eccentric nucleus, which stains deep red with Wright's stain, and an axoneme or rhizoplast running to the margin of the cell from a more or less central kinetoplast (Figure 2).

When blood or tissue containing this leishmania stage is ingested by a sand fly (*Phlebotomus* spp.) or put into a tube of N.N.N. medium, further development of the parasite occurs, to the flagellated leptomonas stage. The leptomonas is a slender spindle-shaped body about twenty microns long by two or three microns wide. Its free flagellum arises from the kinetoplast at the anterior end of the cell and may be as long as the cell body. There is no undulating membrane. The nucleus lies in about the center of the cell. (See Figure 2.)

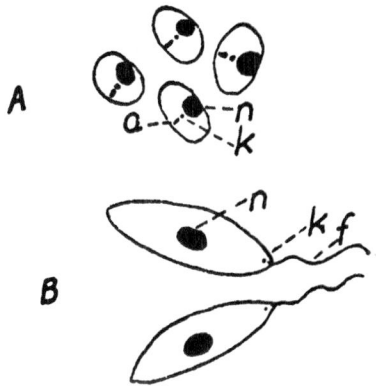

Figure 2. *Leishmania donovani:* A, Leishmania; B, Leptomonas. a = axoneme; f = flagellum; k = kinetoplast; n = nucleus.

The entire life cycle of *Leishmania donovani,* as well as of the other human leishmanias, consists, so far as known, of the two stages just described: the leishmania and the leptomonas stage. The leishmania form occurs in the reticulo-endothelial cells of man and is responsible for the human disease. Less is known about the natural role of the leptomonas stage in the life cycle, for although this stage develops in the sand fly, it has not been proved regularly in nature to pass from the sand fly back to man.

Cultivation.—*Leishmania donovani* was first cultivated by Rogers in 1904. The organism grows readily in N.N.N. medium, and cultures generally reveal many flagellated parasites (leptomonas) usually arranged in rosettes, within ten days or two weeks after infected blood is introduced. Individual organisms, some in longitudinal division, also occur in cultures.

Epidemiology.—The precise mode of infection of man with *Leish-*

mania donovani is as yet obscure. The sand fly (*Phlebotomus argentipes* especially, but others also) and many other bloodsucking insects have long been suspected of transmitting the parasite, but experimental proof of their capacity naturally to do so is as yet lacking. Sand flies become infected if fed on kala azar patients, but natural transmission from the sand fly back to man has only rarely been reported. If an infected sand fly be macerated and its substance injected by syringe into the skin of man, however, infection promptly results.

Recently, other approaches besides insect transmission have been investigated in an effort to explain the epidemiology of kala azar. Since the parasite occurs in the urine and feces of patients, the possibility of the disease being water bourne has been considered, infection of other individuals occurring through drinking water polluted with the feces or urine of kala azar patients. Experiments upon hamsters have shown that infection by mouth is possible, since these animals contract the disease if fed on the tissues of infected hamsters. Droplet infection also is suspected as a means of transmission, since the parasites occur in nasal secretions and could easily be sprayed into the air when the patient coughs or sneezes. Transmission of infection by direct physical contact not only with active human cases but likewise through naturally infected dogs and cats also has been suggested. As yet, however, none of these various possibilities for transmission of the parasite has been established, despite the fact that some epidemiological evidence for all the various routes has been forthcoming from experimental investigations.

The infection is in some countries (e.g., Italy) confined to young children, but in others (India) young adults are most commonly infected. Males are more often infected than females.

Infantile Kala Azar, Case Report.—A female child three years old had been brought to this country from Italy six months before admission to the hospital. She presented few specific symptoms but had continuous fever and an enlarged spleen. Blood culture for bacteria was negative. Finally, largely because other leads failed and because of the history of residence in the Mediterranean basin, it was decided to biopsy the spleen and look for *Leishmania donovani*. The parasite was found in abundance, and treatment with antimony was at once instituted, with resulting recovery. The case was of interest in revealing the long incubation period which is often observed in this infection.

Pathogenicity.—Kala azar is an infection of cells of the reticulo-endothelial system, the organisms proliferating in the reticular syncytium. As these susceptible cells increase in number, those newly formed also promptly become infected with the parasites. The spleen, liver, lymphatic glands, bone marrow, and skin as well as the submucosa of the intestinal wall become infiltrated with numerous macrophage cells and each of these is charged with rapidly multiplying parasites. (See Plate II, A, facing page 94.) The peripheral blood meanwhile reveals a progressive leucopenia, with a marked drop in polymorphonuclear cells but a rise in lymphocytes. Hemorrhage from any part of the body is a frequent symptom. An irregular fever accompanies the infection and is one of the earliest symptoms. Generally this is not so incapacitating as is the fever of malaria, and some patients continue their work unaware of their disease. A most extreme enlargement of the spleen and of the liver is soon noted. Dysentery is common, due in part probably to the leishmania but often to amoebae or to bacteria. Patients finally become severely emaciated and, unless treated, generally die. Acute infections—especially those in the Sudan—may terminate in a few weeks, but some cases last for two or three years before improvement sets in or death occurs. The infantile type of the disease seen in the Mediterranean countries is more severe than, but similar to, the adult infection.

In cases among Caucasians, the feet, hands, and abdomen take on a grey pigmentation which is responsible for the name kala azar ("black disease").

Immunity.—Recovered cases of kala azar are thereafter immune to reinfection with the same disease. Attempts thus far to immunize persons artificially against the infection have failed.

Diagnosis.—*Leishmania donovani* can rarely be demonstrated in stained blood films of the patient. When this method of diagnosis fails, stained smears can be made of the spleen or liver pulp, lymphatic glands, or bone marrow. The stained spleen smear is the method of choice for demonstrating the parasite, although, because considerable danger attends spleen puncture, none but a skilled worker should attempt diagnosis by this method. Examination of the bone marrow is said to reveal about as many positive cases and is less dangerous. Bone marrow is obtained from the sternum in adults and from the tibia in children. Puncture of the lymphatic glands is used chiefly in the

Chinese form of the disease, since in this the lymphatic glands become conspicuously enlarged. Recently, parasites have been shown often to appear in the skin.

Cultivation of any infected tissue in N.N.N. medium is also successfully resorted to as a diagnostic procedure, the parasite growing out in about two weeks after cultures are inoculated. Sterile technique in obtaining material from the patient and in inoculating the media is essential. The injection of hamsters with blood, lymph, or the pulp of the spleen or liver also is useful when the parasite cannot be otherwise demonstrated.

Serological procedures have not proved very useful in diagnosing kala azar. Agglutination and precipitation tests were devised as early as 1913, but the complement fixation test has seemed more useful. These tests are generally applied only when the parasite itself cannot be demonstrated.

Specific therapy.—Any of various antimony compounds serve for the cure of kala azar. Formerly, sodium or potassium antimony tartrate was employed, the freshly prepared solution being given intravenously. Compounds of pentavalent antimony have since come into use because of their lower toxicity. They are administered either intravenously or intramuscularly and generally give excellent results. Intensive treatment is always indicated. Inadequately treated cases often develop subsequently a nodular cutaneous leishmaniasis known as dermal leishmanoid, in which living leishmanias can be demonstrated in the substance of cutaneous nodules.

Prophylaxis.—No specific direction can be given to prevent the contraction of kala azar since the natural mode of spread of the infection is unknown. It is, nevertheless, wise to avoid all possible contact with cases of the disease either in man or in animals, to guard against bites by sand flies, and to avoid possible infection through contaminated water or food.

LEISHMANIA TROPICA AND CUTANEOUS LEISHMANIASIS (ORIENTAL SORE)

Leishmania tropica [2] was probably first observed by Cunningham in 1885 but was first accurately described by Borovsky, a Russian military surgeon, in 1898. It is the cause of cutaneous leishmaniasis,

[2] Common synonyms: *Helcosoma tropica; Herpetomonas tropica.*

which has been called by such different names as Oriental sore, tropical sore, Delhi boil, Aleppo boil, and bouton de Bagdad.

Geographical distribution.—Although *Leishmania tropica* and the disease it causes—generally known as Oriental sore—are present in many countries where *Leishmania donovani* and kala azar also occur, the two parasites seldom occupy precisely the same locality. *Leishmania tropica* is found in many of the countries bordering the Mediterranean Sea, in Ethiopia, the Sudan, the Congo, Nigeria, Mesopotamia and the Near East, southern Russia, India, Indo-China, and northern Australia.

Morphology and life cycle.—*Leishmania tropica* may be slightly larger than, but it otherwise is morphologically identical with, *Leishmania donovani*. The leishmaniform stage of the parasite, which alone is found in man, does not, however, usually occur in the tissues of visceral organs in human beings, as does that of *Leishmania donovani*, but is almost entirely confined to the skin. In the dog, on the other hand, in which *Leishmania tropica* occurs naturally, the leishmaniform stage does sometimes invade the tissues of the viscera.

The life cycle of *Leishmania tropica* is, so far as understood, similar to that of *Leishmania donovani*.

Cultivation.—*Leishmania tropica* can be cultivated in N.N.N. medium, the leptomonas stage developing in the same way as in cultures of *Leishmania donovani*.

Epidemiology.—Nearly all persons who reside for a significant period in endemic areas sooner or later contact infection with *Leishmania tropica*. Natives of such areas almost invariably have been infected at some time, usually while young. Missionaries and others who visit endemic areas likewise generally contract infection.

The parasite can certainly be transmitted by contact with an infected individual, and material from an Oriental sore proves infectious if inoculated into the skin of an uninfected person. Sand flies, particularly *Phlebotomus papatasii*, are considered possible natural vectors of the causal agent, although the vector relationship has not been absolutely proved. The sand fly certainly becomes infected through feeding on an Oriental sore, and if the infected fly is macerated and injected into a normal person, the person contracts a typical lesion. However, the transmission of the disease experimentally through the bite of the infected fly seems seldom or never to occur.

Monkeys and dogs are susceptible to experimental infection. The dog may also serve as a reservoir host.

Pathogenicity.—Oriental sores sometimes are single but often occur multiply. A hundred or more separate sores simultaneously have been observed in some patients. The lesions generally occur on the exposed extremities or the face, seldom on the body trunk, and never on the hairy scalp, palms, or soles. The lesion is characteristically confined to the skin. It begins as a small red papule, which gradually extends. The stratum corneum becomes hypertrophied and infiltrated with macrophages which contain numerous parasites, these macrophages often being disposed as nests or clusters of cells. Sometimes the papule recedes, but commonly it goes on to ulceration. The ulcer is of an undermining type, with its edges raised. It usually reaches one inch in diameter, but, when several sores coalesce, an ulcerating area four inches or so across may result. Secondary bacterial infection of the open ulcer is common. Usually the lesion heals after a few months even if untreated, but often a disfiguring scar results from contraction of the tissue.

Immunity.—It was early noted by the Jews of Bagdad that persons who had recovered from one Oriental sore seldom experienced infection with a second. This fact led to their introduction of vaccination against the disease, a procedure which has since had wide use in endemic regions. Mothers in such areas infect their children on some hidden site and thus safeguard them from the possibility of later contracting disfiguring facial lesions of the disease. Material from an active sore may be inoculated on the thigh, for example, or pure cultures of the organism can be injected. In any case, however, an actual infection with living virulent organisms is necessary, and a characteristic Oriental sore must result. Protection once secured endures for at least several years.

Diagnosis.—Oriental sore is diagnosed by observing the causal parasites in stained smears of material obtained from the edge of the ulcer. (See Plate II, B, facing page 94.) Parasites seldom or never occur in the circulating blood or in visceral organs. Cultures also are helpful in diagnosis, the cultured material coming from the edge of the lesion.

Oriental Sore, Case Report.—A missionary and his family returned to New York in 1940 from Teheran, Iran. A few weeks after arrival, the daughter, age three years, developed a cheek lesion near the corner of the mouth. The history of residence in the Near East, together with the gross appearance of the lesion, suggested Oriental sore. When a film of tissue fluid taken from the margin of the ulcer was stained and examined microscopically, typical *Leishmania tropica* were revealed. The child had evidently been infected abroad, but the lesion appeared many weeks later after the patient returned to this country.

Specific therapy.—Oriental sores are successfully treated with compounds of pentavalent antimony, such as stibosan, given either intravenously or intramuscularly. Tartar emetic, a compound of trivalent antimony, also is used. Often ointments containing antimony (tartar emetic) are applied locally with success. The application of carbon dioxide snow, or the use of X ray, is sometimes advised, as is also the local injection of solutions of berberine sulphate or emetine hydrochloride.

Prophylaxis.—Infection with *Leishmania tropica* is prevented by avoiding contact with either human or animal (dog) cases of Oriental sore or with insects (sand flies) which might have visited such cases. Even indirect contact, as might occur through having an infected person do one's family laundering, is discouraged. Persons who are infected should be treated so as not to expose others; during the course of treatment their sores should be covered, so as to lessen the danger to other persons.

Biological prophylaxis is also possible, as mentioned above in the section on immunity. In this, living cultures of the causal agent are injected in a hidden site. Recovery from the sore resulting from such inoculation protects against reinfection.

LEISHMANIA BRAZILIENSIS AND MUCOCUTANEOUS LEISHMANIASIS (ESPUNDIA)

Leishmania braziliensis [3] was first seen in the mucocutaneous ulcers of espundia in South America by Lindenberg and by Carini and Paranhos in 1909. The parasite is by most authorities considered a distinct species, although some believe that it is a variety of *Leishmania tropica*. The disease has been called by various names: uta, forest yaws, bubas braziliana, espundia, American leishmaniasis, and nasopharyngeal leishmaniasis.

Geographical distribution.—*Leishmania braziliensis* is probably confined to the Western Hemisphere, where it is found almost entirely in

---

[3] Common synonyms: *Leishmania tropica* var. *americana; Leishmania peruviana.*

Central and South America. Endemic cases are known for all the countries of South America, except perhaps Chile, and for Panama, Mexico (Yucatan), and the island of Martinique. Cases resembling the American disease have been reported from Italy, Somaliland, and the Sudan.

Morphology and life cycle.—The morphology and life cycle of *Leishmania braziliensis* are identical with those of *Leishmania donovani*. The leptomonas parasite will develop in the sand fly *Phlebotomus intermedius.*

Cultivation.—*Leishmania braziliensis* can be cultivated in N.N.N. medium, the leptomonas parasites developing within two weeks or so after inoculation.

Epidemiology.—In some endemic areas, infection with *Leishmania braziliensis* is very common. In parts of Paraguay, for example, eighty percent infection has been noted in the general population. Forest workers are most often afflicted. Both natives and strangers in an endemic area are susceptible. Adult males are most frequently infected, perhaps because of their greater exposure while working in rubber tree plantations or while engaged as gum pickers.

The natural mode of transmission of *Leishmania braziliensis* is not established, although a sand fly, *Phlebotomus intermedius,* is believed capable of serving as vector. Direct contact with cases in man or dog is also probably responsible for many infections.

Pathogenicity.—Infection with *Leishmania braziliensis* generally begins with a chancrous papule resembling an Oriental sore. Often this seems wholly to heal, but sometimes, after a variable interval, an extensive series of ulcers containing macrophages filled with leishmanias develops. These may appear on the arms or legs (Plate II, C, facing this page), but are very common on the mucous surface of the nose, mouth, and even the tongue. If untreated, such ulcers often lead to a fatal end. Sometimes the most distressing facial disfiguration is experienced before death, the nose as well as the hard and soft palates being eroded away. The capacity for speech is interfered with, if not lost entirely, from damage to the tongue and larynx. Death usually is precipitated by secondary invaders.

Diagnosis.—The observation of *Leishmania braziliensis* in stained smears of material excised from lesions of espundia suffices to diagnose the disease. Sometimes the parasite can be cultivated from such ma-

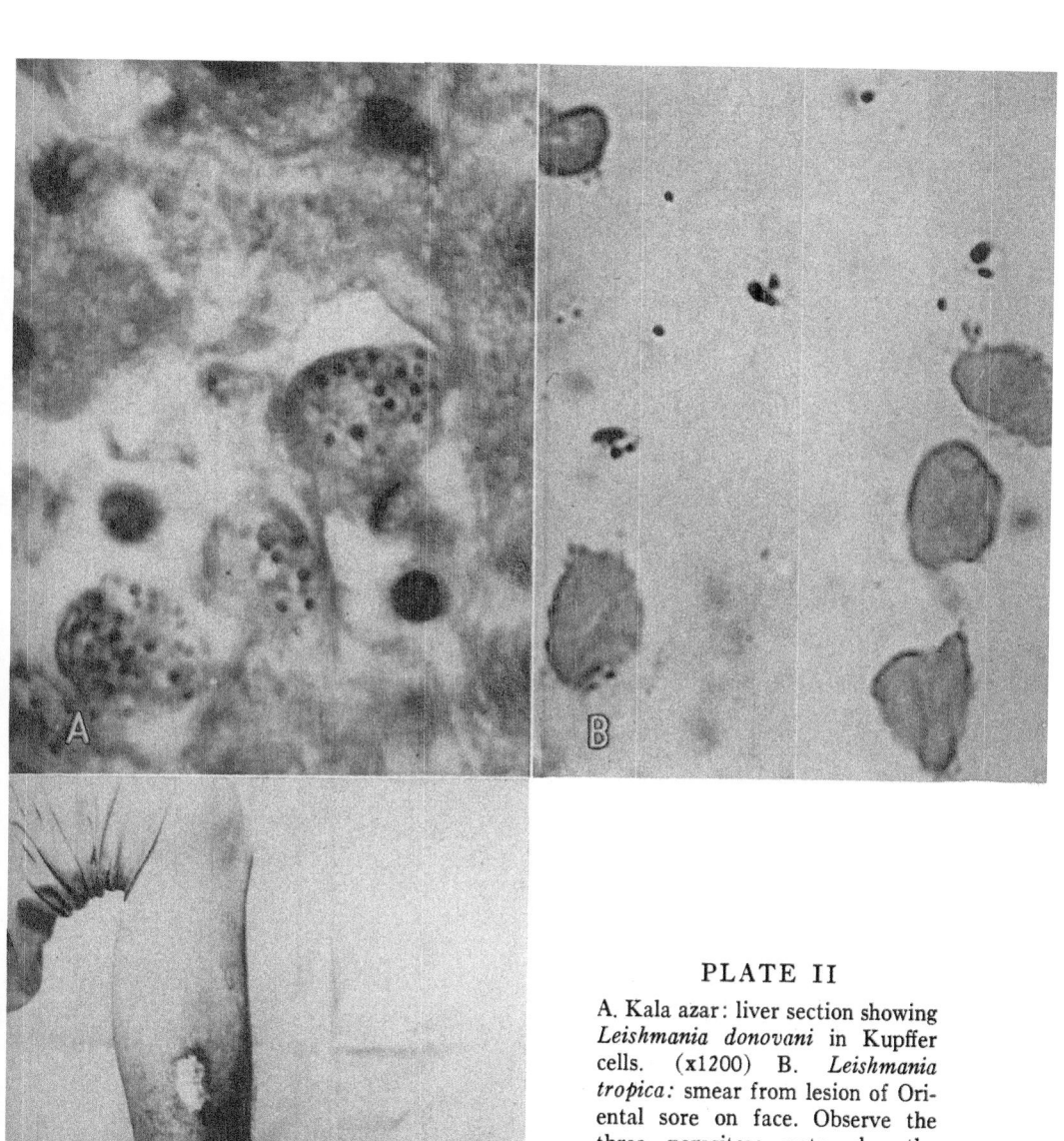

PLATE II

A. Kala azar: liver section showing *Leishmania donovani* in Kupffer cells. (x1200) B. *Leishmania tropica:* smear from lesion of Oriental sore on face. Observe the three parasites; note also the erythrocytes. (x1500) C. Cutaneous leishmaniasis: ulcer near a maleolus; above, scar from healed ulcer.

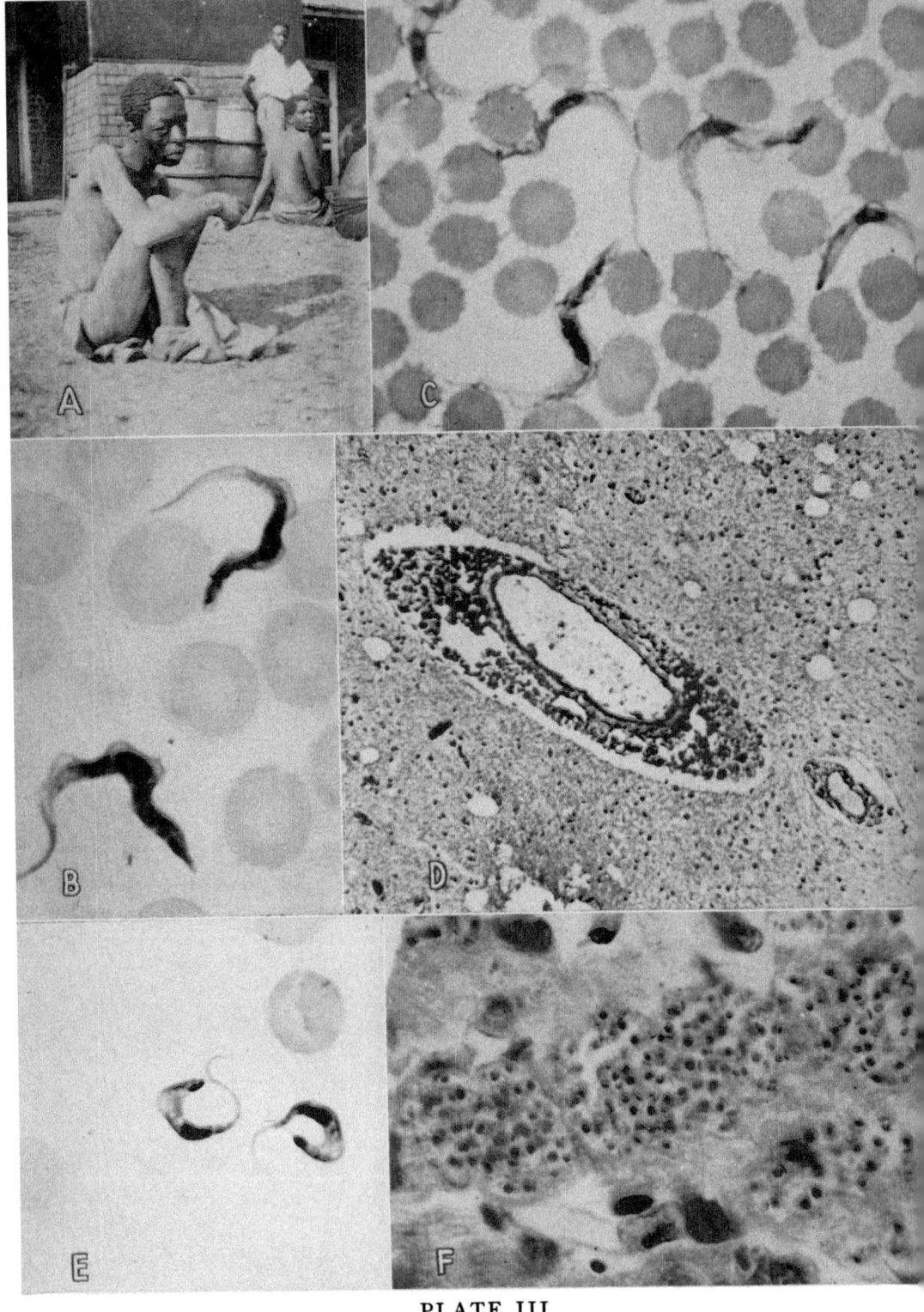

PLATE III

A. African sleeping sickness: advanced stage. B. *Trypanosoma gambiense* in peripheral blood.
(x1200) C. *Trypanosoma rhodesiense* in peripheral blood. (x1200) D. Trypanosomiasis:
section of human brain showing perivascular infiltration with leucocytes. (x100) E. *Trypanosoma cruzi:* trypaniform stage in peripheral blood. (x1200) F. *Trypanosoma cruzi:* leishmaniform stage in heart muscle. (x1200)

terial or even from the juice of regional glands, although the peripheral blood and visceral organs are sterile.

Antigens prepared from cultures of *Leishmania braziliensis* elicit skin reactions in a high percentage of cases of espundia.

Specific therapy.—The intravenous injection of solutions of sodium- or potassium-antimony-tartrate leads to the cure of espundia. External applications of the drug directly to the lesions also is sometimes helpful. Pentavalent antimony compounds, which are given intramuscularly, also are effective therapeutic agents.

Prophylaxis.—Contraction of infection with *Leishmania braziliensis* is generally prevented if one avoids contact with human or animal (dog) cases of infection and protects himself from the bites of sand flies and other insects.

Chapter X

THE TRYPANOSOMIASES

THE TRYPANOSOMES include those protozoans with a single flagellum (order Protomonadina, class Mastigophora), which have typically four developmental stages: leishmania, leptomonas, crithidia, and trypanosome. The leptomonas and the crithidia stages dwell principally in an invertebrate host; the leishmania and the trypanosome stages occur chiefly in a vertebrate. For many species, some of these stages have not yet been described. (See Figure 3.)

Three species of trypanosomes infect man: *Trypanosoma gambiense, Trypanosoma rhodesiense,* and *Trypanosoma cruzi.* The first two of these forms are found exclusively in Africa, where they cause a form of sleeping sickness, transmitted by tsetse flies. The third species is found exclusively in the Western Hemisphere, where it causes Chagas's disease, transmitted by any of several species of hemipteran insects.

TRYPANOSOMA GAMBIENSE AND GAMBIAN SLEEPING SICKNESS OF AFRICA

Although the sleeping sickness stage of trypanosomiasis had been known as a disease of man since shortly after the year 1800, the fact that trypanosomes were responsible for this condition was not established until about one hundred years later. In 1901, Forde found in the blood of a European suffering from fever in the River Gambia colony of Africa a strange organism which Dutton concluded from further observations in 1902 to be a trypanosome. In the next year Castellani found the trypanosome in the spinal fluid as well as in the blood of a case of sleeping sickness in Uganda. During subsequent years the causal relationship of the trypanosome to the disease and its transmission by the tsetse fly, *Glossina palpalis*, were fully established.

Geographical distribution.—*Trypanosoma gambiense* occurs in numerous isolated communities of Senegal, Sierra Leone, Nigeria, and the Cameroons of West Africa, and in the Belgian Congo, Angola, and

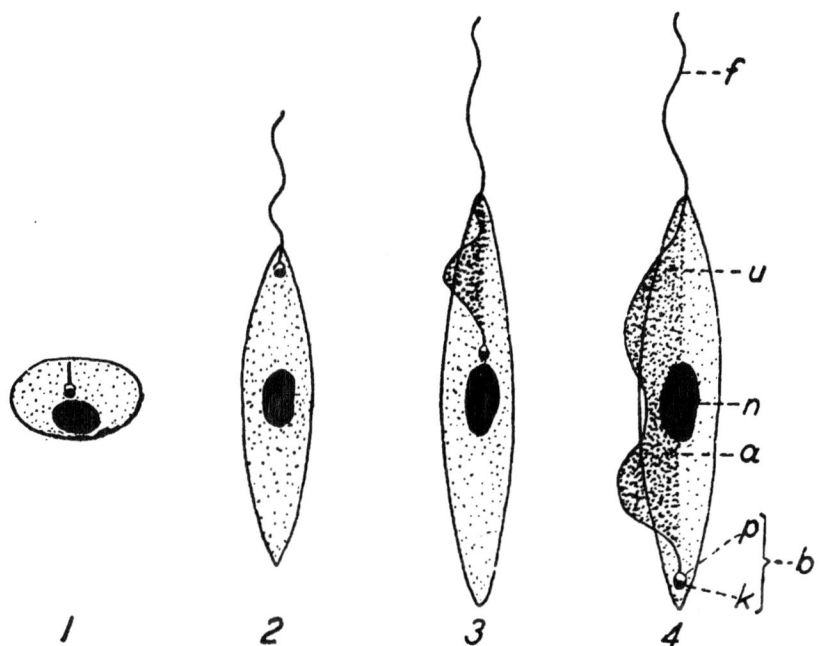

Figure 3. Developmental stages of typical trypanosome: 1, leishmania; 2, leptomonas; 3, crithidia; 4, trypanosome. a = axoneme; b = blepharoplast; f = flagellum; k = kinetoplast; n = nucleus; p = parabasal body; u = undulating membrane.

Uganda, of Central Africa. Its distribution coincides quite perfectly with that of its natural vector, *Glossina palpalis*. Generally this vector is confined to the underbrush bordering streams, and infection is greatest in communities near such streams.

Morphology and life cycle.—*Trypanosoma gambiense*, as it occurs in the blood of man, is a polymorphic trypanosome: a long slender, flagellated form, a short stumpy aflagellar form, and an intermediate form all are known. In the fresh blood, the cells exhibit constant motion and might easily be mistaken for large spirochetes. In blood films stained with Wright's stain, they appear as spindle-shaped bodies fifteen to thirty microns long, with an undulating membrane running nearly the full length of the cell. A nucleus is located about the mid-length, and at the posterior end is a kinetoplast from which rises an axoneme which runs anteriorly along the border of the undulating membrane. Usually the axoneme terminates as a free flagellum. Reproduction of the cells occurs in the peripheral blood, by longitudinal division. Sexual forms are unknown. (See Plate III, B, facing page 95.)

When blood containing trypanosomes is swallowed by the tsetse fly (*Glossina palpalis*), the trypanosomes lose their infectivity after two days. They proceed to reproduce by longitudinal division in the midgut and hindgut, some of those forms seen having the morphology of crithidia. Between the tenth and fifteenth days, exceptionally long, slender trypanosomes with poorly developed undulating membranes appear in the proventriculus of the insect. These migrate anteriorly to the hypopharynx of the fly, and thence go on to the salivary glands. Crithidial forms develop here between the fifteenth and thirtieth day after the fly becomes infected and reproduce rapidly by division. Finally, in from twenty to forty days after the fly infection, infective adult trypanosomes develop in the salivary glands. These are ejected along with saliva into the bite wound just before a blood meal is taken from the next individual who is bitten. About ten days later the polymorphic parasites can be seen in the blood of this person.

Cultivation.—If blood from a person infected with *Trypanosoma gambiense* is inoculated into N.N.N. medium (see Appendix p. 262), the parasites persist for five or six weeks with little change. Reproduction is limited and sometimes may not even occur. Subcultures in N.N.N. medium are not usually obtained.

Epidemiology.—Man is the natural reservoir of *Trypanosoma gambiense*, but many game animals also serve as alternate reservoirs. Many kinds of antelopes, including waterbuck, reedbuck, bushbuck, and situtunga, as well as most domesticated animals, such as ox, goat, and sheep, and laboratory animals (except baboon and fowl) serve as hosts. The natural transmitter of *Trypanosoma gambiense* is the tsetse fly, *Glossina palpalis*. Other types of bloodsucking flies are not believed involved in the natural transmission of this species of trypanosome. The tsetse fly apparently can act either as a mechanical or as a biologic transmitting agent. If a tsetse fly is interrupted while feeding on an infected person, it may attack a second individual while living trypanosomes remain on its proboscis. These may be introduced into the second individual and result in the infection of that person. If the fly is not interrupted in its first feeding, it will not be likely to attack a second individual until after any trypanosomes on its proboscis are dead by drying. Since those parasites which are swallowed soon lose their infectivity for man, the fly will then be unable to convey the parasite to another individual until after the twenty to forty days during which the parasites must develop through the fly to reach the infective stage in the fly salivary gland.

By no means all the tsetse flies found in nature—even of the appropriate species—are infected with *Trypanosoma gambiense*. Indeed, only about 0.2 percent of those caught in the field harbor the parasite. Among laboratory-bred flies which are fed upon infected captive animals, only from three to five percent usually become infected, although the percentage is improved if, after a first feeding, the flies are starved. Both male and female flies become infected and can transmit the parasite back to the vertebrate host.

The natural transmitting insect lives characteristically in shaded areas, which are to be found only around native villages or along streams. It is here, however, that contact with man is most likely. The infection in man often occurs epidemically, almost the entire population of a small village becoming infected. It is found quite commonly also in boatmen, fishermen, and others whose occupation is associated with watercourses. The flies generally travel only two hundred feet or so from their natural haunts, seldom molesting persons aboard river craft in midstream or individuals in open fields a few hundred feet from the river bank. However, they frequently follow into the open country a person who has passed through the underbrush where they dwell.

Pathogenicity.—In the early stages of infection with *Trypanosoma gambiense* the lymphatic glands become swollen, congested, and even hemorrhagic, especially those in the posterior cervical and submaxillary regions and in the mesentery. The spleen becomes hypertrophied. The meninges may be congested, and the cerebrospinal fluid may become turbid and of increased amount. Throughout the brain, cord, and meninges, but most conspicuously in the medulla and cerebral cortex, the perivascular tissue becomes infiltrated with small round cells. (See Plate III, D, facing page 95.) Trypanosomes, sometimes in small nests, may be found in the nervous tissue. They occur also in the cerebrospinal fluid, which they enter through the choroid plexus. Often nests of parasites also occur in the myocardium, at least in animals infected experimentally with the organism.

Generally a comparatively severe local reaction lasting for several days occurs in the skin immediately after a tsetse fly has bitten the individual. Symptoms of the trypanosome infection proper usually develop within about two weeks after the bite by an infected fly, fever which sometimes lasts for weeks before remission, patchy erythema or even a pustular eruption, and generalized edema first being noted. Trypanosomes may appear in the peripheral blood as early as ten days after infection, but usually are found only after about three weeks. Sometimes they are abundant, perhaps two or three appearing in every microscope field, but more often they are so rare that it is impractical to demonstrate them in blood films. Kerandel's symptom —fear of striking any object, and delayed extreme local pain following contact—develops early in the disease. Anemia, tachycardia, and, as previously mentioned, enlargement of the lymph glands especially in the posterior triangle of the neck (Winterbottom's sign) soon appear, and, unless treated, the patient gradually declines to the sleeping sickness stage of the disease.

The duration of the sleeping sickness stage of trypanosomiasis varies from a few months to several years. In this, there is gradual disinclination to any activity, mental dullness, and a chronic tendency to lapse into sleep even while walking or eating. Responses to any stimulus are made slowly. Conversation lags and usually is incoherent. If the patient can be induced to take food, however, he assimilates it, and emaciation may thus be postponed. Finally, however, there is general wasting, little but convulsive movement, and a tendency to opisthotonos. Bedsores develop along with a severe pruritis of the skin. The saliva dribbles, the sphincters relax, and paralysis spreads. Death generally is precipitated by any of various secondary infections. (See Plate III, A, facing page 95.)

Immunity.—If human beings contract infection with *Trypanosoma gambiense*, they eventually succumb to the disease if untreated, although often they prove comparatively resistant and die only after infection for several years. Man has not been shown to acquire immunity as a result of infection, even though he survives by reason of specific drug therapy. Among experimental animals, however, immunity to *Trypanosoma gambiense* results if an initial infection is aborted by the administration of drugs, and it seems not unlikely that eventually a similar immune response, perhaps of some limited effectiveness in preventing reinfection, will be shown to develop in man. It is well known that man is absolutely resistant naturally to the trypanosomes of animals. Indeed, the fresh blood serum of man is markedly trypanocidal both in vitro and in vivo upon the different trypanosomes pathogenic for animals. It is, however, without effect upon *Trypanosoma gambiense* even after this form is passed through laboratory animals for many years.

Diagnosis.—The early diagnosis of trypanosomiasis is a matter of the utmost concern to patients harboring the parasite, in order that therapy can be instituted before the parasite is established in the nervous tissue. Often early clinical symptoms of trypanosomiasis are masked by the more prominent symptoms of other tropical infections which may have been contracted previously.

The direct microscopic demonstration of the parasite in blood, lymph gland juice, or cerebrospinal fluid is the first diagnostic procedure attempted with any suspected case. The lymph gland juice is a particularly favorable site for observing the parasite, since the organism is recoverable from this juice in about eighty-five percent of cases. Smears of the spleen or liver substance also are sometimes useful for demonstrating the parasite. The parasite may be seen in fresh preparations but can be recognized most conclusively in stained films. Thick blood films generally are used by those skilled in their examination.

Where direct demonstration fails, the parasite can often be revealed by inoculating animals with blood, lymph gland juice, or other material from the patient. The rat, guinea pig, dog, and *Macacus* monkey are the most suitable animals for such tests.

Specific therapy.—Two compounds are most useful for treating trypanosomiasis: germanin (Bayer 205) and tryparsamide. Germanin is a colorless water-soluble compound of great complexity (urea of acid dimeta-aminobenzoyl-meta-aminoparamethylbenzoyl-1-naphthylamino-4-6-8 trisulfonate of sodium) which has proved particularly valuable in treating cases early in their course. It is relatively atoxic, and individuals can tolerate intravenous injections of one gram of the drug every few days. Usually complete recovery, in early cases, follows a few doses. Sometimes, after a number of doses, a nephritis lasting six weeks or so is noted.

Tryparsamide (sodium salt of N-phenylglycineamide-p-arsonic acid) is widely used in trypanosomiasis, even for advanced cases in which nervous tissue involvement has begun. Some patients, however, are sensitive to tryparsamide, as they are to other arsenic compounds, and atrophy of the optic nerve with resulting blindness must be guarded against in those given tryparsamide. Other older arsenic compounds have largely been replaced by tryparsamide for treating trypanosomiasis, because of the lesser toxicity of this substance.

Prophylaxis.—After germanin is inoculated it is only slowly secreted from the body, since the drug fixes itself to the tissues and cells of the injected individual. Use has been made of this fact to protect man from infection with *Trypanosoma gambiense*. The injection of one gram of germanin suffices to protect adult persons for a period of about three months thereafter.

Community measures also are helpful in protecting against trypanosomiasis. Underbrush in which tsetse flies live can be cleared from along streams, especially at boat landings. The tsetse flies themselves or their larvae or pupae can be caught. Infected persons can be treated or, if beyond aid by treatment, they can be segregated so as not to lead to infection among flies. Potential animal reservoirs can be exterminated. Persons should be advised not to enter fly belts. Those who must do so should wear white clothing, since this seems to repel the tsetse fly.

TRYPANOSOMA RHODESIENSE AND RHODESIAN SLEEPING SICKNESS OF AFRICA

Cases of sleeping sickness contracted in Rhodesia were quite early recognized to be generally more severe and more rapidly fatal than those contacted in West and Central Africa. This difference was shown in 1910 by Stephens and Fantham to result from the occurrence in the Rhodesian cases of a distinct species of trypanosome, which these investigators called *Trypanosoma rhodesiense*. Many authorities feel that, although the organism is properly distinct from *Trypano-*

soma gambiense, it is a variant of *Trypanosoma brucei*, which causes nagana, a disease of animals.

Geographical distribution.—*Trypanosoma rhodesiense* is confined to the territory around Lake Nyasa in southeast Africa, including northeastern Rhodesia, southwestern Tanganyika, Portuguese East Africa, and Nyasaland. Its distribution is essentially the same as that of the animal trypanosome, *Trypanosoma brucei,* and that of the insect vector common for the two species, *Glossina morsitans.*

Morphology and life cycle.—*Trypanosoma rhodesiense* is indistinguishable in any of its stages, either in the vertebrate host or in the insect vector, from the corresponding stages of *Trypanosoma gambiense* and *Trypanosoma brucei.* When *Trypanosoma rhodesiense* is injected into rats or guinea pigs, a considerable percentage of posteriorly nucleated forms will appear. In this respect *Trypanosoma rhodesiense* resembles *Trypanosoma brucei* rather than *Trypanosoma gambiense,* for very few such forms are developed in rodent infections with the Gambian parasite. (See Plate III, C, facing page 95.)

Cultivation.—*Trypanosoma rhodesiense* can be grown with difficulty in N.N.N. medium. Subcultures usually cannot be obtained.

Epidemiology.—It seems probable that man is merely an occasional or sporadic host of *Trypanosoma rhodesiense,* the parasite residing naturally in game animals—especially various antelopes—of the endemic regions. The infection differs epidemiologically from the Gambian disease in that it occurs more as an infection of the field, away from native villages. The parasite is transmitted among game animals, and from them to domesticated animals (cattle, sheep, horses, etc.) and to man by *Glossina morsitans.* Transmission may be mechanical, but cyclical transmission, requiring development in the insect body, also takes place. Mechanical transmission may occur with many biting insects, and cyclical development is possible in some species of *Glossina* other than *morsitans.* Usually only a small percentage of the *Glossina morsitans* found in nature are infected, and even when laboratory-bred flies are fed on a known case of trypanosomiasis, comparatively few become infected. Of these still fewer can transmit the infection back to man. Epidemics of the infection in man are rare.

Pathogenicity.—Human infection with *Trypanosoma rhodesiense* is essentially the same as that with *Trypanosoma gambiense,* although the course of the disease with the Rhodesian parasite is shorter and the symptoms are more acute. Death in untreated cases usually comes within one year after infection. Nervous symptoms and evidence for glandular enlargement usually are less prominent than in the Gambian disease, but febrile paroxysms are more frequent and weakness and emaciation are striking.

Diagnosis.—The same methods are used for diagnosing infections with the Rhodesian parasite as with the Gambian trypanosome form. The organism occurs in the juice of the lymphatic glands and in the blood, possibly in greater number than does the Gambian parasite.

Specific therapy.—Germanin (Bayer 205) is the drug of choice for *Trypanosoma rhodesiense* infections. It is more effective in this disease than in *Trypanosoma gambiense* infection. Tryparsamide is said to be much less satisfactory for treating the Rhodesian infection than it is for the Gambian disease.

Prophylaxis.—The same prophylactic measures are used for the Rhodesian infection as for the Gambian disease. The segregation and treatment of human cases, the elimination of potential reservoir animals, and the eradication of the tsetse fly so far as possible by clearing underbrush are community measures always advised. The wearing of white clothing is probably helpful in protecting individuals who enter the fly belt. The use of germanin prophylactically may also be helpful in protecting individuals who must reside for short periods in endemic areas.

TRYPANOSOMA CRUZI AND CHAGAS'S DISEASE OF SOUTH AMERICA

Trypanosoma cruzi was first found by Chagas in 1909 in Brazil in the intestine of a hemipteran insect, *Triatoma megista*. It was seen later in the blood of a monkey some days after this animal was bitten by an insect infected with the parasite. Finally, the trypanosome was observed in the blood of a Brazilian child with symptoms of fever, anemia, and lymphatic gland involvement. The parasite has since been proved to be the cause of the infection now called Chagas's disease.

Geographical distribution.—*Trypanosoma cruzi* has a widespread distribution in the Western Hemisphere. It has been recorded from practically all the countries of South America, although it occurs chiefly in Brazil and Venezuela. It is known in Panama, Honduras, and Guatemala of Central America, in Mexico, and in California, Arizona, New Mexico, Texas, and Utah of the United States. Human infection with this parasite has not, however, as yet been reported from the United States, although animal infections are known.

Morphology and life cycle.—*Trypanosoma cruzi* has several distinct morphologic stages in its development. In man, two trypanosome stages—one long and slender and the other short and broad—occur in the blood. In the muscle and endothelial tissue, as well as elsewhere, a leishmania form is found. In stained blood films, the parasites, which measure twenty microns or less, generally are sharply curved, as the letter C. (See Plate III, E, facing page 95.) A nucleus occupies the center of the cell, and a large kinetoplast is found at the posterior end. The poorly developed undulating membrane is bordered by an axoneme which rises from the kinetoplast and extends to the anterior end of the cell. At the anterior tip, the axoneme becomes the free flagellum. In the tissue cells, in which all reproduction goes on by repeated division, leishmanias are observed as oval parasites three or four microns in greatest dimension. (See Plate III, F, facing page 95.) They finally fill the invaded cell and, on growing into small trypanosomes, disrupt the cell and enter the peripheral blood or other tissue cells. Often the parasite seems to propagate itself continuously in the tissue cells without appearing in the peripheral blood except rarely. The blood-stream infection is seldom intense.

In the insect, the crithidial stage appears in the posterior intestine within a few days after the insect has fed on an infected host. After ten days or so, a metacyclic trypanosome stage is found in the insect rectum. When passed in feces, these forms lead to infection through contaminating the bite wound. Rather characteristically these insects defecate by passing a bloody, fluid mass, during or soon after feeding, not uncommonly depositing the feces directly on the identical part of the skin from which the proboscis has just been drawn. Contamination of the wound, especially if this be rubbed, is, therefore, almost assured. The trypanosome stage will appear in the blood of the infected person about two weeks later.

Cultivation.—*Trypanosoma cruzi* can be quite easily cultivated on N.N.N. medium. Growth is slow, often requiring three or four weeks, but is rather sure. Many rosettes as well as isolated organisms are noted after this interval. Earlier, great clumps of leishmanias are usually seen in cultures.

Epidemiology.—*Trypanosoma cruzi* is probably not primarily a human parasite but a form natural to the armadillo and some other native animals. It can infect a wide range of hosts, including nearly all the mammalian laboratory or domesticated animals. Infections of man are comparatively rare and evidently sporadic, following occasional bites of infected hemipteran bugs. Many reduviid hemipterans (especially the genera *Triatoma, Rhodnius,* and *Erathyrus*) have been found naturally infected and are capable of transmitting the parasite. Bedbugs and certain ticks also are susceptible to infection and can pass the parasite experimentally to laboratory animals. In all cases, evidently, infection of the vertebrate follows contamination of the bite wound by the vector feces.

Human infections occur chiefly among the very poor, who sleep on the earth floor of their huts possibly on straw beds. Persons are generally infected at night, when the vector leaves crevices in the floor or wall and searches for a blood meal. Children are the ones usually bitten, and they suffer decidedly more severe infections than older persons.

Pathogenicity.—Infected endothelial and muscle cells are destroyed by *Trypanosoma cruzi,* the parasite multiplying within these cells. The symptoms usually reflect the extent to which these cells are damaged. In acute infections, found mostly in children one year or so old, death may occur in two or three weeks, with enlargement and congestion of the thyroid, the lymphatic glands and spleen, and the liver. The eyelids may be swollen and one eye closed. Trypanosomes generally are found in the blood of such cases. In the chronic infection, found mostly in adults, symptoms are often absent. When noted, they suggest involvement of the heart, nervous system, or endocrine glands. Trypanosomes are few in the peripheral blood of chronic cases.

Diagnosis.—The demonstration microscopically of the parasite in the blood or tissues is conclusive evidence of infection with *Trypanosoma cruzi.* The culture of the organism in N.N.N. medium is also a satisfactory diagnostic procedure, although one not yet widely used. The detection of antibody in the serum of patients either by complement fixation or the agglutination method is employed by some workers.

Xenodiagnosis—observing the parasite in insects fed on the patient —also is occasionally resorted to.

Specific therapy.—No drug is effective upon *Trypanosoma cruzi,* and cases of Chagas's disease are not improved by treatment with germanin (Bayer 205), tryparsamide, or other drugs used for the African trypanosomiases.

Prophylaxis.—Prophylaxis against Chagas's disease consists in protecting persons from bites by potential vectors of *Trypanosoma cruzi.*

Chapter XI

THE INTESTINAL FLAGELLATE INFECTIONS

THE INTESTINAL FLAGELLATES belong to the order Polymastigina of the class Mastigophora. All of these forms bear more than one flagellum, and are thus easily distinguished from the leishmanias and the trypanosomes, of the order Protomonadina.

Five species of flagellated protozoa are found in the intestine of man. These forms are *Giardia lamblia, Chilomastix mesnili, Trichomonas hominis, Embadomonas intestinalis,* and *Enteromonas hominis.* Two other presumably distinct species of flagellates, *Trichomonas buccalis* and *Trichomonas vaginalis,* are found, respectively, in the mouth and in the vagina or the prostatic secretion. None of these organisms is known to be pathogenic, despite the association of symptoms with the presence of some. The identification of the organisms by medical men is nevertheless essential, if only to exclude the forms from consideration during search for the true cause of disease presented by a given patient.

GIARDIA LAMBLIA

Although probably observed by Leeuwenhoek in 1681 in his own stool, *Giardia lamblia* [1] was not described until 1859, when Lambl found it in a patient's feces.

Geographical distribution.—*Giardia lamblia* has cosmopolitan distribution but occurs more frequently in the tropics than in the temperate zones. In the United States, its incidence is greater in southern than in northern states.

Morphology and life cycle.—*Giardia lamblia* occurs as a trophozoite

---

[1] Common synonyms: *Giardia intestinalis; Lamblia intestinalis.*

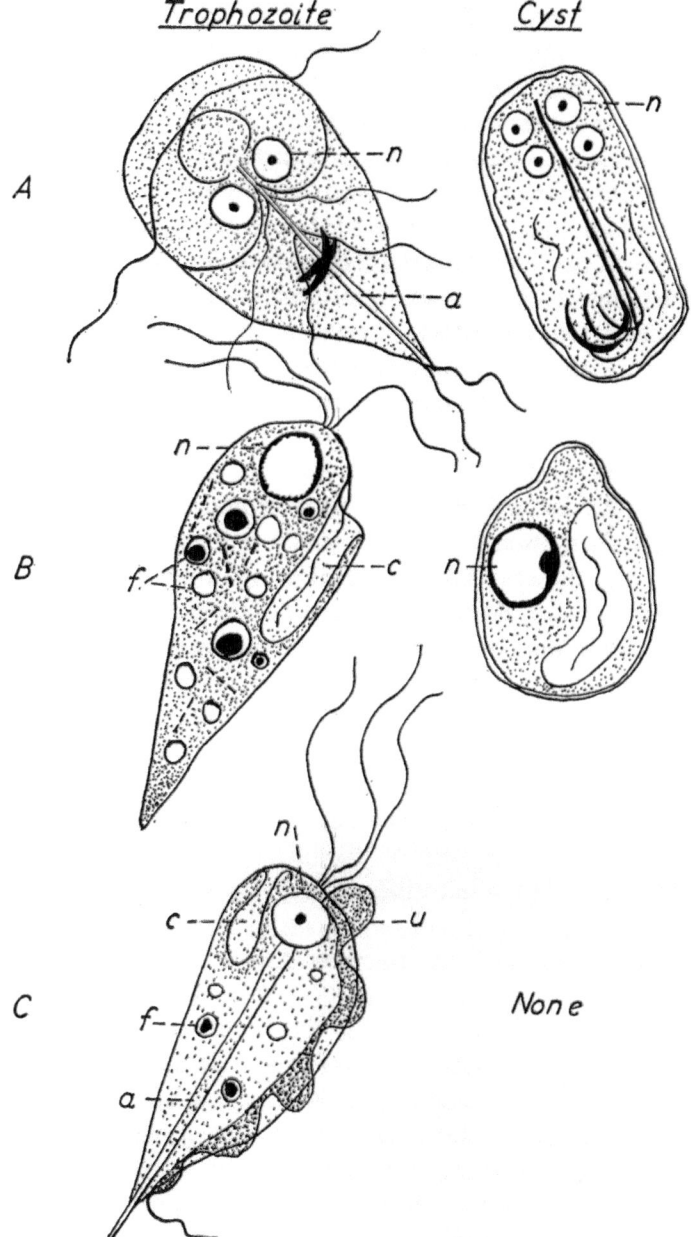

Figure 4. Common intestinal flagellates of man: A, *Giardia lamblia;* B, *Chilomastix mesnili;* C, *Trichomonas hominis.* a = axostyle; n = nucleus; c = cytostome; f = food vacuole; u = undulating membrane.

and as a cyst. The trophozoite is usually confined to the small intestine but may appear in the diarrheic stool. The cyst is found regularly in the feces of infected persons. (See Figure 4, A.) The *Giardia* trophozoite is a pear-shaped structure, rounded at its anterior end and pointed posteriorly. It measures from ten to twenty microns long by five to fifteen microns broad, the size often varying considerably in a single patient. On its ventral surface is a sucking disk by which it commonly adheres to the intestinal epithelium. When the organism is stained, two nuclei, two axonemes, and four pairs of flagella are distinguished, these structures being disposed with striking symmetry. One or more deeply stained parabasal bodies occur just behind the sucking disk. No cytostome is present, and food vacuoles do not appear in the cytoplasm.

The *Giardia* cyst is an oval body measuring about twelve microns long by eight microns broad. Usually four nuclei can be seen toward one end of the cyst, and running through the central axis toward the opposite end of the cyst are several short, curved, deeply stained fibrils. Remnants of flagella and axonemes sometimes occur in young cysts. Generally, the mature cyst appears to be shrunken back from the cyst wall.

The trophozoite of *Giardia lamblia* lives in the small intestine, where it reproduces by longitudinal division into two cells. If the trophozoite is passed, it soon dies, but the cyst which is developed in the intestine survives when eliminated with feces. When such cysts are swallowed by other persons, they lead to infection. The ingested parasite excysts in the intestine, each cyst giving rise to two trophozoites.

Cultivation.—*Giardia lamblia* has not as yet been cultivated in artificial media.

Epidemiology.—*Giardia lamblia* is the commonest intestinal flagellate. Many reports indicate its presence in at least from twelve to fifteen percent of the general population of warmer regions. Sometimes infections persist for several years. The organism occurs more frequently in children than in older persons, the incidence in children being about three times that in adult persons.

Infection with *Giardia lamblia* usually follows the ingestion of food or drink contaminated with the feces of an individual carrying the parasite. Flies, roaches, and other insects which visit human fecal deposits as well as food stores of man are probably instrumental in the distribution of the cysts of *Giardia*. Thus far, man is the only recognized vertebrate host, although a number of related species of *Giardia* parasitize lower animals.

Pathogenicity.—Although *Giardia lamblia* is by some authorities considered the cause of certain forms of dysentery as well as of some forms of gall bladder inflammation, no conclusive proof of its etiological relationship has yet been presented. Its presence in the diarrheic stools of persons suffering with abdominal pain as well as in the inflamed gall bladder is unquestioned, but generally it occurs in the intestine in association with other organisms, such as *Endamoeba histolytica*, which are probably responsible for the pathology or symptom. At the present time, therefore, *Giardia lamblia* is usually considered nonpathogenic.

Diagnosis.—The presence of *Giardia lamblia* is established by observing the cysts or, rarely, the trophozoites of the parasite in the feces. The trophozoites occur naturally only in diarrheic stools but can be caused to appear by administering a purgative. They can be found readily in the duodenal contents of those infected.

Specific therapy.—The drug most effective for the permanent elimination of *Giardia lamblia* is atebrin. When 0.2 or 0.3 gram of atebrin is given daily in divided doses for five days, the parasites generally disappear from infected individuals.

Giardiasis, Case Report.—The patient was a female twenty-five years old. She had diagnosed her own infection six years earlier, observing cysts in the stool during an exercise in a parasitology class. During the interval, parasites were seen whenever the stool was examined. There were occasional periods of diarrhea, at which times trophozoites appeared. The patient was troubled with digestive disturbances, and believed these caused by her giardia infection. A physician had administered carbarsone three years earlier, without cure of the giardiasis. After the infection had continued for six years, atebrin was administered, two 0.1 gram tablets being given daily for five days. Parasites could not be demonstrated on the day after treatment was suspended or during the next six weeks while the case was followed. Evidently complete cure had resulted from the single course of atebrin. Unfortunately, the digestive disturbance continued.[2]

Prophylaxis.—Prevention of infection with *Giardia lamblia* consists in protecting food and drink from contamination with feces contain-

[2] J. T. Culbertson, *Journal of Laboratory and Clinical Medicine*, 26: 1465 (1941).

ing cysts of the parasite. Known carriers of the organism should be treated so that they cannot transmit it to others.

Chilomastix mesnili [3] was first observed by Davaine in 1854 in the feces of cholera patients. It was carefully described by Wenyon in 1910 and given its present name by Alexieff in 1912.

Geographical distribution.—*Chilomastix mesnili* has been found in practically all parts of the world.

Morphology and life cycle.—*Chilomastix mesnili* exists as a trophozoite and as a cyst. As yet it is not established whether the trophozoites dwell in the large or the small intestine of the host. The cysts are found in the feces. (See Figure 4, B.)

The trophozoites are pear-shaped bodies ten to twenty microns long by three to ten broad, which move with a characteristic jerky motion usually while revolving slowly about the long axis. They are asymmetrical, with a large cleftlike cytostome and a spiral groove which encircles the body. There are three free flagella, coming from blepharoplasts near the anterior end. A fourth flagellum turns posteriorly into the cytostome. The rather large nucleus is located near the anterior end. Numerous rather conspicuous food vacuoles generally are visible. The food consists chiefly of bacteria. The cells reproduce by longitudinal fission.

The cysts are lemon- or pear-shaped bodies about ten microns long by six microns broad. They contain the nucleus and blepharoplasts, as well as remnants of the cytostome.

When the cysts, which are passed in formed stools, are swallowed by another person, they excyst and the resulting trophozoite becomes established in the intestine of the individual. Later cysts are eliminated in the feces of this person and these lead to the infection of still others.

Cultivation.—*Chilomastix mesnili* can be grown in Boeck's medium, which is commonly employed for the cultivation of *Endamoeba histolytica*. Cultures must be transplanted every two or three days.

Epidemiology.—Man becomes infected with *Chilomastix mesnili* by swallowing food or water polluted with feces containing cysts of the parasite. Insects such as flies may facilitate the dissemination of the

---

[3] Common synonyms: *Chilomastix hominis; Cercomonas intestinalis.*

cysts. The incidence of human infection is not high. From 1.4 to 7.5 percent of the general population in the southern United States has been reported to harbor the organism.

Pathogenicity.—*Chilomastix mesnili* is believed to be a harmless commensal. Quite often it is found in large number in diarrheic stools, but other acknowledged pathogens generally are also present.

Diagnosis.—Infection with *Chilomastix mesnili* is established by observing the cysts of the parasite in the feces. Trophozoites frequently are found in diarrheic stools but cysts alone occur in formed stools. When organisms are few, methods of cultivation aid in establishing the diagnosis.

Specific therapy.—No specific therapeutic treatment is available for infections with *Chilomastix.*

Prophylaxis.—If food and drink are protected from contamination with feces harboring the cysts of *Chilomastix mesnili,* infection with the organism can generally be prevented.

TRICHOMONAS HOMINIS

Trichomonas hominis [4] was first observed by Davaine in 1854. In 1879, Leuckart ascribed to the organism the name it now bears.

Geographical distribution.—*Trichomonas hominis* has a cosmopolitan distribution, although its incidence is greater in the warmer parts of the world.

Morphology and life cycle.—Trichomonads differ from all other intestinal flagellates in that only the trophozoite stage is known. The trophozoite is peculiarly resistant to unfavorable environment and evidently carries on the function of transmission which in other intestinal species is reserved for the cyst. (See Figure 4, C.)

Trichomonas hominis is a pear-shaped form measuring about twelve microns in length by five microns in breadth. It is actively motile, bearing from three to five flagella and an undulating membrane bordered by a flagellum which becomes free toward the posterior end of the cell. The nucleus lies near the anterior end of the cell, and, on its anterior side, three or more blepharoplasts—often appearing as a single mass—can be seen. The flagella, the undulating membrane, and the axostyle all originate from the blepharoplasts. The rodlike axostyle usually protrudes from the posterior end of the body. A

[4] Common synonyms: *Trichomonas intestinalis; Cercomonas hominis.*

cytostome occurs near the anterior end of the cell, and food vacuoles —sometimes containing red corpuscles—often are visible in the cell cytoplasm. Cysts are unknown for the species.

The trophozoites, which represent both the infecting stage and the transmitting stage, multiply by longitudinal division. New individuals become infected by swallowing trophozoites passed in the feces by infected persons. These trophozoites evidently can resist the stomach acids as they pass to the large intestine, where they usually take up final residence.

Cultivation.—Trichomonas hominis can be cultivated in Boeck's medium. Transplantation every two or three days is required.

Epidemiology.—Trichomonas hominis is evidently transmitted through food or drink polluted with feces containing trophozoites of the organism. Its incidence appears low, for several careful surveys in the southern United States indicate less than five percent of the general population harbors the parasite. House rats and cats may aid in disseminating the organism.

Pathogenicity.—Trichomonas hominis is not known to cause disease in man, although it is found in greatest number in persons suffering with diarrhea.

Diagnosis.—The observation of motile *Trichomonas hominis* in the fresh feces or in cultures of feces establishes the diagnosis of this infection.

Specific therapy.—No drug is regularly effective for eliminating trichomonads. Those used in amoebiasis and those employed in giardiasis are without effect in trichomoniasis.

Prophylaxis.—Measures which protect food or water from contamination with feces containing cysts of *Trichomonas hominis* prevent infection with this parasite.

TRICHOMONADS IN OTHER SITES

Two other presumably distinct species of *Trichomonas* infect man in sites other than the intestine. *Trichomonas buccalis* is found in the mouth and *Trichomonas vaginalis* in the vagina of women or the prostatic secretion of men.

TRICHOMONAS BUCCALIS

Trichomonas buccalis [5] was first discovered in the human mouth

[5] Common synonyms: *Trichomonas elongata; Tetratrichomonas buccalis.*

by Steinberg in 1862. Its distribution is probably world-wide, and its incidence, as indicated by several reports from the United States, approximates twenty percent of the general population.

Morphologically the organism is identical with the intestinal form, *Trichomonas hominis*. Cysts are unknown. Its transmission is probably often directly from mouth to mouth, as in kissing, although it may also be spread through common utensils, such as drinking glasses. Transmission by droplet infection also seems possible, at least for very short distances.

The parasite is not believed to be pathogenic, although it occurs more often in mouths with caries, pyorrheal pockets, or other dental pathology than in healthy mouths. The presence of the form is determined by direct microscopic observations of the tartar or other material from about the teeth. Cultures of such material in Boeck's medium is also a useful aid in diagnosis. No specific treatment is available to eradicate the parasite. Generally the organism cannot survive or become established in well-kept mouths.

TRICHOMONAS VAGINALIS

Trichomonas vaginalis was the first trichomonad found in human beings, it having been discovered in vaginal secretions by Donné in 1837. Apparently the organism has a cosmopolitan distribution, and some reports suggest its occurrence in fifty percent or more of women with vaginitis. It is found likewise in the prostatic secretion of men and in the urine of both men and women. Its mode of transmission is not established, although probably sexual intercourse accounts for a part of its dissemination.

In the opinion of most authorities, the parasite is morphologically identical with, but possibly larger than, *Trichomonas hominis*. It seems distinct from *Trichomonas hominis*, however, in its physiological adaptation to residence in the vagina. Cysts are not known. The organism can be cultivated in Boeck's medium.

Despite the fact that *Trichomonas vaginalis* occurs only among women with an abnormal vaginal secretion and is frequently found in cases of vaginitis, most authorities believe the parasite to be a harmless commensal. Its presence is established by direct microscopic observation of the organism in the vaginal secretion or by the cultivation of this secretion. No specific treatment is available, but the parasite usually disappears following symptomatic medication. Generally infection with the organism can be avoided by due care in matters of personal hygiene.

OTHER INTESTINAL FLAGELLATES

The following species are exceedingly rare parasites, with little medical significance. They will be discussed briefly.

EMBADOMONAS INTESTINALIS

Embadomonas intestinalis[6] was discovered in 1917 by Wenyon and O'Connor in Egypt.[7] It has since been found in the Far East, Brazil, and the United States of America. It is small, measuring less than ten microns in length. There are two flagella, one directed anteriorly and the other posteriorly after passing through the lateral cytostome. The pear-shaped cysts measure five to seven microns in length. The nucleus and, often, remnants of the cytostome are found in the cyst. The organism is cultivable, both trophozoites and cysts occurring in Boeck's medium. Reproduction evidently goes on only in the trophozoite, which divides longitudinally.

Although the organism is found usually in persons suffering with diarrhea, it is considered a harmless commensal. Its presence is determined by microscopic examination or cultivation of the feces. No treatment is available and none is necessary. Infection is prevented by protecting food or drink from fecal contamination.

ENTEROMONAS HOMINIS

Enteromonas hominis[8] was discovered in 1915 in Brazil by Da Fonseca. It has since been observed in Egypt, the Far East, and the United States. The trophozoites are pear-shaped, but flattened on one side. The nucleus is located anteriorly. There are three anterior flagella and one other which extends along the flattened side finally to become free posteriorly. The cysts are round or oval in outline, measuring about eight microns in greatest dimension. They contain from one to four nuclei arranged, in the multinucleate forms, at op-

[6] Common synonym: *Waskia intestinalis*.

[7] Another species, *Embadomonas sinensis*, was discovered in 1921 by Faust and Wassell in China but has never been found outside that country. It resembles *Embadomonas intestinalis* in many respects but differs in having its two flagella both project anteriorly, neither passing through the cytostome. The organism is cultivated in Wenyon's medium. It is not believed to be pathogenic.

[8] Common synonym: *Tricercomonas intestinalis*.

posite ends of the cell. Both trophozoites and cysts appear in cultures prepared in Boeck's medium. Reproduction is by longitudinal division in the trophozoite. Each cyst probably yields four trophozoites.

Infection follows the ingestion of cysts of the organism. The parasite causes no pathology or symptoms. Its presence is determined by microscopic examination or by cultivation of the feces. No treatment is available or needed. Infection is prevented by protecting food from fecal contamination.

Chapter XII

THE MALARIAS

THE SPOROZOAN PARASITES of man are found in two suborders of the order Coccidiida: Eimeriidea and Haemosporidiidea. The species of Eimeriidea are intestinal parasites and cause a rare disease known as coccidiosis. The species of Haemosporidiidea are parasites of circulating blood cells and cause the very important human infection, malaria. The Haemosporidiidea require an invertebrate host in which to complete their sexual development, since in man only asexual reproduction occurs; the species of Eimeriidea, so far as is known, undergo both sexual and asexual development in the human host.

HUMAN MALARIA

Malaria is the most important disease of man in the tropics. More persons suffer from the infection in warm climates than from any other disease, and no one living in or visiting endemic areas can expect to remain free of malaria. Fortunately, specific therapeutics for malaria, the bark of the cinchona tree and its derivatives, have long been known. Indeed, these substances have been in general use since long before the causal agents of the disease were described and before the natural mode of transmission of these agents was determined.

Malaria has been known as a disease of man since ancient times. Hippocrates recognized and differentiated certain fevers of the tertian, quartan, and quotidian types which undoubtedly were caused by malarial parasites. The disease represented a hazard to the progress of all the great conquests by armies and the mass migrations in the world's history, and it was one of the most important obstacles in the colonization of the New World. Many settlements in North America, especially along the coast of the southeastern United States, were necessarily given up soon after their founding because of the ravages of malaria.

A cure for malaria was discovered in the Americas. In the first years of the seventeenth century, Jesuit missionaries in Peru began to adopt the native method of treating malaria by the use of the bark of a Peruvian tree. The precise circumstances of the introduction of this method to Europe are obscure. According to one school of historians, Don Francisco Lopez Canazares, the Corregidor of Loxa, who had himself been cured by the treatment, sent a supply of the bark to Lima in 1638, where Francesca de Ribera, the second wife of the Viceroy of Peru, lay ill with malaria. Her infection also was cured. So impressed was Francesca de Ribera with the curative potentialities of the bark that she carried a quantity back to Spain where, in 1640, it was employed for the treatment of persons ill of malaria on her husband's estate. Cinchona bark,[1] as it later came to be called, and its alkaloid derivative quinine, which was first prepared in 1820, have been used ever since as specifics for the malady.

The parasite which causes human malaria was not discovered until 1881, when Alphonse Laveran, then a French military physician, observed it while examining blood films of troops in Algeria. Virchow and others had earlier noted the deposit of pigment in the organs of patients dead of malaria, and some workers, who had seen such pigment circulating in the blood, considered it diagnostic of the disease. Following Laveran's first observations of the parasites, intensive studies undertaken at once by Italian investigators established the facts that at least three distinct species of protozoan cause malaria in man and that the clinical symptoms of infection with each species differ from that with the others.

It was proved by Gerhardt in 1884 that malaria could be transferred by inoculating into a normal person blood from a patient with the disease. The natural mode of spread of the disease was not understood, however, until the end of the nineteenth century. Sir Patrick Manson had shown earlier (1879) in China that the human filarial worm *Wuchereria bancrofti* developed in mosquitoes, and he suggested to one of his associates, Ronald Ross, in England that the mos-

---

[1] The name Cinchona was applied erroneously by Linnaeus in 1742, in honor of the Countess of Chinchon, the first wife of the Viceroy of Peru, who had died in 1625 without visiting America. She had nothing to do with the discovery of the treatment for malaria.

quito might also be responsible for the transmission of malaria. Ross went to India in 1894 and began investigations first in the malaria of birds. By 1898 he had proved that the parasites of bird malaria are carried among the birds by a *Culex* mosquito. In the same year (1898) two Italian workers, Grassi and Bignami, proved that anopheline mosquitoes are the vectors of human malaria and that the disease is spread naturally through the bites of these insects. Tremendous controversy ensued as to who should receive the chief honor for the discovery of the mosquito role in malarial transmission. Finally, Ross was given the greater recognition, receiving for his contributions the Nobel prize in 1902.

At the present time, four distinct species of sporozoan are known to cause human malaria: *Plasmodium vivax, Plasmodium malariae, Plasmodium falciparum,* and *Plasmodium ovale. Plasmodium vivax* and *Plasmodium ovale* cause a benign tertian form of malaria, infections with the *ovale* parasite being particularly mild. *Plasmodium malariae* causes a quartan form of malaria, and *Plasmodium falciparum* causes a malignant form of subtertian or quotidian malaria.

PLASMODIUM VIVAX, THE CAUSE OF BENIGN
TERTIAN MALARIA

Although probably seen earlier by Laveran, *Plasmodium vivax* was first described in 1886 by Golgi, an Italian investigator.

Geographical distribution.—*Plasmodium vivax* is a widely distributed parasite, being found through much of the world lying between 60° N. and 40° S. latitude.[2] In the tropics, its incidence is substantially greater and its distribution more widespread than in the cooler areas.

Morphology and life cycle.—The morphology and life cycle of *Plasmodium vivax* are, in their essentials, similar to those of other human malarial parasites. The same stages occur, and the same alternation of generations—the schizogonous development in the vertebrate host and the gametogonous and sporogonous development in the invertebrate host—goes on in all. The morphology and life cycle of *Plasmodium vivax* are discussed in considerable detail below. The differences from *Plasmodium vivax* are accentuated in the discussion of the other species.

[2] Occurs indigenously as far north as the vicinity of Lake Ladoga, near Leningrad, Russia; and as far south as southern Argentina.

When seen in fresh blood, *Plasmodium vivax* generally exhibits greater amoeboid movement within the red cell than do other species of human malarial parasite, hence the application of its specific name. Its characteristic morphology can be well seen, however, only in stained preparations. If blood films are prepared at various times during the course of an infection and well stained, many developmental stages of the parasite can be observed. Most of these go to make up the schizogonous or asexual cycle. After the infection has gone on for some time, sexual stages also appear. The sexual phase of development can be followed, however, only in the mosquito. It should be noted that *Plasmodium vivax*—in distinction from *Plasmodium malariae* and *Plasmodium falciparum*—preferentially infects reticulocytes. (See Figure 5.)

Schizogony.—Natural infections with malaria begin when sporozoites are introduced under the skin of an individual by an infected mosquito. These sporozoites soon enter erythrocytes in which they develop to trophozoites. The young trophozoite is ring-shaped, the rings enclosing what is probably a vacuole. When these rings are stained with Wright's stain, the cytoplasm is blue, but has a conspicuous red-staining dot of chromatin at one point of its periphery. The infected erythrocyte, which is larger than the uninfected cells, is stained pink. Gradually this "ring stage" develops to the "amoeboid stage," its cytoplasm growing out irregularly over the red cell. The chromatin dot and the vacuole generally persist in the amoeboid form. By this time, some small red dots, known as Schüffner's dots, can also be observed, dispersed over the erythrocyte. Malarial pigment likewise appears in the parasite body, finally becoming concentrated toward the center of the cell. (See Plate IV, A and B, facing page 126.) Gradually the parasite grows to fill the entire cell, it then being called the "schizont." The original single mass of chromatin in the parasite body breaks up into from twelve to twenty-four masses of granules which are distributed over the schizont. The schizont then splits into an equal number of units called "merozoites," each of which contains one chromatin granule. These merozoites are freed into the plasma by rupture of the infected erythrocyte, but they promptly invade new erythrocytes. The malarial pigment, which is also liberated into the plasma when the enclosing erythrocyte is ruptured, becomes deposited in the cells of some of the fixed tissues, which finally become deeply pigmented.

The process of schizont development and segmentation is repeated many times, until finally many cells are parasitized. The complete schizogonous cycle requires forty-eight hours.

Gametogony and sporogony.—After the schizogonous cycle has gone on for several days, some of the merozoites experience a different development and grow directly into sexual cells—male or female gametocytes. These are round or oval masses which eventually very nearly fill the infected erythrocytes. The cytoplasm of the male cell, or "microgametocyte," stains pale blue with Wright's stain, whereas that of the female cell, or "macrogametocyte," is deep blue. The nucleus of the male cell is larger and its chromatin rather diffuse, whereas that of the female cell is smaller and its chromatin more compact. Pigment is scattered throughout the cytoplasm of the male cell but is mostly near the periphery of the female cell. These gametocytes float about in the plasma without further development until they are swallowed by an appropriate mosquito host. In the mosquito "stomach," the male cell exflagellates, a procedure characterized by the liberation of slender, flagellalike male gametes, which with Wright's stain appear to be essentially pure chromatin, since they take a deep red color almost throughout. These male gametes promptly search out the female cells, and the fertilization of the female cells ensues. The resulting zygote or "oökinete" migrates to the wall of the mosquito stomach, which it penetrates. On the outer surface of the stomach a cyst, the "oöcyst," is formed. (See Plate IV, C, D, E, and F, facing page 126.) This soon becomes filled with sporozoites. The oöcyst ruptures after some time, and the sporozoites are liberated into the body cavity of the mosquito. They swim through the contained fluid of the body cavity to all parts, and some reach the salivary glands. They penetrate these glands and finally come to lie in the salivary ducts. Here the forms rest until the mosquito feeds. Just prior to withdrawing blood from its next victim, the mosquito ejects into the tissue a quantity of saliva which mixes with blood prior to its removal and prevents its coagulation. With this saliva are passed some of the sporozoites which are in the salivary ducts or glands. It is these sporozoites which lead to the infection of the bitten person. Within an hour or so they have penetrated his erythrocytes.

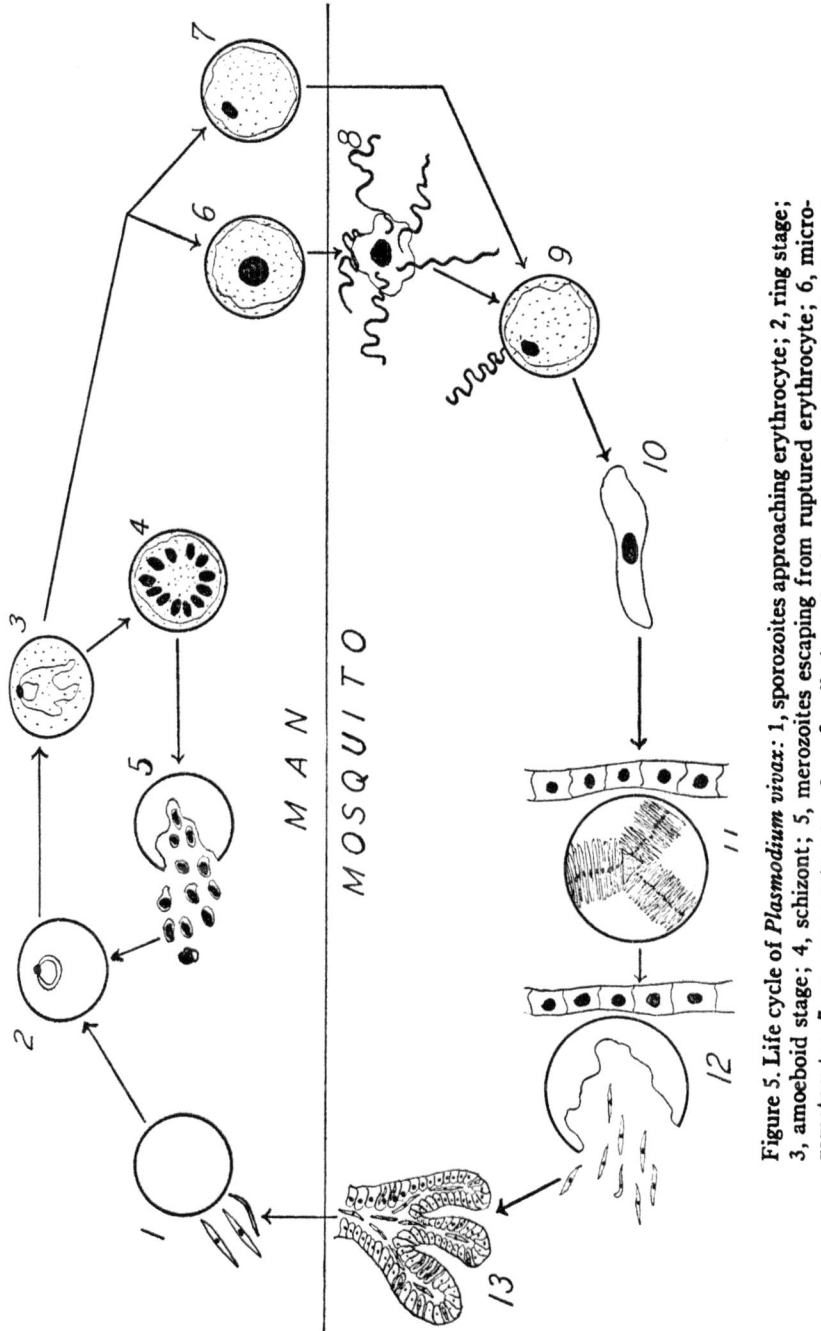

Figure 5. Life cycle of *Plasmodium vivax*: 1, sporozoites approaching erythrocyte; 2, ring stage; 3, amoeboid stage; 4, schizont; 5, merozoites escaping from ruptured erythrocyte; 6, microgametocyte; 7, macrogametocyte; 8, exflagellation of microgametocyte; 9, fertilization of macrogametocyte; 10, oökinete; 11, sporozoites developing in oöcyst on outside wall of mosquito stomach; 12, sporozoites escaping from ruptured mature oöcyst; 13, sporozoites in salivary gland cells and in salivary ducts.

PLASMODIUM MALARIAE, THE CAUSE OF QUARTAN MALARIA

Plasmodium malariae was first observed by Laveran in 1881 but was first fully described as a distinct species of malarial parasite by Golgi in 1886.

Geographical distribution.—*Plasmodium malariae* is a widely dispersed species of malarial parasite, the limits of its distribution coinciding largely with those of *Plasmodium vivax*. It is probably a commoner parasite in temperate than in tropical regions, although in both it is rare. In some intensely malarious localities, its incidence in low, and from many it is wholly absent. In India, Malaya, and parts of Africa, however, severe epidemics of infection with this organism have been reported.

Morphology.—Erythrocytes infected with *Plasmodium malariae* are not larger than uninfected cells. Furthermore, they contain no Schüffner's dots, although Zieman's dots, which are smaller, less intensely staining forms, are brought out by special staining methods. The "ring stage" is very similar to that of *Plasmodium vivax*, but often in place of the amoeboid form which develops in *vivax* infections, there is a "band" form, which stretches across the central part of the erythrocyte. These band forms are distinctive of *Plasmodium malariae* and diagnostic of infection with that parasite. The schizont approximately fills the infected red cell and, when mature, splits into from six to twelve (usually into from eight to ten) merozoites. Prior to its segmentation, the schizont generally exhibits a rather intense pigmentation, granules of dark brown or black pigment being collected near the center of the parasite. The asexual development of *Plasmodium malariae* is slower than that of *Plasmodium vivax*, seventy-two hours being required. (See Plate IV, G, H, I, and J, facing page 126.)

The gametocytes of *Plasmodium malariae* are similar to those of *Plasmodium vivax*, although they do not fill the infected erythrocyte despite the fact that this is no larger than a normal red cell. Furthermore, Schüffner's dots are absent.

PLASMODIUM FALCIPARUM, THE CAUSE OF MALIGNANT
SUBTERTIAN MALARIA

Laveran first observed the crescent-shaped gametocytes of *Plasmodium falciparum* in 1881. Eight years later, Marchiafava and Celli adequately described the parasite and differentiated it from the other species of malarial organisms.

Geographical distribution.—Natural infections with *Plasmodium falciparum* are largely confined to the tropics, and in these regions this parasite is the prevailing species of *Plasmodium*. It occurs also in the warmer parts of the temperate zones, as in the southern United States and in southern Europe (Greece), where the winters are not severe.

Morphology.—Infections with *Plasmodium falciparum* are distinctive in that usually only the ring stage of the schizogonous cycle and the gametocytes appear in the peripheral blood. Other stages of schizogony are confined to the tissues or, rather, to the capillary beds. They are found in material obtained by spleen puncture, in the bone marrow, or in maternal blood from the placenta post partum.

The ring stage is quite like that of *Plasmodium vivax*, although frequently two chromatin granules occur either side by side or on opposite sides of the ring of cytoplasm. Very tiny rings or marginal (appliqué) forms are rather often seen. Very commonly more than one ring—often three or four—are found in the same infected erythrocyte despite the fact that the infected red cell is not larger than uninfected cells. The schizonts are compact forms, considerably smaller than the enclosing red cells. They segment usually into from eighteen to twenty-four small merozoites, although more or less are often reported. The time required for completion of the schizogonous development is more variable than that of other species. Sometimes it is completed only after forty-eight hours, but sometimes after thirty-six hours. (See Plate IV, M, facing page 126.)

The mature gametocytes of *Plasmodium falciparum* are crescent-, bean-, or kidney-shaped bodies and are quite distinctive for the species. They are generally enclosed by the wall of an erythrocyte, although often this is much distorted and difficult to detect; sometimes it is absent. The male cell or microgametocyte is recognized by the more extensive distribution of its chromatin and pigment over the cell body. In the female cell or macrogametocyte which usually is longer than the male cell and has pointed tips, the chromatin as well as the pigment is collected in a compact mass toward the center of the cell. Generally, comparatively few of the gametocytes make their way into the peripheral blood. (See Plate IV, N and O, facing page 126.)

PLASMODIUM OVALE, THE CAUSE OF OVALE TERTIAN MALARIA

Plasmodium ovale, although observed by Craig in 1900 and by others subsequently, was not fully recognized as a new and distinct species of malarial parasite until 1922, when Stephens described the organism. The name is derived from the fact that the infected erythrocyte, as well as the schizont and the gametocytes, of the parasite is often of oval shape.

Geographical distribution.—*Plasmodium ovale* occurs naturally in the Philippine Islands and in Africa. It has also been reported in Russia, Persia, and South America.

Morphology.—In some respects *Plasmodium ovale* resembles both *Plasmodium vivax* and *Plasmodium malariae* morphologically, although absolute differences from both species are readily noted. Schüffner's dots appear in the infected cells, the *ovale* infection thus resembling the *vivax* rather than the malariae form. In the *ovale* development, however, the dots appear in large number even as early as the ring stage (Plate IV, K, facing this page), whereas with *Plasmodium vivax*, they usually occur only in erythrocytes containing later stages. The schizont stage of the *ovale* parasite, however, resembles that of *Plasmodium malariae*, since only from six to twelve merozoites are generally found. In distinction from both the *vivax* and the *malariae* parasites, the *ovale* schizonts as well as some of the amoeboid forms occur in oval erythrocytes of which the edges are ragged or fimbriated. The schizogonous development of the *ovale* parasite requires forty-eight hours, as does that of *Plasmodium vivax*.

The *ovale* gametocytes are in most respects similar to those of *Plasmodium vivax* but are smaller and occur in oval cells with more intense development of Schüffner's dots. (See Plate IV, L, facing this page.)

Cultivation.—*Plasmodium vivax*, as well as *Plasmodium malariae* and *Plasmodium falciparum*, were cultivated in 1912 by Bass and Johns. Other workers have since confirmed their findings many times, although in no case have cultures ever been maintained for more than a few generations. Only asexual stages occur in cultures. The merozoites which result from the segmentation of schizonts generally seem unable, or at best only poorly able, to infect new erythrocytes.

Epidemiology.—The occurrence of malaria endemically in any region

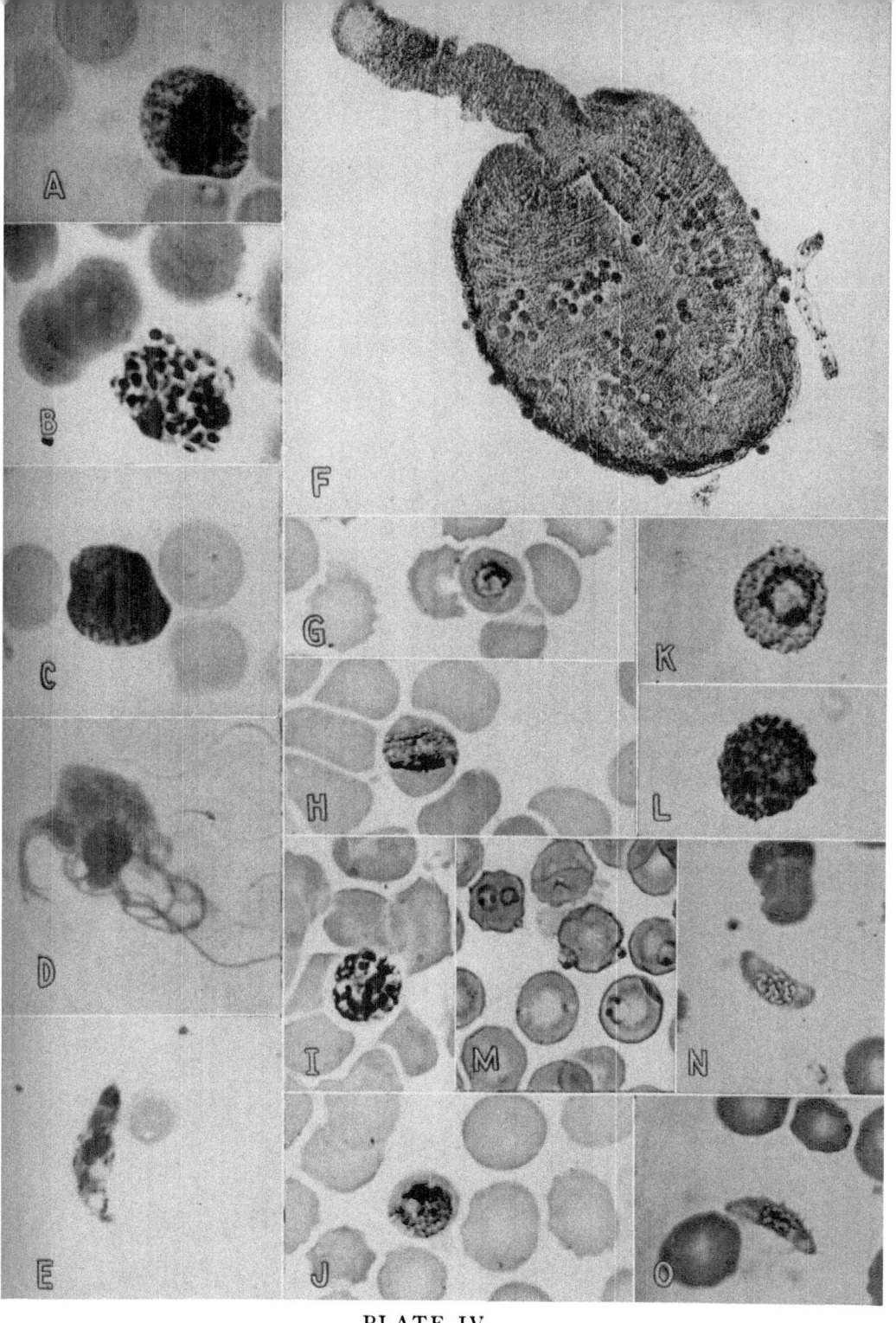

PLATE IV

Plasmodium vivax: A. amoeboid. (x1450) B. schizont. (x1450) C. microgametocyte. (x1450) D. exflagellation of microgametocyte. (x1450) E. oökinete. (x1450) F. oöcysts on ventriculus ("stomach") of *Anopheles* mosquito. (x100) G. ring, with some extension. (x1200) H. band form. (x1200) I. schizont. (x1200) J. amoeboid. (x1200) K. ring. (x1200) L. macrogametocyte. (x1200) M. ring. (x1200) N. microgametocyte. (x1200) O. macrogametocyte. (x1200)

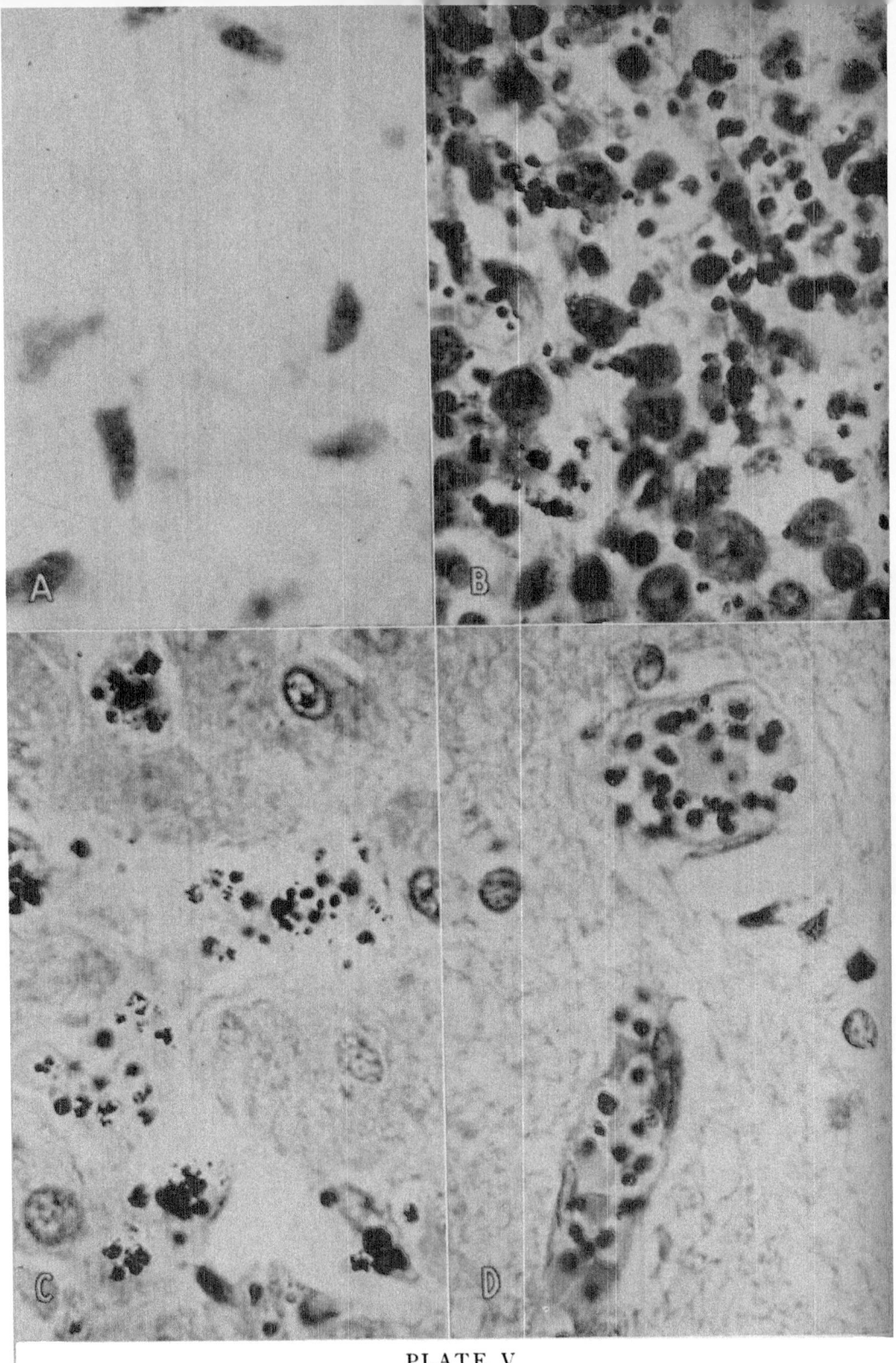

PLATE V

A. *Plasmodium falciparum*: gametocytes in thick blood film. (x1500) B. Malignant malaria: section of spleen. (x1000) C. Malignant malaria: section of liver. (x1000) D. Malignant malaria: section of brain. (x1500)

depends upon (1) the presence of susceptible human cases, (2) the presence of susceptible mosquito vectors, and (3) an environment favorable both to the propagation of the mosquito transmitter and the development of the parasite in the mosquito.

(1) The human factor.—Man is the only known vertebrate reservoir of the human malarial organisms. A few of the higher monkeys can be infected experimentally, but none of these is responsible for the continuation of the disease as a medical or public health problem. Among natives in the tropics, the disease is principally one of children, who may suffer repeated severe infection for the first several years of life, especially with the tertian parasite, *Plasmodium vivax*. Negro children generally, and indeed all persons of the Negro race irrespective of age, appear more resistant than those of the white race. Nevertheless, previously unexposed persons of all races are usually susceptible at any age. On the other hand, persons of all races who are or who recently have been infected with malarial organisms resist reinfection by the same strain of parasite for some time because of a specific immunity acquired from the initial infection. The predominance of such persons in any community would, of course, tend to limit the development of epidemics of malaria. Occasionally a presumably naturally immune individual who has never been previously infected is encountered.

The presence of gametocytes in the blood is essential before an individual can lead to the infection of the mosquito vector. Usually, gametocytes of the malarial organisms appear in the blood within five to ten days after asexual parasites are first noted, but many infected individuals develop few or no gametocytes. Such persons are, of course, not infective for mosquitoes and are, therefore, not truly carriers of malaria in an epidemiological sense. Indeed, a considerable number of gametocytes must usually occur in his blood before a person is able to infect a mosquito. According to one investigator working with *Anopheles maculatus*, these infections must equal, for *Plasmodium vivax*, one gametocyte per 1000 leucocytes; for *Plasmodium malariae*, one per 330 leucocytes; and for *Plasmodium falciparum*, one per 200 leucocytes. The gametocytes are not infective for mosquitoes when first produced but become so within a few days.

(2) The mosquito factor.—Malarial parasites of all species are naturally transmitted through the bite of infected female mosquitoes

of the genus *Anopheles*. Not all anophelines are suitable vectors of these parasites, and in most communities there are only two or three species which can act as vectors. Some species of mosquitoes are quite susceptible to experimental infection by *Plasmodium*, and can even experimentally transmit the organism back to man, but they are nevertheless insignificant as natural vectors either because they do not frequent human habitation or else because they prefer the blood of other animals. In the southern United States, the most important vector of malaria is *Anopheles quadrimaculatus*, whereas along the Pacific coast *Anopheles maculipennis* is most significant. *Anopheles maculipennis* is also the most important transmitter in Europe. In the West Indies and in Central and South America *Anopheles albimanus* has the greatest significance as a vector. *Anopheles gambiae* is the most serious transmitter in tropical Africa. This form has recently been found also in Brazil, where it promises likewise to become a significant vector. In the East Indies, several species, including *Anopheles culicifacies* and *Anopheles ludlowi*, have great importance.

(3) The factor of environment.—It is often very difficult to explain why, in a given community where malaria is endemic, one species of malarial parasite is prevalent. Sometimes one form will occur intensely and all other forms will be wholly absent, so far as can be determined. Special requirements of temperature, moisture, altitude, or other elements of climate sometimes seem to furnish the most satisfactory explanation. The fact that certain species of anophelines are better transmitters of one species of malarial parasite than of another also helps to explain the problem.

The availability of water for the propagation of the mosquito is, of course, entirely essential in order that vectors be available, and when swamps or sluggish streams and canals with grassy banks are near by, malaria can be expected in most tropical places. Indeed, the proximity of mosquito breeding grounds and the abundance of mosquitoes govern to a large extent the intensity which malarial infection may attain in any community.

The time required for development of the parasite to the infective stage in the mosquito (the sporogonic phase) varies with the temperature of the given locality. Optimum development of *Plasmodium vivax* goes on at 25° C. and then is completed in about eleven days. *Plasmodium malariae* prefers a temperature of 22° C., under which development will be completed in eighteen days. *Plasmodium falciparum*, the tropical species, requires a much higher temperature: 30° C. At this temperature, development is completed in ten days. When the temperature falls severely below the optimum given for a species, development of the parasite is arrested, although when a favorable temperature is reëstablished, growth is resumed. On the other hand, if the parasites have previously developed to the sporozoite stage in the salivary ducts, the mosquito will transmit the organism even in the winter season, if it bites a susceptible person. The parasite is unable to establish itself in the mosquitoes of a community if the mean temperature is below 16° C.

In the subtropics and warmer temperate zones, malaria has a seasonal periodicity. Cases of *Plasmodium vivax* infection occur chiefly in the spring and early summer, and those of *Plasmodium malariae* usually in the late summer. Cases of *Plasmodium falciparum* infection are generally encountered in the late summer and fall, hence the name of this type—aestivo-autumnal malaria.

Pathology and symptoms.—Following a preliminary period during which the patient may complain of vague aches and pains, typical symptoms of malarial infection are initiated, these being characterized usually by periodic fever which may reach 105° F. Symptoms begin after variable intervals, depending on the species of parasite involved. They are noted about ten days after infection with *Plasmodium falciparum*, about twelve to fourteen days after *Plasmodium malariae* infection, and from fourteen to seventeen days after *Plasmodium vivax* infection. The febrile paroxysms occur with a periodicity characteristic for each species of parasite, the period equaling the interval required by each parasite to complete its schizogonous cycle. For *Plasmodium vivax* and *Plasmodium ovale* this interval is forty-eight hours; for *Plasmodium malariae* it is seventy-two hours; and for *Plasmodium falciparum* it is a less constant period, although usually forty-eight hours or less (thirty-six hours). (See Figure 6.) The febrile paroxysm begins coincidentally with the rupture of the erythrocyte containing the merozoites of the parasite and may be caused by the liberation of "toxins" of the parasite or possibly by the liberation of potassium from the ruptured erythrocyte. Within a few hours after the fever peak is attained, the temperature drops, often below normal, and no further fever is experienced until the parasite

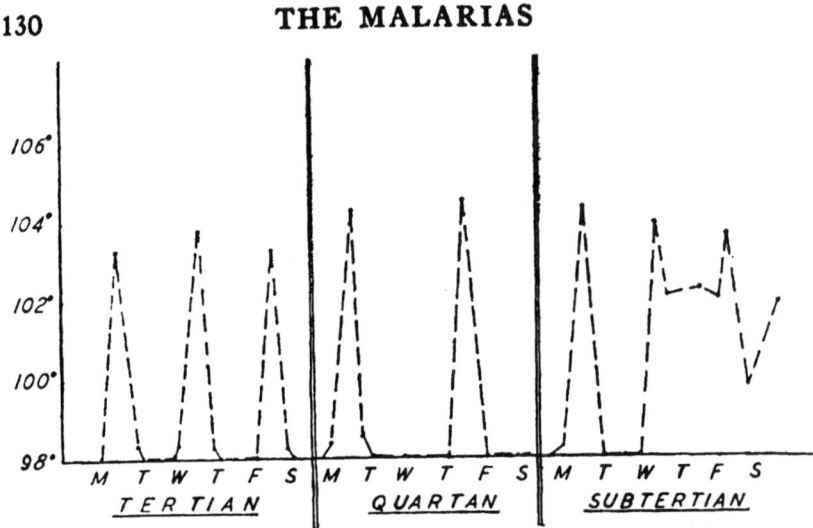

Figure 6. Temperature curves in tertian, quartan, and subtertian malaria.

completes the schizogonous cycle once more. In the subtertian infection, however, one paroxysm may be so prolonged as to overlap with the next. False crises between paroxysms are rather common in the subtertian infection.

The malaria paroxysm actually can be divided into three stages: the stage of coldness, which lasts about an hour, the hot stage, which lasts three or four hours, and the sweating stage, which lasts two to four hours. All of these indicated times are highly variable, although usually they last collectively about six hours. Oddly, most paroxysms occur between midnight and noon, or else in the early afternoon. This is a point of significance clinically to differentiate malaria from fevers caused by other infectious agents.

Not infrequently, mixed infections with two species of malaria or double infections with two strains of a single species occur. In such cases, paroxysms may occur with greater frequency, a febrile attack being experienced whenever the schizogonous cycle is completed for either species or strain.

Severe malarial infection always involves the destruction of many red blood cells, with a resulting anemia. Symptoms usually appear only after one erythrocyte per 100,000 is infected. The anemia is principally of a secondary character, although it may become of pernicious type in prolonged infections. There is some evidence for the in vivo action of a hemolysin, perhaps the malarial pigment derived from the parasite, since some erythrocytes are destroyed without being infected. The haemoglobin of surviving cells is also reduced. Leucopenia is marked, although monocytic cells are relatively increased.

Enlargement of the spleen and liver characteristically occurs in malaria, the spleen particularly often finally filling the abdominal cavity. Early in the disease, the enlargement takes place only during accessions of the fever, but chronic persistent enlargement eventually develops. The enlargement occurs chiefly among children in the tropics. Adult native persons, infected for long periods and relatively immune, commonly reveal a spleen of normal size. Should the enlarged spleen rupture spontaneously, as it sometimes does, or from trauma (e.g., from a blow in the abdomen), death will usually follow, unless operation is undertaken at once.

Following malignant malarial infection, essentially all organs, when sectioned, reveal capillaries charged with infected erythrocytes which seem to adhere to the blood-vessel walls. The tissues themselves contain large amounts of malarial pigment, and in prolonged infections, the bone marrow, the brain, and particularly the spleen may be black from the pigment deposition. Some of the circulating phagocytic cells also contain malarial pigment, its detection being diagnostic of the disease. In infections with the quartan parasite, the patient not uncommonly develops nephritis. (See Plate V, B, C, and D, facing page 127.)

Relapse.—Relapse in malaria is the recurrence of clinical malaria after apparent cure of a first infection, without exogenous reinfection. The tendency to relapse after apparent cure is one of the chief characters of malaria. Often a change of climate, such as removal from the tropics to a cold northern latitude, is sufficient to cause relapse. Extended fatigue or inadequate food also may cause exacerbations of the disease. Apparently the disease, prior to the relapse, has lain dormant or latent, and only when the patient experiences an unusual strain does the infection light up.

Tertian Malaria, Case Report.—A man thirty years old, born in London, had lived on a tea plantation in India for ten years. Following this period in India, he began a year's vacation trip around the world. He reached New York city in September, some three months after leaving India. After residing in New York for six weeks, during which time the temperature dropped very considerably with approaching winter, the patient experienced a febrile attack, which he himself recognized as a malarial paroxysm. Examination of his blood in the laboratory revealed the *vivax* organism. Because of his history, the patient seems almost certainly to have been infected prior to his arrival in New York. Since he lived for six weeks in New York before symptoms appeared, his infection was probably not newly acquired while he was en route to the city, but was the relapse of an old infection, the relapse being brought on by the colder climate.

Relapses may be divided into those following latency for a short term (e.g., six weeks) and those following latency for long periods. Relapses from *Plasmodium falciparum* are almost always of the short-term variety. Relapses from *Plasmodium vivax* and *Plasmodium malariae* are often of the long-term variety, occurring even after two years or more.

Blackwater fever.—Blackwater or hemoglobinuric fever is a serious and often fatal complication which is observed in some cases of prolonged infection with *Plasmodium falciparum*. It is an anaphylaxislike reaction, of sudden onset, which presumably results from the sensitization of the patient to the antigens of the malarial parasite. An attack is precipitated by, or at least occurs together with, a malarial paroxysm, although often malaria has not been previously suspected clinically. Characteristically, tremendous numbers of erythrocytes are lysed in the circulation of the patient within twenty-four hours or so during the attack, red cell counts often at the end of this time being less than one million per cubic millimeter of blood. The urine becomes of mahogany color from the liberated hemoglobin of these cells, and this, together with the febrile character of the disease, confers the name blackwater fever.

The disease is found chiefly in or near low, swampy areas, where the subtertian parasite exists. It is known along both the east and the west coast of Africa and along the Congo, Zambezi, and other rivers. It occurs in the Balkan States in Europe, in the southern United States, the West Indies, Central and South America, India, and the Far East. The disease is also sometimes encountered in northern latitudes (England, Canada, etc.) among persons who have been in the tropics and whose malarial infection has relapsed on return to the North.

Negroes of the tropics seldom experience blackwater fever, and Europeans or Americans experience it only after residing in an endemic area for at least one year, this interval evidently being required for sensitization. Arabs and Hindus are about as susceptible as white persons, and Negroes who have never suffered malarial infection before entering an endemic region likewise are readily susceptible. As a result of an attack of blackwater fever, the malaria infection which leads to the attack is generally miraculously cured. Individuals usually survive the initial attack, but less often live through a second experience. Some persons, who suffer particularly mild attacks, amounting to little more than a transitory hemoglobinuria, may survive from six to ten attacks. Mortality varies greatly from place to place and from time to time, yet on the average is about twenty-five percent. The recovery of those who survive is generally astonishingly rapid.

Immunity.—Most persons recover from any of the malarias except that caused by *Plasmodium falciparum* even without treatment, although often, especially in the very young, the initial infections are severe and symptoms are serious. Yet second and third infections with the same strain of malaria as that which caused the first infection are much milder and may not cause symptoms or even lead to the appearance of parasites in the blood stream. The continuation of this acquired immunity depends on the persistence of the parasite in the body of the patient in latent form. Soon after the parasite is eliminated either spontaneously or by drug treatment, the immunity is lost. Likewise, unless natural reinfections by the same strain of parasite occurs with some frequency, the resistant state is lost, for the infection will finally become eradicated by the host's defensive mechanisms. With *Plasmodium vivax*, immunity, by reason of a persisting latent infection, may last for two years in the absence of exogenous reinfection, but with *Plasmodium malariae*, it may persist for very much greater periods. There is but little experimental evidence yet available for the development of any immunity against *Plasmodium falciparum* consequent upon latent infection, and a patient is susceptible to reinfection within a few days or weeks after recovery from a previous attack.

Quartan Malaria, Case Report.—The longevity of latent infection with the quartan malarial parasite is well revealed in the following experience which occurred in 1938. A native American woman, thirty years of age, who had been in the hospital wards for one week, was given a transfusion. The blood came from her husband, who was in good health. Twenty-eight days later, symptoms of quartan malaria appeared in the recipient and the quartan parasite was subsequently identified in her blood cells. When the history of the husband was taken, he was found to have suffered with quartan malaria in 1920, when he served in the Italian army. He had been treated in 1921 just before coming to the United States, and had suffered no symptoms since. Unfortunately, the parasite could not be demonstrated directly in the husband's blood but, since no other source of infection for the wife was apparent, and since the number of days since transfusion till symptoms appeared represented a possible incubation period of quartan malaria, the husband was considered the source of the wife's infection. The quartan infection had evidently been latent in the husband for seventeen years—from 1921 to 1938.[3]

The necessity of constant reinfection to fortify an existing immunity to malaria is revealed by those who leave an endemic area where they have developed an immunity for a sojourn of several years in a nonmalarial community. On return to the endemic area, such persons prove just as susceptible as persons not previously immunized to the infection. While resident in the nonmalarial community, these persons experienced no reinfection and consequently soon lost their latent infection and, with it, the immunity which they previously had acquired.

The immunity to malaria is not merely species-specific but actually strain-specific. Often, therefore, an individual who travels from one area where *Plasmodium vivax* is endemic to another will suffer infection in both, provided immunologically distinct strains of *Plasmodium vivax* occur in the two areas. Even a persisting or latent infection with one strain of *Plasmodium vivax* will not protect against an immunologically distinct strain of the same species. There is, likewise, no immunity whatsoever against a wholly different species of malaria.

The acquired immunity in malaria depends on the action of the phagocytic cells and, perhaps to at least an equal extent, on the presence of humoral antibody. The antibody first sensitizes or opsonizes the parasites, and the phagocytic cells then remove the sensitized organisms from the circulating blood. The centers of most active phagocytosis are the spleen and liver.

As stated earlier in this chapter under "Epidemiology," different

[3] W. A. Gardner and L. Dexter, *Journal of the American Medical Association*, 111: 2473 (1938).

races manifest a marked difference in natural susceptibility to malaria. Negroes are relatively resistant at least to the symptoms of infection with *Plasmodium vivax* and *Plasmodium ovale* and suffer comparatively little from infection with *Plasmodium falciparum*. They have about the same susceptibility as white persons to the effects of *Plasmodium malariae*. White persons, in contrast, are almost invariably susceptible to all the malarial parasites and generally suffer severe symptoms or even death. Children, particularly, experience severe disease, are most likely to succumb, and, after apparent cure, are most prone to relapse. Adult persons often overcome their infections without specific treatment.

Diagnosis.—Any person with fever who is or has been in the tropics must be suspected of having malaria. If this fever is periodic, the likelihood of malaria is very great, indeed. Symptoms of malaria are protean, and fevers of unusual course, or even infections without fever in the event of past exposure, always must be suspected as malaria. The disease is capable of lying dormant for months, so that unless the past history of the patient is carefully taken, malaria may occur when least suspected.

Malaria is most satisfactorily diagnosed by observing microscopically the parasite in the blood. Thick blood films (Plate V, A, facing page 127) are best for this purpose if the observer is experienced in their use, and for survey purposes they are decidedly preferred. A very considerable experience is usually required by most persons, however, before the separate species of parasites can be recognized in thick films. The parasites can most clearly be seen for purposes of identification in thin blood films.

Whenever possible the blood must be examined before treatment is begun, for most antimalarial drugs quickly drive the organism out of the peripheral blood. The presence of leucocytes containing pigment in blood films can usually be taken as presumptive evidence of malarial infection. Smears of spleen pulp also reveal large quantities of pigment as well as many parasites. Often parasites can be forced into the peripheral blood, when none can otherwise be found there, by the intravenous administration of adrenalin hydrochloride (2 cc. in a volume of 300 cc. of salt solution).

Immunological tests have had little use as yet for diagnosing malaria. Antibody is nevertheless present in the blood within a few weeks after infection, and its detection by the precipitin test or by the complement fixation test is possible. Henry's flocculation test, depending on the greater precipitability by water of serum globulin in malaria patients also has had some trial in diagnosis.

Surveys to find the number of presumptive cases of malaria in a given community are often conducted by determining the "spleen rate"—that is, the percentage of enlarged spleens in the general population. The method is quite satisfactory, except in areas where kala azar or schistosomiasis is endemic.

Specific therapy.—Three drugs are available for treating malaria: quinine, atebrin, and plasmochin. Quinine and atebrin are useful against all stages of *Plasmodium vivax, Plasmodium ovale*, and *Plasmodium malariae*. They likewise affect the asexual or schizogonous stages of *Plasmodium falciparum* but are without effect upon the gametocytes of this species. Plasmochin alone among the available substances will act upon the *Plasmodium falciparum* gametocytes. Therefore, persons infected with *Plasmodium falciparum* should be treated with two drugs: quinine or atebrin, for the elimination of the schizogonous stages, and plasmochin, for the elimination of the gametocytes.

Quinine is the oldest of these several drugs and is still the one most widely used in malaria. Its use must be continued for months before an infection can be certainly cured, and relapse after quinine therapy is usual, particularly with *Plasmodium vivax* and *Plasmodium malariae* infections, since most individuals drop the treatment before absolute cure. Atebrin has the distinct advantage of being effective within a shorter time, often within a week or so, and according to some observers, relapse less frequently follows atebrin treatment. Other investigators, however, have noted relapse after atebrin therapy about as frequently as after the administration of quinine. Some subjects, furthermore, do not tolerate atebrin very well.

It is a fortunate fact that the most dangerous malaria parasite, *Plasmodium falciparum,* is the species most amenable to treatment by drugs and is the one which, after treatment, is least likely to persist and cause relapses of malaria. Relapses of *falciparum* infections usually occur after a few weeks, if at all, and are rare after one year, if the patient has left the endemic area. The complete elimination of *Plasmodium vivax* or *Plasmodium malariae* by drugs is decidely more difficult, although the organisms are readily driven from the peripheral blood. Indeed, usually, if quinine or atebrin is administered during the sweating stage of the paroxysm, the next attack will be decidedly less severe, and the one scheduled to follow thereafter may fail to develop. Yet absolute cure of these infections is never a simple procedure.

At the present time the point of view is taken that the drugs themselves seldom cure malaria. They seem instead merely to check the development of the parasite. The final eradication of the causal organism results from the action of the immune mechanism of the host upon the parasite. Hence, present practice dictates, particularly in endemic areas where reinfection is probable, that drug treatment be withheld until the patient has suffered five or six severe attacks of fever and has thus had opportunity to develop immunity. Once an immune response has been made, the danger of relapse when treatment is discontinued is less. However, persons who live outside endemic areas generally are given intensive drug treatment at once, since such individuals need not be protected from subsequent reinfection with malarial organisms.

Prophylaxis.—Prophylaxis against malaria may be directed toward protecting the individual or toward protecting the community. Individual or personal prophylaxis is generally attempted through administering antimalarial drugs. Five grains of quinine given daily is often advised and has, indeed, long been relied upon, as it still is, by those in endemic areas to afford protection against the contraction of malaria. In recent years, the value of quinine prophylaxis has been greatly questioned, by reason of experimental findings. It is pointed out that quinine does not prevent infection with malarial parasites but merely checks the symptoms of disease by holding down the number of parasites. Atebrin prophylaxis seems potentially better, since prolonged administration is evidently not necessary. However, after prophylaxis with atebrin, too, infection occurs, although it may not be manifest until some weeks or months later when the effect of the drug has worn off. Some authorities feel, therefore, that the wiser method is to withhold these drugs until after the infection is contracted, since there will then be no danger of the parasite being "drug-fast," and the drugs will possibly have a higher level of therapeutic activity.

Malignant Malaria, Case Report.—One of the disadvantages of chemoprophylaxis is revealed by the following cases. Three men were sent by steamship to West Africa to lay out an airplane base. En route all received five grains of quinine daily. For appropriate reasons, the men were returned to the United States after only several days in Africa. The drug was continued not only while the men were ashore but also during the first week of the return trip. A few days after the drug was suspended, however, all the men, as well as several shipmates, developed febrile attacks suggestive of malaria. The drug was resumed at once without the formality of proving malarial parasites the cause of the fever. The men were brought to the hospital on reaching New York. The greatest difficulty was encountered in the hospital in proving the cases actually to be malaria, for all parasites had been driven from the peripheral blood by the quinine. Within a few days, however, parasites of the *falciparum* type were observed, and the etiology of the disease was thus established.

If an individual dwelling in the tropics sleeps beneath mosquito netting, keeps his house well screened, and avoids native villages, especially in the early evening hours, he will be somewhat less likely to contract the disease.

Protection of the community from malaria involves two principal objectives: (1) the sterilization of human carriers and (2) the elimination of mosquito transmitters. The sterilization of carriers involves treating these individuals with antimalarial drugs so that the mosquito population cannot become infected. The elimination of the mosquito usually is a formidable task, yet notable success toward this objective has been achieved in many parts of the world. The construction of the Panama Canal and of the naval base at Singapore in Malaya was possible only after the mosquito was controlled. The elimination of mosquito breeding places through the drainage of swamps is always advised. The spraying of Paris green or the oiling of water which cannot be drained but which serves for mosquito breeding is also helpful. When none of these measures is possible, such waters may be stocked with fish (*Gambusia* sp.) which feed on the mosquito wrigglers or may be planted to *Chara* or other plants which may repel adult mosquitoes and prevent their laying eggs in such water.

In addition to large bodies of water, however, that in small receptacles in the immediate vicinity or even within dwellings may serve as a breeding place for mosquitoes. Indeed, the "malaria houses" in the tropics, in which all the members of the family and their visitors contract malaria, often owe their reputation to the fact that mosquitoes breed in poorly draining gutters, uncovered water barrels and cisterns, flower urns, tin cans, or holes in tree stumps in the dooryard of the dwelling, and thus have opportunity to bite every person entering or leaving that house.

MALARIA-INDUCED THERAPY IN NEUROSYPHILIS

Since 1917, certain types of nervous disease which follow syphilis have been treated by infecting the patient with malaria. After the individual has experienced a number of severe paroxysms which attain 104° F., his nervous affliction is often cured, the spirochetes evidently being eradicated. The malaria can then be treated with any of the usual antimalarial drugs. The severity rather than the number of paroxysms determines the success of treatment. *Plasmodium vivax* or *Plasmodium ovale* are most commonly used in white persons. Recently, *Plasmodium knowlesi,* a malarial parasite from an Asiatic monkey, has been employed for the purpose in Caucasians. In the Negro, however, none of these benign parasites is effective, and the use of the malignant form, *Plasmodium falciparum,* or of *Plasmodium malariae* generally must be resorted to.

MALARIA IN DRUG ADDICTS

In recent years, epidemics of malaria among drug addicts have been reported in Cairo, Egypt, and in New York city, New Orleans, and elsewhere in the United States. The addicts use a common syringe without the precaution of sterilizing it between successive persons. Eventually, it appears, all in the group using the instrument become infected with malaria if one member introduces the parasite. In most cases in which the parasite has been identified, *Plasmodium falciparum* has been revealed, although *Plasmodium vivax* and *Plasmodium malariae* also have appeared in some patients. The usual antimalarial drugs are effective in therapy, although, because of the advanced state of the infection when most patients are seen, the intravenous administration of quinine dihydrochloride is often necessary.

Chapter XIII

THE COCCIDIOSES

THE INTESTINAL SPOROZOANS belong to the suborder Eimeriidea of the order Coccidiida. The organisms are commonly referred to as the coccidia, and the disease they cause is called coccidiosis.

A number of species of coccidia have been described from time to time as human parasites, their transmitting stages (oöcysts) being observed in human feces. Generally these forms later have been shown properly to be parasites of animals, the oöcysts having been seen as they passed through the intestine of man after their ingestion with food. For example, three species of the genus *Eimeria* which were once described as parasites of man were found later to be coccidia of fish, the oöcysts of these forms merely occurring in feces of persons who ate the fish. At present only two or three species of coccidia are believed capable of establishing themselves in human beings, and of these only one, *Isospora hominis,* is a well-authenticated human parasite. Many different species are known to infect animals, and some of these cause severe diseases in these hosts.

ISOSPORA HOMINIS AND COCCIDIOSIS

Isospora hominis [1] was first found in 1860 by Kjellberg in the intestinal villi of a patient who came to autopsy. The oöcysts of the parasite were first found in human feces in 1890 by Railliet and Lucet.

Geographical distribution.—Human cases of coccidiosis have been reported from nearly all countries bordering the Mediterranean, from many parts of Africa, from the Near East, India, the Philippines, the East Indies, and China, as well as from South America and the United

---

[1] Common synonym: *Isospora belli.*

States. The disease thus has essentially a cosmopolitan distribution. Its incidence, however, is so low that it is not a significant public health factor: up to 1935, only about 200 cases altogether had been reported.[2]

Morphology and life cycle.—The only stages of *Isospora hominis* which have as yet been studied are the oöcyst and those which develop immediately from the oöcyst. The oöcysts measure from twenty to thirty microns long by ten to twenty microns broad. They contain a central granular mass of cytoplasm representing the parasite proper. In a favorable environment this central mass divides into two sporo-

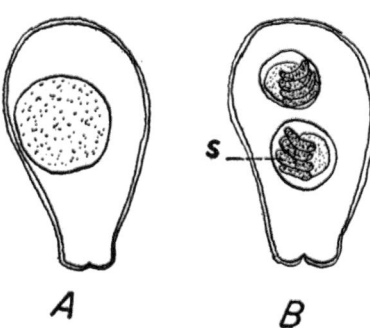

Figure 7. *Isospora hominis:* oöcyst. A, freshly passed in feces; B, germinated oöcyst showing eight sporozoites.

A   B

blasts each of which is contained in a spore wall. If swallowed by an appropriate host, these sporoblasts each divide twice to yield, in all, eight sporozoites, four being found in each of the spore walls. (See Figure 7.) As yet, nothing further of the life cycle or of the morphology of its various stages is known, although it seems very probable that these stages do not significantly differ from those of animal species of *Isospora.*

Cultivation.—Coccidia have not been cultivated artificially beyond the sporozoite stage which results from the oöcyst.

Epidemiology.—*Isospora hominis* is a very rare parasite of man. At the Mayo clinic, for example, a survey of 60,000 persons over many years failed to reveal a single case of infection.[3] This paucity of human cases of *Isospora hominis* infection creates doubt that man is the only host, or even the preferred host, of this parasite. Although the species is not known regularly to infect any animal, its survival

[2] T. B. Magath, *American Journal of Tropical Medicine*, 15: 91 (1935).
[3] *Ibid.*

through infecting man alone seems unlikely. Its transmission, in any case, goes on through the ingestion of the oöcysts as contaminants of food or drink.

Pathogenicity.—The oöcysts of *Isospora hominis* are sometimes found in apparently healthy persons. Other individuals, however, reveal symptoms of diarrhea or dysentery. Often other parasites such as *Endamoeba histolytica* are present, and in some cases these forms may be responsible for the observed symptoms. Lesions must occur, however, probably in the intestine, although these have not yet been described.

One case of accidental laboratory infection has been reported, with symptoms setting in after eight days. Oöcysts were found in the feces twenty-eight days after the infection.[4]

Diagnosis.—The observation of oöcysts, usually unsegmented, in the feces suffices to diagnose infection with *Isospora hominis*. Charcot-Leyden crystals sometimes appear in the feces of infected persons.

Specific therapy.—No specific therapy is available for coccidiosis. None is generally required, since most cases are self-limiting.

Prophylaxis.—Prevention of the contamination of food or drink with feces of infected individuals provides adequate prophylaxis.

[4] A. Connal, *Transactions of the Royal Society of Tropical Medicine and Hygiene*, 16: 223 (1922).

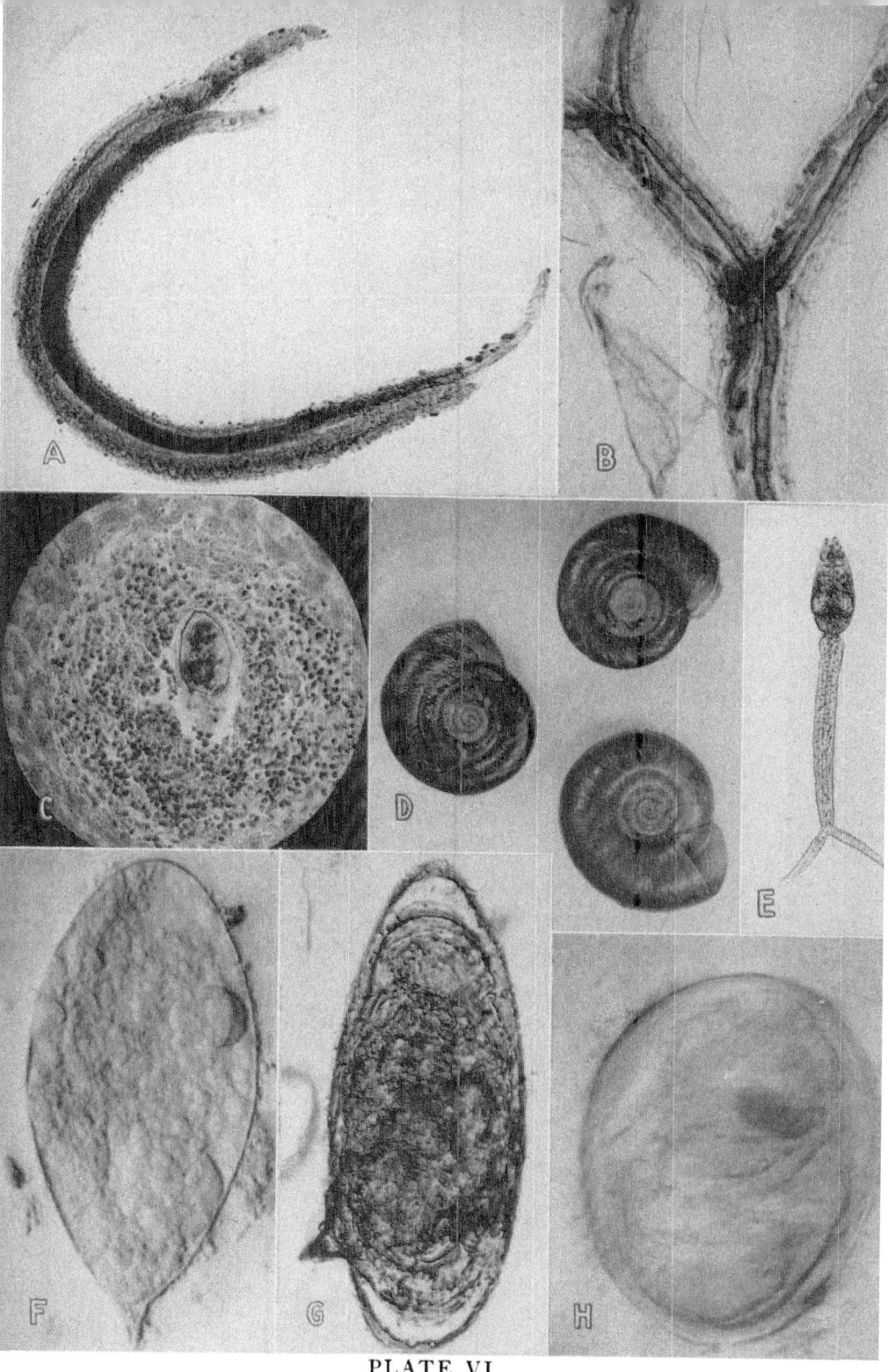

PLATE VI

Schistosoma mansoni: A. adults in copulation. Female (slender form) enclosed within gynecophoral canal of male worm. (x30) B. adults in mesenteric veins. (x5) C. egg in pseudotubercle of liver. (x300) D. *Australorbis glabrata:* snail host in West Indies. (x1) E. cercaria. (x100) F. *Schistosoma haematobium:* egg. (x600) G. *Schistosoma mansoni:* egg. (x450) H. *Schistosoma iaponicum:* egg. (x600)

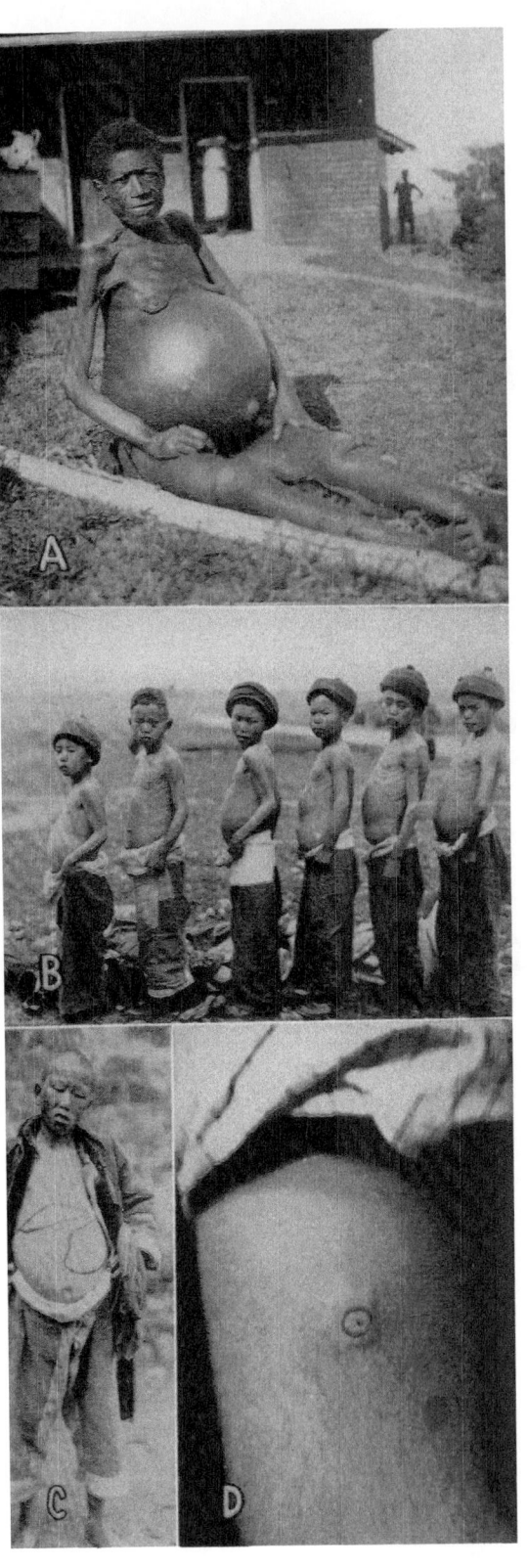

PLATE VII

A. Schistosomiasis *mansoni:* advanced stage in native of Belgian Congo. B and C. Schistosomiasis *japonicum:* patients with enlarged abdomens caused by liver cirrhosis and splenomegaly. D. Schistosomiasis *mansoni:* positive immediate skin test in patient following intradermal injection of antigen. Note wheal and pseudopodia. Circle represents outline of initial bleb immediately following injection of antigen.

Chapter XIV

THE CILIATE INFECTIONS

THE ONLY CILIATED PROTOZOAN of significance in human infection is *Balantidium coli*. This form was first observed in two patients with dysentery in 1857 by Malmsten, who considered it to be a species of *Paramoecium*. Within a few years, however, other investigators showed it to be distinct from the paramoecia, and it has since been designated by the name it now bears.

BALANTIDIUM COLI AND BALANTIDIASIS

Geographical distribution.—*Balantidium coli* has a cosmopolitan distribution. It is found especially in areas where pigs are raised and occurs primarily in those persons whose work or other experience brings them in close contact with pigs. It is said to occur with some frequency in the Philippine Islands, as well as in Europe, and has been recorded from man also in the United States, Puerto Rico, Brazil, the smaller islands of the Pacific, China, Indo-China, Siberia, and some other regions.

Morphology and life cycle.—*Balantidium coli* exists as two distinct forms: the trophozoite and the cyst. The trophozoite is the active growing stage responsible for the disease which the species causes. It is found in the tissue of the colon wall of man, or in the patient's stool when this is of fluid consistency. The cyst is the inactive, resistant, transmitting stage, responsible for the dissemination of the parasite and for its survival during unfavorable periods. It is found in the formed stools of patients. (See Figure 8.)

The trophozoite of *Balantidium coli* is ovoid in outline, and measures from fifty to seventy microns in length by from forty to fifty microns in breadth. The entire cell is covered with short, fine cilia arranged in longitudinal rows. Near the pointed anterior end of the cell is a cytostome into which, largely by the movement of special, longer cilia, food particles such as blood cells, bits of tissue, and fecal debris are passed. At the posterior rounded end of the cell is the egestion pore, through which wastes are eliminated. Food vacuoles are usually seen circulating in the endoplasm. Two contractile vacuoles are disposed, one toward each end of the cell. When the organism is

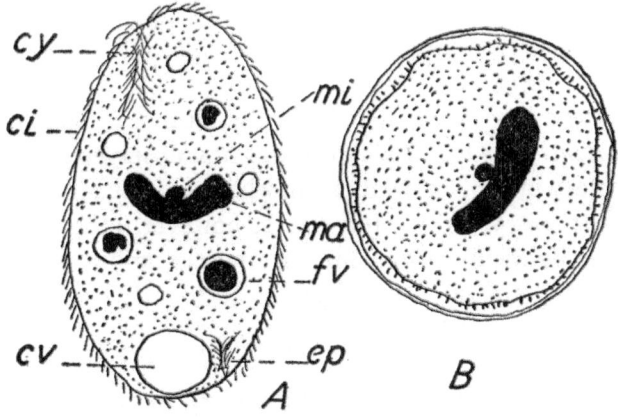

Figure 8. *Balantidium coli:* A, trophozoite; B, cyst. ci = cilia; cy = cytostome; cv = contractile vacuole; ep = egestion pore; fv = food vacuole; ma = macronucleus; mi = micronucleus.

stained appropriately, two nuclei are visible. The larger macronucleus is kidney-shaped; the smaller micronucleus is more or less spherical and lies in the concavity of the macronucleus. Reproduction takes place by transverse fission of the cell.

The spherical cyst measures from forty-five to sixty microns in diameter. Usually a single parasite occurs in each cyst, but often two forms are present. Sometimes the living parasite is seen to move freely within the cyst wall. Usually both the macronucleus and the micronucleus are visible in the stained cyst, and cilia also can be seen when the newly encysted parasite is at rest inside the cyst wall. Food vacuoles are absent from the encysted parasite.

Cysts which have been ingested by an individual excyst in the intestine, one trophozoite usually coming from each cyst. After several transverse divisions, they enter the tissue of the intestinal wall, their entry probably being facilitated by a cytolysin emanating from the parasite. Nests of parasites soon develop in the tissue. Some of the parasites later become encysted and are passed out of the intestine with the feces. It is these forms which must be swallowed by the next individual if the parasite life is to continue.

Cultivation.—*Balantidium coli* was first cultivated in 1921 by Barret and Yarbrough in a mixture of inactivated human serum (one part) and 0.5 percent salt solution (sixteen parts). Mediums now used for the purpose generally consist of from five to ten percent horse serum in Ringer's solution plus a small amount of rice starch. Often, enough agar is added to give the mixture a semisolid consistency. Feces containing the *Balantidium coli* is seeded into the medium warmed to 37° C. If transfers are made every few days, strains can be preserved for many months. The organism can also be cultivated in Boeck's medium.

Epidemiology.—Man appears usually to contract infection with *Balantidium coli* from pigs carrying the parasite. About two thirds of all pigs are said to harbor the organism. One quarter of all human cases give a history of contact with pigs, such as that experienced by pig raisers or by workers in pig-slaughtering houses. Infection from human carriers also is known, however. Infection takes place following the ingestion of food or drink polluted with infected feces, although direct infection through hands soiled with the feces also is possible. Flies may act as mechanical transmitters.

The incidence of human infection with *Balantidium* is very low, usually substantially less than one percent of the general population. In one survey of 142 inmates of a mental hospital in South Carolina, however, five percent were found infected (seven cases).[1] It seems possible that, especially in warmer regions, the incidence of infection is higher than is now appreciated at least in poorly sanitated communities. The human parasite probably can be transferred from man to the cat or to certain monkeys. Man has not as yet been infected experimentally with the pig parasite despite the epidemiological evidence that such transmission occurs naturally.

Pathogenicity.—Infection with *Balantidium coli* is manifested in twenty percent or so of those infected by a chronic diarrhea or dysen-

---

[1] M. D. Young and C. Ham, *Journal of Parasitology*, 27: 71 (1941); M. D. Young, *Journal of the American Medical Association*, 113: 580 (1939).

tery. Lesions containing numerous balantidia can generally be found in the mucosa or submucosa of the colon and sometimes in the posterior small intestine of those who harbor the parasite. The ulcers are of an undermining character, and their serpigenous channels may interconnect as do those in amoebic infection of the colon wall. While the lesions in balantidiasis are usually smaller than those in amoebiasis, they may extend over the entire colon and finally account for the patient's death. The patient commonly presents blood and mucus in his diarrheic stools, but some cases are constipated. The parasite does not usually invade other organs, although it has been recovered on one occasion from mesenteric glands. (See Plate I, E, facing page 78.)

Immunity.—Most persons appear to be refractory to infection with *Balantidium coli*, as the low incidence of infection suggests. Individuals who do contract infection generally bring the disease under control with little trouble. Among animals, the diet appears to influence profoundly the natural resistance, those on a high protein diet quickly eradicating the parasite.

Diagnosis.—The observation of the trophozoite stage in the fluid stool, or of the double-walled cyst stage in the formed stool, provides unequivocal diagnosis of balantidiasis. Usually the diagnosis can be made on the fresh untreated specimen, without resort to staining procedures. When parasites are very scarce, the stool may be cultivated in an appropriate medium.

Specific therapy.—No special treatment is generally required in balantidiasis, the infections usually clearing spontaneously. For those infections which persist, methylene blue, carbarsone, and stovarsol are often recommended. Certain silver compounds (protargol) are sometimes useful as enemata. Emetine, widely employed in amoebic infection, is of no value in balantidiasis.

Prophylaxis.—Prevention of infection with *Balantidium coli* consists in preventing the ingestion of the cysts of the parasite. If food and drink are protected from contamination by feces containing these cysts and if pigs or other possible sources of infection are avoided, little danger of infection remains.

Chapter XV

THE TREMATODE INFECTIONS

THE TREMATODE PARASITES or "flukes," are those flatworms (class Trematoda, phylum Platyhelminthes) which have, in the adult stage of development, an unsegmented body, with a simple food tube which ends blindly. Many trematodes have been found in man. Of these, relatively few are primarily human forms, however, and most species are merely sporadic or accidental invaders of the human host. The life history of many human trematodes has been completely known only in comparatively recent years, and that of some species is still obscure.

TYPE MORPHOLOGY OF ADULT

Adult trematodes characteristically have two suckers for attachment to the host. One of these, the anterior or oral sucker, is at the anterior end of the body and surrounds the mouth. The other, the ventral sucker or acetabulum, occurs on the ventral surface of the worm along the mid-line.

The oesophagus is short, and soon divides into two caeca, which end blindly. A bladder, which opens at the posterior end of the body, receives excretory products from the tissues of the worm through a system of branched collecting tubules which originates in flame cells dispersed through the tissue. The nervous system is primitive: there are ganglion cells grouped about the pharynx, and, from these, anastomosing nerve trunks proceed posteriorly.

Most species of trematodes are hermaphrodites, although one group (the schistosomes) have separate sexes. There are usually two testes, and sperm cells pass from these through the seminal ducts and the vas deferens to the male genital pore. The single ovary is connected with an oötype by an oviduct. As the egg passes along the oviduct, it is fertilized by a sperm cell from the seminal receptacle. In the oötype, which is surrounded by shell glands, the eggs are provided with a shell and are supplied with food. The food comes through the vitelline ducts from the vitellaria, which usually occur in the lateral fields. The fertilized encapsulated egg is then passed into the uterus and eventually discharged through the female genital pore. A vestigial vagina (Lauer's canal) opens to the exterior from the seminal receptacle. This structure may once have functioned for cross-fertilization. (See Figure 9.)

TYPE LIFE HISTORY

The human trematodes all experience part of their larval development in a mollusk, and some must undergo additional larval life in second intermediate hosts, such as arthropods or lower vertebrates. In all, following the egg stage, four or five distinct larval stages characteristically can be identified.

The egg, which escapes in feces, urine, or sputum, is usually oval in outline, with an operculum at one end. The first larval stage, known as a miracidium, may be developed within the egg by the time it is passed from the host, but sometimes eggs are immature and require additional weeks for maturation. Eventually, however, if the egg reaches water, the miracidium escapes and by means of its cilia swims actively through the water in search of a suitable molluscan host, which usually is a snail. It penetrates the foot, gills, or tentacles of the snail, aided by lytic glands which open at the cephalic tip. Within the snail "liver," it metamorphoses to the sacklike second larval stage, known as the sporocyst. Inside the sporocyst, the third stage is formed. This is either a second sporocyst or a redia which differs from the sporocyst in having a pharynx and intestine. These intramolluscan stages are important because of the asexual or parthenogenetic reproduction that occurs. Eventually, within the third-stage larvae, many fourth-stage larvae, known as cercariae, are developed. These leave the molluscan host and swim actively through water until they find either a suitable primary host or a second intermediate host, whereupon they change to the metacercarial larval stage. Those forms which require a second intermediate host—which is for some an animal and for others a plant host—generally become encysted and remain thus

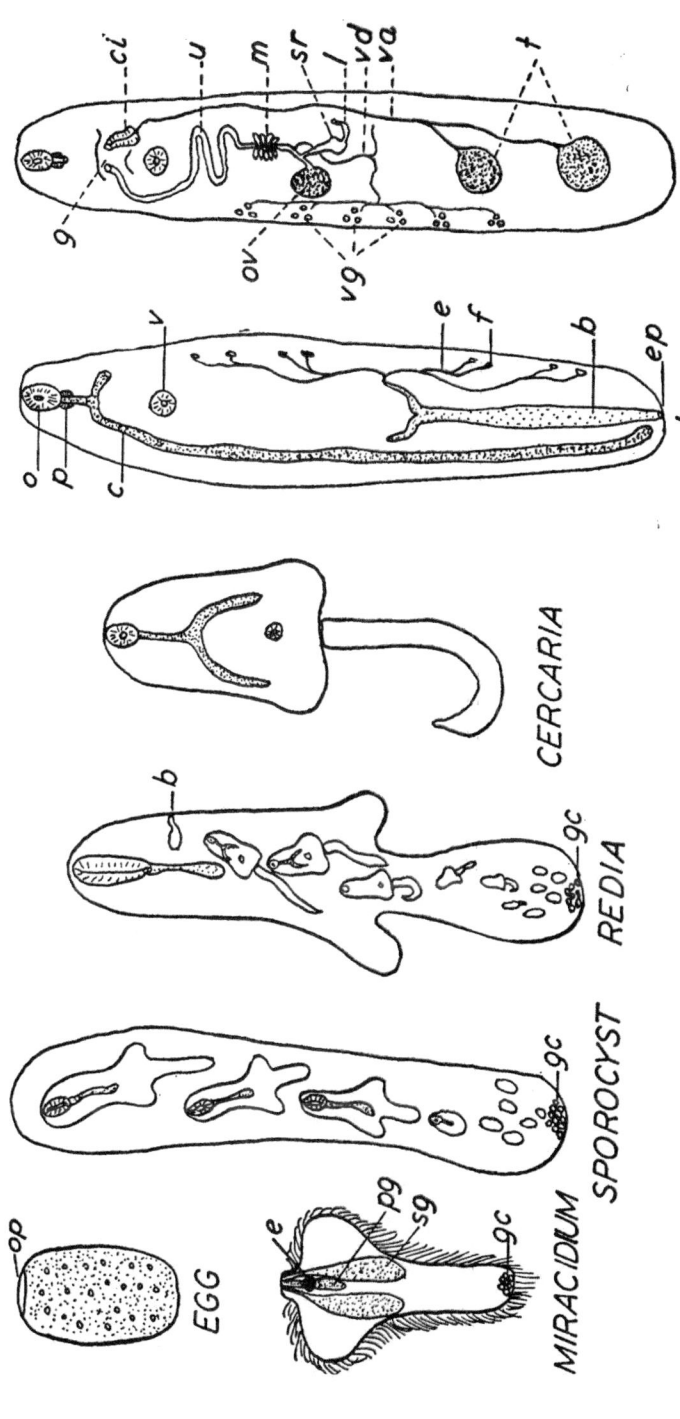

Figure 9. Stages in life cycle of typical trematode. b = birth pore; c = caeca; ci = cirrus; e = eye-spot; ex = excretory tubules; ep = excretory pore; f = flame cell; g = genital pore; gc = germinal cells; l = Lauer's canal; m = Mehlis's gland; op = operculum; ov = ovary; o = oral sucker; p = pharynx; pg = primitive gut; sg = secretory glands; sr = seminal receptacle; t = testis; u = uterus; v = ventral sucker (acetabulum); va = vas deferens; vd = vitelline duct; and vg = vitelline glands.

until the intermediate host tissue is ingested by a suitable primary host. On reaching the primary host, the metacercarial stage soon grows to become an adult form. (See Figure 9.)

CLASSIFICATION

The human trematodes, all of which occur in the subclass Digenea and the order Prosostomata, can conveniently be placed in one of three suborders: Strigeata (schistosomes), Distomata (distomes), and Amphistomata (amphistomes). These groups differ from each other in the following important characters:

	Strigeata	*Distomata*	*Amphistomata*
Position of acetabulum	anterior	anterior or central	posterior
Sexes	separate	united	united
Eggs operculated	no	yes	yes
Cercariae with pharynx	no	yes	yes
Cercarial tail bifurcate	yes	no	no

The more important human trematodes of each of these suborders follow. All of these forms will be discussed in brief detail.

Order	*Representative*
Strigeata (schistosomes)	Schistosoma haematobium Schistosoma mansoni Schistosoma japonicum
Distomata	Paragonimus westermani Clonorchis sinensis Fasciola hepatica Fasciolopis buski Heterophyes heterophyes Metagonimus yokogawai
Amphistomata	Gastrodiscoides hominis

INFECTIONS WITH THE SCHISTOSOMES
(THE BLOOD FLUKES)

The schistosomes are the only trematode parasites which infect the blood of man. They are dioecious forms which dwell in the portal system. Their eggs, in distinction from those of other trematodes, are nonoperculate, and their cercariae are apharyngeal and have a bifurcated tail. Infection of man takes place by the cercariae penetrating the human skin directly. The metacercarial stage does not encyst but proceeds at once to develop into an adult worm which resides in the blood stream. Three species are important in medicine: *Schistosoma haematobium, Schistosoma mansoni,* and *Schistosoma japonicum.* The three forms can be differentiated by the characteristics of Table 5.

TABLE 5

DIFFERENTIATION OF HUMAN SCHISTOSOMES

Characteristics	Schistosoma haematobium	Schistosoma mansoni	Schistosoma japonicum
Eggs			
Size (microns)	120–160 x 40–60	140–165 x 60–70	80–100 x 50–60
Where laid	veins of bladder wall	veins of intestinal wall	veins of intestinal wall
Where found	urine	feces	feces
Distinction	terminal spine	lateral spine	lateral knob
Adult			
Skin bosses	present	present	absent
Male			
No. of testes	4	7–9	7–9
Female			
Length of single caecum	posterior third of body	posterior two-thirds of body	posterior half of body
No. eggs in uterus	20–30, single file	one or very few	over 100, not in single file
Important molluscan hosts	*Bulinus contortus, Physopsis africana*	*Planorbis* spp., *Australorbis* spp.	*Oncomelania nosophora*

SCHISTOSOMA HAEMATOBIUM

Schistosoma haematobium [1] was first recovered from the mesenteric veins of an Egyptian native in Cairo by Bilharz in 1851. The life cycle was first fully described by Leiper between 1915 and 1918. The parasite is the cause of vesical schistosomiasis.

Geographical distribution.—The parasite is found in the Nile valley, along the Mediterranean coast of North Africa, along the entire east coast of Africa, and along the west coast of Africa from Senegal to the Congo. It occurs also in southern Europe (Portugal, Spain, Greece) and in the Near East.

Morphology and life cycle.—The adult male *Schistosoma haematobium* measures 1 to 1.5 centimeters in length by 0.8 to 1.0 milli-

[1] Common synonyms: *Distoma haematobia; Bilharzia haematobia.*

meters in breadth. There are two suckers, the ventral one (acetabu-lum) being the larger. The pharynx divides into two caeca which fuse two thirds of the way toward the posterior end of the body to form a single tube which ends blindly. Usually four testes are present, which lead into a common vas deferens opening on the ventral surface just posterior to the acetabulum. The sides of the body are flaplike and form the gynecophoral canal in which the female worm is found during copulation.

The adult female worm is longer than the male, often attaining twenty-five millimeters in length. The suckers are small. Eggs from the ovary are fertilized, are supplied with food and a shell in the oötype, and are then passed into the uterus. Often twenty or so eggs occur simultaneously in single file in the uterus.

The egg of *Schistosoma hematobium* is an oval form, with a ter-minal spine. (See Plate VI, F, facing page 142.) When passed from the female worm it is not mature, but by the time it is eliminated with urine (several days later) by the infected person, it encloses a miracid-ium. On reaching water, the egg hatches to yield the free-swimming miracidium. The miracidium searches for and must invade within a few hours certain snails, chiefly of the genera *Bulinus* and *Physopsis*. In the ensuing six weeks or more within the snail, two parthenogenetic generations of sporocysts are developed, and in the second of these, fork-tailed cercariae are formed. The cercariae leave the snail host and search during the ensuing two or three days for a vertebrate host, which they infect by directly penetrating its skin. They are equipped for this penetration by lytic glands which open at the anterior end. By the action of this lytic secretion as well as by their muscular move-ments, the cercariae succeed in burrowing into the skin within a few minutes. The head or the body only of the cercaria penetrates the skin, the forked tail being dropped off before or during penetration. The small cercaria body—a metacercaria—makes its way into the small venules and is carried by the blood to the liver, where development takes place. The adults, which develop within approximately one month, generally are found in the vesical or pelvic plexuses, which they reach by traveling against the blood current of the portal sys-tem.

Epidemiology.—The infection of man with *Schistosoma haematobium* follows contact with water containing the cercariae of the parasite.

Persons whose work or other activity brings them into water harboring infected snails regularly become infected. Farmers cultivating inundated or irrigated fields, women who wash clothes in streams, and children who play in the streams are especially likely to contract infection. Religious practices and popular customs often increase the level of infection in a given community. In the chief endemic centers of infection, as along the Nile River in Egypt, seventy-five percent or more of the native population may be infected.

Transmission of the parasite directly from man to man, or from any other vertebrate to man, is impossible. The transmission occurs only through the molluscan host, and only a few species of non-operculated snails, chiefly of the genera *Bulinus* and *Physopsis*, are known to serve as the intermediate host for this trematode. Man is the only vertebrate host significant as a reservoir of the parasite, although certain monkeys are also sometimes naturally infected. A number of domesticated or laboratory animals are susceptible to experimental infection, but these are not of consequence as natural transmitters of the parasite.

Pathogenicity.—Early symptoms in vesical schistosomiasis consist of headache, loss of appetite, pain in the back and extremities, fever, and night sweating. The liver and spleen are hypertrophied, and the abdomen is enlarged. There is a leucocytosis and an eosinophilia which may reach fifty percent of the total leucocyte number. After about one month, toxic symptoms develop, and an urticarial rash appears.

During the time that eggs are passing through tissue and before they make their appearance in the urine, symptoms may not be marked. Thereafter, however, blood will often be noted in the voided urine, and micturition may be painful. The desire to urinate occurs with greater frequency, and the volume of urine passed each time will gradually diminish. The mucous surface of the urethra becomes inflamed, perhaps from secondary infection, folded, and covered with papillomata which are built around the eggs of the parasite. Pseudotubercles occur around the eggs in the neighboring tissue as well as in the liver and lung, whence many eggs are carried by blood. Often, in the male, the urethra will be occluded, and elephantiasis of the penis may develop from blocking of the lymphatics. Secondary infection may develop and death may occur. Pathology in the female is usually less pronounced.

Diagnosis.—The presence of terminally spined eggs, especially in the last portion of the voided urine as well as, sometimes, in the feces, establishes the diagnosis of *Schistosoma haematobium* infection. (See Plate VI, F, facing page 142.) The presence of blood in the urine affords presumptive evidence of infection in endemic areas, especially where the blood count reveals also an eosinophilia.

The complement-fixation test and the skin test are positive in infected persons. Antigen for these tests is usually derived from the "livers" of snails which are infected with the parasite.

Specific therapy.—Antimony compounds, such as tartar emetic and sodium-antimony tartrate, are useful in treating vesical schistosomiasis, the drugs being given intravenously. Another synthetic antimonial, fuadin, is likewise efficacious in treatment and is somewhat more easily tolerated. It is given intramuscularly. Radical surgery must be resorted to and is sometimes helpful in advanced cases.

Prophylaxis.—Persons will not contract infection with vesical schistosomiasis so long as they avoid contact with water which contains the infective stages of the parasite. Not only is it necessary that the individuals not wade in or otherwise expose their skin to the water, but also water must be boiled or let stand for several days before being used for drinking purposes.

The elimination of schistosomiasis from a community, however, is a matter of considerable difficulty and is possible only through instructing the general population as to the relationship of snails to the disease and in the necessity of avoiding snail-infested water in order to prevent infection. The proper means of disposal of infected human feces must also be taught, so that the snail host does not become parasitized. The destruction of the snail host itself has been widely tried as a community measure, chiefly by treating snail-infested water with copper sulphate or by draining for long periods the irrigation canals in which they propagate and subsequently treating the beds with copper sulphate. Drainage alone is usually of little benefit, however, since the snails survive by burrowing into the mud and resume their usual activity when the canals are once more flooded.

SCHISTOSOMA MANSONI

Schistosoma mansoni [2] was probably first observed by Bilharz in

[2] Common synonyms: *Distoma haematobium; Schistosomum americanum.*

1852. Its egg was first described by Manson in 1903, and its identity as a species distinct from *Schistosoma haematobium* was proved by Leiper between 1915 and 1918.

Geographical distribution.—*Schistosoma mansoni* occurs endemically in the Nile delta, in the Sudan, in Central and South Africa, possibly in Arabia, in northern Brazil, Dutch Guiana, and Venezuela, and in many of the Caribbean islands. Cases of schistosomiasis are seen in many other areas to which persons from endemic regions have migrated. The infection is potentially almost cosmopolitan in its disposition, since suitable molluscan hosts for the parasite have very broad dispersal.

It is believed that the infection in the New World resulted from the importation of infected slaves from the Congo basin, Angola, Mozambique, Zululand, and Basutoland in Africa. The parasite has never established itself within the United States.

Morphology and life cycle.—Grossly both the males and females of *Schistosoma mansoni* resemble the adults of *Schistosoma haematobium,* although those of the *mansoni* form are smaller. The testes of the male are more numerous in *Schistosoma mansoni*, numbering up to nine. The caeca in the female unite to form a single tube about one third the body length from the head end. The uterus seldom contains more than a single laterally spined egg at one time.

The adult worms are found chiefly in mesenteric venules from the wall of the large bowel, although sometimes they occur in the vesical plexus or in the liver. Characteristically, the adults are observed together, the female enveloped by the male until shortly before she lays her eggs. (See Plate VI, A, facing page 142.) The eggs, which differ from those of *Schistosoma haematobium* in having a lateral rather than a terminal spine, are often flushed back into the liver, but may break out of the venules and traverse the tissue of the bowel wall until discharged into the bowel lumen. The miracidium must invade snails, chiefly of the general *Planorbis* or *Australorbis* (Plate VI, D, facing page 142), within sixteen hours or so after leaving the egg. After two generations of sporocysts, cercariae are produced which are similar to but smaller than those of *Schistosoma haematobium*. These invade man by penetrating his skin, in the same manner as do the cercariae of *Schistosoma haematobium*. After several circulations these smaller worms collect in the liver, and the adult forms are subsequently found in the mesenteric veins. (See Plate VI, B and E, facing page 142.)

Epidemiology.—Man is the usual reservoir host of *Schistosoma mansoni.* Monkeys have occasionally been found naturally infected with the parasite, and several domesticated and laboratory animals can be experimentally infected. Transmission occurs only through infected snails, and human infection follows contact with water harboring infected snails. Infection is most common among persons in low-lying, irrigated areas, who contract infection from the sluggish waters of irrigation canals. In some endemic areas of intense infection, practically the entire native population (ninety percent or more) is infected by the age of ten years.

Pathogenicity.—Symptoms and pathology in *Schistosoma mansoni* infections are similar to those seen in the *haematobium* disease, except that the bowel wall is affected rather than the urogenital tract. A dysentery is common in the *mansoni* disease. There is abdominal pain, bloody mucus in the frequent stool, the development of papillomata and general fibrosis in the bowel wall. Eggs lodge in the liver, spleen, lymph glands, and elsewhere, and pseudotubercles are seen about them in tissue sections (see Plate VI, C, facing page 142.) Often the bowel is prolapsed, and ulceration of the wall is extensive. The spleen is greatly enlarged, and anemia develops. The liver is often damaged by cirrhosis, and fluid not uncommonly collects in the peritoneum. (See Plate VII, A, facing page 143.) A leucocytosis with an eosinophilia develops, and an urticaria is common.

Schistosomiasis mansoni, Case Report.—A Puerto Rican woman, age thirty years, who had lived in New York city for thirteen years, was admitted to hospital with pain of eleven days' duration in the lower abdomen. The spleen was enormously enlarged. The patient suffered alternately from constipation and diarrhea. She appeared undernourished and had lost eight pounds in recent weeks. Blood count showed a leucopenia, 3,000 white cells being present per cubic millimeter of blood, with twelve percent eosinophiles. After observation for five days, the patient was considered to present Banti's syndrome as a result of schistosomiasis, although no schistosome eggs were detected in the feces. Splenectomy was advised, and a spleen five or six times normal was removed. The liver at operation was observed to be cirrhotic, with a rough nodular surface. There was no fluid in the peritoneum and no engorgement of the portal system, except in the splenic vein. Section of liver biopsy revealed an immature parasite which, unfortunately, the attendant could not identify. Within a few days after operation, the white cell count rose to normal, although the eosinophilia persisted. The patient was dismissed, apparently in an improved condition.

Hepatic symptoms developed about five years later, and the patient returned to hospital. A skin test for schistosomiasis was performed, with a strongly positive result. Subsequently, after many stool examinations, a few eggs of *Schistosoma mansoni* were found. Drug therapy (fuadin) was then instituted, and after two weeks eggs disappeared from the stool. The patient was dismissed, apparently cured of schistosomiasis, several weeks later.

The case was of some interest in indicating the long incubation period which often is seen in schistosomiasis. It also indicates the usefulness of the skin test for the diagnosis of the disease.

Diagnosis.—Laterally spined eggs appear in the feces of patients infected with *Schistosoma mansoni*. (See Plate VI, G, facing page 142.) In a small percentage of cases, the eggs also appear in the urine. In infections by male worms alone, however, no eggs are found. Complement-fixation and skin tests are useful diagnostic aids. (See Plate VII, D, facing page 143.) Eosinophilia, dysentery, and intestinal pathology are indicative of infection in endemic areas.

Specific therapy and prevention.—The treatment of infection with *Schistosoma mansoni* is the same as that with *Schistosoma haematobium*. Similar measures are effective in protecting persons from infection with the two parasites.

SCHISTOSOMA JAPONICUM

Schistosoma japonicum was first observed in Japan by Fujinami in 1904 and was described in the same year by Katsurada. Its life cycle was determined by several Japanese workers between 1909 and 1914.

Geographical distribution.—The parasite is found only in the Far East. Endemic foci occur in China, where millions are infected, and in Formosa, Japan, the Philippine Islands, and Celebes.

Morphology and life cycle.—The adult worms are about the size of those of *Schistosoma haematobium*. They differ from both *Schistosoma haematobium* and *Schistosoma mansoni* in lacking bosses or tuberculations on their integument. The males have seven testes. In the females, the caeca unite at about mid-length of the body. Over 100 eggs may occur in the coiled uterus, these not being in single file. The eggs are nearly spherical bodies, with a knoblike process near one end. Eggs are laid in the mesenteric venules near the bowel and must pass into the bowel lumen for expulsion. The miracidium hatches from the egg and promptly invades any of several species of snail belonging chiefly to the genera *Katayama* and *Oncomelania*. Two generations of sporocysts develop, and these are followed by the formation of fork-tailed cercariae similar in general appearance to those of the other human schistosomes. The cercariae invade man by directly penetrating his skin. Ultimately, after a complete circulation, many of these lodge in the intrahepatic portal circulation. After growing to maturity, the worms migrate to the mesenteric venules where they mate and begin oviposition.

Epidemiology.—Not only man, but also dogs, cats, cattle, horses, water buffaloes, and field rodents are naturally infected with *Schistosoma japonicum* in the endemic areas. Human infection is largely confined to those who dwell or work in rural areas. Workers in paddy fields or fishermen searching for edible eels in such fields are commonly infected. The use of human feces as fertilizer contributes largely to the continuation of the infection in the endemic regions. Congenital infection with this worm has also been reported.

Pathogenicity.—An intense urticaria is usually observed and diarrhea invariably develops as an early symptom in infections with *Schistosoma japonicum*. The spleen and liver become greatly enlarged. Later, damage to the bowel wall develops, as in *Schistosoma mansoni* infection. Pseudotubercles form about eggs in the bowel wall, as well as in the liver and other organs. More eggs usually are formed than by *Schistosoma mansoni,* and the effect of the Oriental infection is consequently more pronounced. Cirrhosis of the liver is common, resulting from obstruction of blood flow by egg masses, and ascites collects in the peritoneum. (See Plate VII, B and C, facing page 143.) Papillomata are common on the large bowel wall surface.

Diagnosis.—The diagnosis of *Schistosoma japonicum* infection is accomplished by finding the characteristic laterally knobbed eggs in feces of patients. (See Plate VI, H, facing page 142.) Usually the egg has more or less fecal debris attached. When the eggs cannot be found, other diagnostic measures are often helpful. One simple method is to dilute the feces with water and let it stand for a day or so. Miracidia, which are visible to the unaided eye, will be seen in the water if the feces contains viable eggs of the parasite. Complement

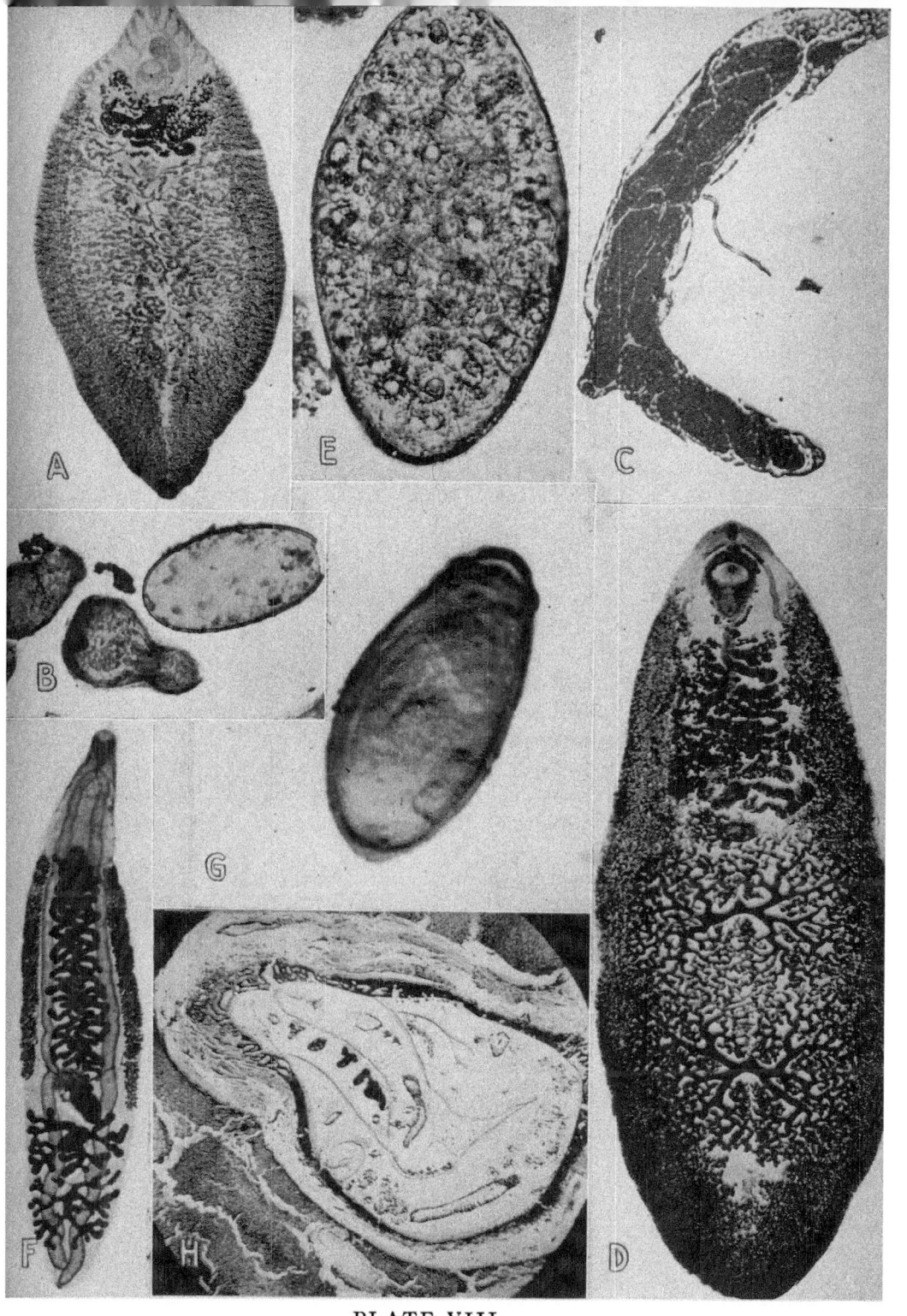

PLATE VIII

A. *Fasciola hepatica:* adult. (x2)   B. *Fasciola hepatica:* egg and miracidia. (x250)   C. *Fasciola hepatica:* redia with cercariae inside. (x40)   D. *Fasciolopsis buski:* adult. (x2)   E. *Fasciolopsis buski:* egg. (x500)   F. *Clonorchis sinensis:* adult. (x3)   G. *Clonorchis sinensis:* egg (x1000)   H. Clonorchiasis: section of bile duct showing *Clonorchis sinensis.* Note folding of bile duct epithelium. (x4)

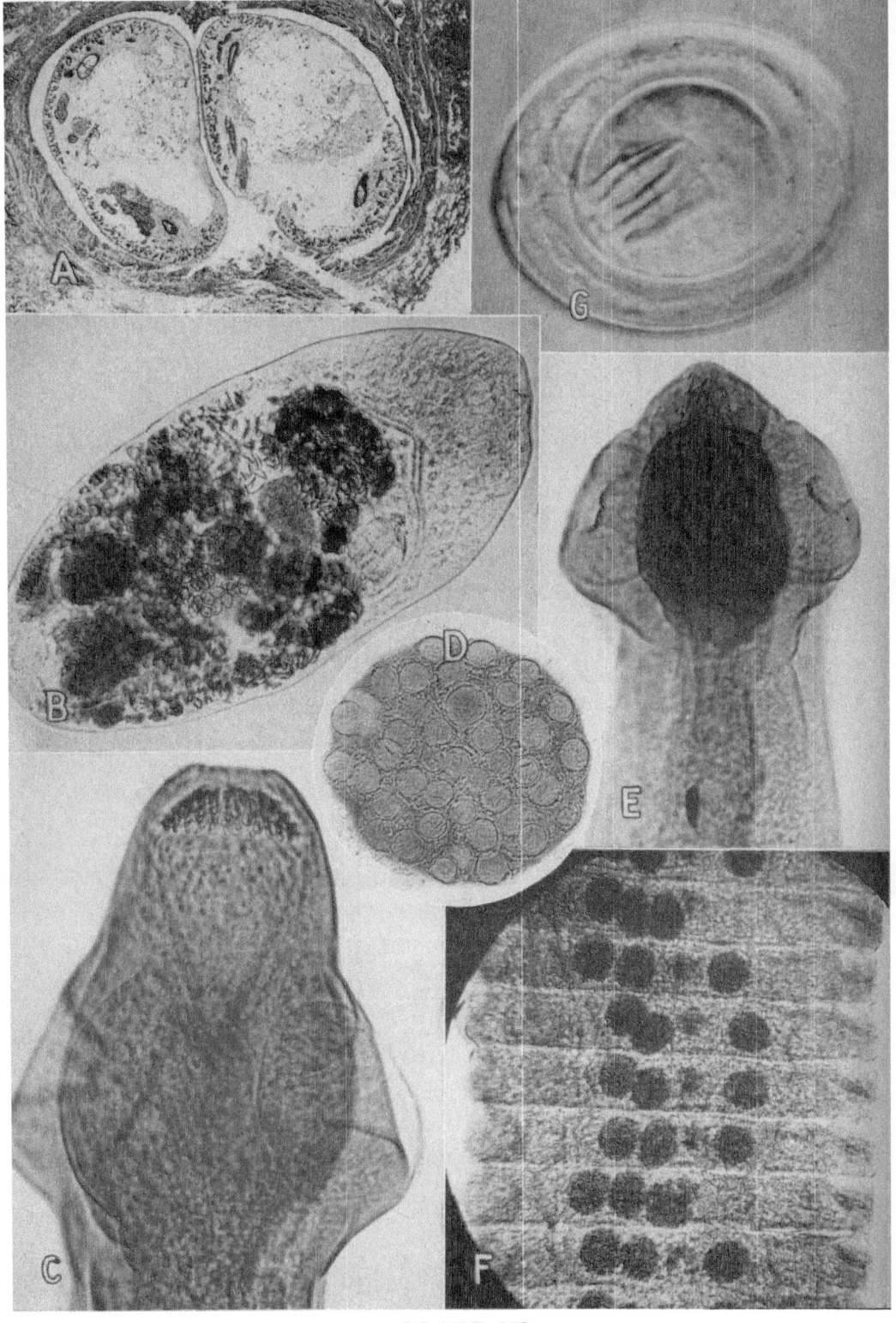

PLATE IX

A. Paragonimiasis: section of lung cyst showing two adult *Paragonimus westermani*. (x3)
B. *Heterophyes heterophyes*: adult. (x50)   C. *Dipylidium caninum*: scolex. (x175)   D. *Dipylidium caninum*: egg nest. (x100)   E. *Hymenolepis diminuta*: scolex. (x175)   F. *Hymenolepis diminuta*: mature segments. (x40)   G. *Hymenolepis nana*: egg. (x600)

fixation and skin tests become positive in this disease, and eosinophile counts generally are high.

Specific therapy.—Treatment is the same as in infections by other species of schistosome, sodium antimony tartrate and fuadin generally being administered.

Prevention.—The prevention of human infection with *Schistosoma japonicum* is a difficult problem in endemic areas, particularly since not only man but many domesticated animals also are susceptible and serve as natural reservoirs. The general use of human feces as fertilizer in the Orient aids in the dissemination and the maintenance of the parasite. Nevertheless, the accepted methods of prophylaxis of man are the same with *Schistosoma japonicum* as with the other schistosomes. These consist primarily in educating the general population to avoid contact with water harboring snails infected with the larval parasites and in storing human feces for several days before using it as fertilizer, in order to kill the eggs of the parasite and the miracidia which hatch from them. The use of copper sulphate to kill the snail host can be employed in control where the body of water is of small size.

CERCARIAL DERMATITIS

When the cercariae of any of several species of schistosomes which infect exclusively the lower animals come in contact with man, they penetrate his skin but develop no further. A definite dermatitis is often noted, with intense itching. A papule or pustule not uncommonly appears in a day or so, but this subsides soon and usually leaves no serious effects. The reaction is most severe in those persons who have been reinfected many times. Several species of schistosome cercariae evidently can cause the dermatitis, but the one most widely concerned in the United States is *Cercaria elvae*. Apparently, the local reaction to the cercariae of the human schistosomes is much less, if it develops at all.

The elimination of snails from lakes and beaches used for bathing purposes is the only method of protecting those who enter infested waters against schistosome dermatitis. When copper sulphate is added to such waters in a concentration of a little more than one in 500,000 parts, snails are usually killed. The waters will be safe for bathing for some time after such treatment.

DISTOMATE INFECTIONS (FLUKES OF THE INTESTINE,
THE LIVER AND BILE DUCTS, AND THE LUNG)

The various flukes of the suborder Distomata infect the lung, the liver and bile ducts, and the intestine of man. Only one species—namely, *Paragonimus westermani*—occurs in the lungs, but a rather large number of forms have been recovered at different times from the liver and bile ducts or from the intestine. Of these, two species occur with some frequency in the bile ducts: *Clonorchis sinensis* and *Fasciola hepatica*. Three forms have some importance as intestinal parasites: *Fasciolopsis buski*, *Heterophyes heterophyes*, and *Metagonimus yokogawai*.

PARAGONIMUS WESTERMANI

The lung fluke of man, *Paragonimus westermani*,[3] was first observed by Ringer in 1879, in a Portuguese living in Formosa. It is an Oriental parasite and is found chiefly in China, Japan, Korea, Siam, India, and the Philippine Islands. It has been reported from Central Africa and parts of South America. It is a comparatively rare parasite of man in many of these areas, but in some parts of China is found in thirty percent or more of the general population.

Morphology and life cycle.—The adult lung flukes live usually in pairs in cystlike dilatations or pockets of the bronchioles of the lung. The fleshy, oval parasites measure from eight to twelve millimeters in length by five millimeters in breadth and taper toward each end. They are covered with a spinose integument. There are two suckers, the ventral one being at about the mid-length of the body. The caeca are not branched. The testes and ovary are lobed, and the vitellaria extend along nearly all of both sides of the body. The uterus is a tightly coiled mass on the side of the acetabulum opposite the ovary. The bladder is large and conspicuous, extending nearly the full length of the mid-line.

The eggs of the lung fluke, which are immature when passed, escape from the cystlike lung pouch into the bronchial tubes and often can be observed in the sputum, which commonly is of rusty color. If the patient swallows his sputum, the eggs then also appear in the feces.

---

[3] Common synonyms: *Distoma westermani*; *Distoma ringeri*.

They are rather distinctive among trematode eggs, because of their slight but definite asymmetry (Figure 16). The eggs mature in from three to several weeks, and the free-swimming miracidia then invade snails chiefly of the genus *Melania*. One sporocyst and one redia generation occur, and microcercous (very short-tailed) cercariae then develop. The cercariae invade the muscles or other tissues (gills) of crayfish (*Astacus* spp.) or crabs (*Potamon* spp.), and there the metacercariae become encysted. When the infected tissue is swallowed by man or other susceptible vertebrate, the organism excysts in the duodenum, and migrates presumably directly through the intestinal wall, diaphragm, and pleural cavity into the lung, where the cystlike pouches are formed about them.

Epidemiology.—Human infection with the lung fluke follows the ingestion of raw crabs or crayfish or the drinking of raw water infested with the encysted metacercarial stage of the parasite. Man is probably less responsible than are lower animal reservoirs for the perpetuation of the parasite in any given area. The parasite has been found in tiger, wildcat, panther, cat, wolf, fox, weasel, mink, pig, and some other forms.

Pathogenicity.—The symptoms in lung-fluke infection are almost entirely pneumonic and might easily be confused with those in early tuberculosis. A cough is usual, with blood-stained sputum. The lung cysts are about one centimeter in diameter. They begin as a leucocytic infiltration of the host tissue about the parasite, with ultimately the formation of a fibrous wall. Cysts occur also in the liver, brain, and lymphatic glands and, indeed, may be found in nearly any organ. (See Plate IX, A, facing page 159.)

Diagnosis.—The diagnosis of lung-fluke infection is generally established by observing the parasite egg in the sputum or the feces. Complement-fixation antibodies for the worm antigen are present in the blood serum. The cysts are generally not revealed by X-ray photographs.

Specific therapy.—No specific drug is available for lung-fluke infection, although emetine and antimony compounds are sometimes used to relieve the pulmonary symptoms.

Prophylaxis.—Infection with the lung fluke can be avoided by eating neither crabs nor crayfish unless these are thoroughly cooked and by boiling all drinking water.

CLONORCHIS SINENSIS

The Chinese liver fluke, *Clonorchis sinensis*,[4] was first observed by McConnell in 1874 in the bile passages of a Chinese autopsied in Calcutta.

Geographical distribution.—*Clonorchis sinensis* is confined to the Orient. The heaviest centers of infection are in Japan, Korea, southern China, and French Indo-China.

Morphology and life cycle.—The adult *Clonorchis sinensis* measures 1.5 to three centimeters in length by 0.5 centimeter in width. It is tapered somewhat toward the anterior end. The caeca are simple. The tandem testes are branches, and the ovary is rather superficially lobed. The vitellaria are restricted to the lateral fields in the middle third of the worm. The uterus also lies mostly in the middle third of the body. It is compactly coiled and holds many eggs. (See Plate VIII, F, facing page 158.)

The operculated eggs are of oval shape, the operculum fitting into a rimlike extension of the shell. At the opposite end of the egg, a hooklike protuberance is generally noted. The greatest breadth of the egg is beyond mid-length, slightly toward the hooked end. The eggs are mature when laid. (See Plate VIII, G, facing page 158.) They hatch only after being ingested by snails, chiefly of the genera *Bithynia* and *Parafossarulus*. One sporocyst and one redia generation precede the development of lophocercous eye-spotted cercariae. Soon after leaving the snail, the cercariae encyst as metacercariae on the scales or in the tissue of any of many species of fresh-water fish, which thus serve as the second intermediate hosts. If these fish are ingested without adequate cooking, infection results. The parasites excyst in the duodenum and migrate up the bile duct to its capillaries, where they grow to adults. The adults may live for twenty years or more in this site.

Epidemiology.—Many fish-eating vertebrates besides man, including especially dogs and cats, are susceptible to infection. In China, the pollution of artificial fish ponds with human feces leads to infection first of the snails which usually abound in such ponds, and finally of the fish themselves.

Pathogenicity.—Heavy infections with *Clonorchis sinensis* leads to

[4] Common synonyms: *Clonorchis endemicus; Distoma sinense; Distoma endemicus.*

serious hepatic disturbance. The bile ducts may be blocked, with consequent jaundice, and cirrhosis of the liver is not uncommon. The pancreatic duct also may be invaded. Milder infections are often symptomless. Usually, about each worm in the bile ducts, the epithelium is proliferated and thrown into folds which often completely entrap the parsites. An intensive leucocytic infiltration of the area generally is noted. "Graves" of the parasite eggs are seen in the liver parenchyma. (See Plate VIII, H, facing page 158.)

Diagnosis.—The observation of the parasite eggs in the feces of the patient establishes the presence of this infection.

Specific therapy.—Tartar emetic, emetine, and gold salts have all been used in clonorchiasis, but with little or no success. The administration of gentian violet is much more effective. This drug often appears first to stimulate egg production by the parasite, but it eventually eliminates the worm.

Prophylaxis.—The thorough cooking of all fresh-water fish before these are ingested protects against possible infection with *Clonorchis sinensis*. Control of the snail host or of other vertebrate hosts besides man is extremely difficult.

FASCIOLA HEPATICA

The sheep liver fluke, *Fasciola hepatica*,[5] was described by Jehan de Brie in 1379. It was the first trematode shown to be the cause of disease. The parasite has been reported from essentially all parts of the world and occurs in all the important sheep-raising areas.

Morphology and life cycle.—*Fasciola hepatica* was the first trematode whose life cycle was completely described, Leuckart accomplishing this is 1883. The leaflike adult worm measures up to three centimeters long by one and one-half centimeters broad. There is a characteristic conelike process at the anterior end. The caeca are branched. The two testes and the ovary are likewise branched. The branched vitellaria extend along the lateral fields to the posterior end. The coiled uterus generally is short and contains relatively few eggs, considering the size of the fluke (see Plate VIII, A, facing page 158).

The brownish eggs are rather perfectly oval. They are immature when laid. The eye-spotted miracidium which develops in two weeks or so invades many species of snail, chiefly of the genus *Lymnaea*.

[5] Common synonym: *Distomum hepaticum*.

(See Plate VIII, B, facing page 158.) One sporocyst generation and two redia generations lead to the formation of the free-swimming cercariae. (See Plate VIII, C, facing page 158.) The cercariae as metacercariae become encysted (adolescaria) usually on the leaves of water vegetation (e.g., water cress). When man, or more commonly an herbivorous animal, consumes such vegetation the parasite is swallowed and excysts in the duodenum of the host. The young adult form migrates through the intestinal wall to the peritoneum, thence through the liver capsule and liver parenchyma to the bile ducts.

Epidemiology.—Sheep are the principal vertebrate host of *Fasciola hepatica,* and man is little more than an accidental host for the parasite. Only with the greatest infrequency is man responsible for transmission of the infection to the snail host. Man is naturally infected only from food or drink carrying the metacercarial cyst. In some parts of the world, especially in Syria, where raw sheep liver is eaten, laryngeal infection of man with the adult worms is sometimes reported.

Pathogenicity.—Human infections are so rare that little is known of symptoms of this disease in man. In the sheep, the liver parenchyma is so severely eroded in heavy infections that toxic symptoms are usual. Obstruction of the bile duct by the worms also commonly occurs. In man an eosinophilia up to sixty percent is generally observed.

Diagnosis.—The infection is diagnosed by finding eggs of the worm in the feces. Antibodies for the antigens of the parasite can be detected, at least in the serum of infected animals. Skin tests have also been used successfully in diagnosing the disease in animals.

Specific therapy.—Emetine, carbon tetrachloride, and oleoresin of *Aspidium* all have been used in therapy, often with success.

Prophylaxis.—The destruction or treatment of infected sheep, or the elimination of the snail host, will, if practicable, eradicate this parasite from a community. Water cress or other aquatic plants should not be eaten if grown in endemic areas.

FASCIOLOPSIS BUSKI

Fasciolopsis buski,[6] the largest trematode parasitic in man, was

---

[6] Common synonyms: *Distomum crassum; Fasciolopsis fülleborni; Fasciolopsis goddardi; Fasciolopsis spinifera.*

discovered by Busk in 1843, in the intestine of a lascar sailor autopsied in London.

Geographical distribution.—*Fasciolopsis buski* is common in central and south China, Formosa, Malaya, Thailand, India, Borneo, and Sumatra.

Morphology and life cycle.—The adult worm measures from two to seven centimeters long by five-tenths to two centimeters broad. (See Plate VIII, D, facing page 158.) The two suckers are close together. The caeca are unbranched. The tandem testes and the ovary are branched. The vitellaria are disposed along the lateral and posterior margins. The uterus is loosely coiled and appears small for so large a worm.

The eggs which are essentially identical with those of *Fasciola hepatica* are immature when laid. (See Plate VIII, E, facing page 158.) The miracidium develops within a few weeks, and invades snails, chiefly of the genera *Planorbis* and *Segmentina*, in which one sporocyst and two redia generations develop. The cercariae become encysted as metacercariae on the outer leaves, roots, or pods of any of various water plants (water chestnut, water caltrop, water bamboo). If man swallows the cysts, the parasite excysts in his duodenum and becomes fixed to the wall of the intestine where, within about one month, it develops into the adult worm.

Epidemiology.—Man, pig, and dog are the chief hosts of *Fasciolopsis buski*. All are infected by ingesting cysts which occur on the surface parts of water plants and nuts which are commonly used as food. Man becomes infected when he peels back with his teeth the outer leaves in order to expose the edible parts.

Pathogenicity.—At the point of attachment of the adult parasite to the intestinal wall, an area of inflammation develops, and in some cases this may even ulcerate. In heavy infections, symptoms suggestive of gastric ulcer are usual, with diarrhea, anorexia, and facial edema. Many worms may cause intestinal stasis. Eosinophiles usually increase, and sometimes a lymphocytosis occurs.

Diagnosis.—Infection with *Fasciolopsis buski* is established by finding the eggs of the parasite, or occasionally the adult worm itself, in the feces of the patient.

Specific therapy.—Several drugs, including carbon tetrachloride, beta-naphthol, oil of chenopodium, thymol, and hexylresorcinol, have been used evidently with good success in *Fasciolopsis* infections of man.

Prophylaxis.—In any program of prophylaxis, the general population of endemic areas must be instructed not to eat those plant foods which carry the encysted metacercariae without first cooking them or immersing them in boiling water. In some centers of the Orient, street vendors of water nuts are required by law to immerse their products in boiling water just before selling them.

HETEROPHYES HETEROPHYES

The very small intestinal fluke, *Heterophyes heterophyes*,[7] was first seen in an Egyptian by Bilharz in Cairo in 1851. It is found chiefly in the Nile delta and the Far East.

Morphology and life cycle.—*Heterophyes heterophyes* is a minute, egg-shaped fluke about 1.5 millimeters long by 0.4 millimeter broad. It is somewhat tapered anteriorly and broadly rounded posteriorly. There are the usual two suckers, and also a third, the genital sucker. The caeca are simple. The testes and the ovary are smooth. The vitellaria are few in number, but large. (See Plate IX, B, facing page 159.)

The eggs when laid resemble those of *Clonorchis sinensis* in size but differ from them in being broadest about mid-length, in having no conspicuous rim on the shell at the operculated end, and in having no distinct hook at the end opposite that with the operculum. They are mature when laid, but hatch only after ingestion by an appropriate snail (*Pironella* spp.; *Tymphonotomus* spp.) A sporocyst and one or two generations of rediae develop prior to the formation of cercariae. The cercariae encyst as metacercariae on fish, which serve as second intermediate hosts. Man is infected by eating the infected fish. The parasite excysts in the duodenum and attaches to the intestinal wall often deep in the crypts of the small bowel.

Epidemology.—Man and other fish-eating mammals (dog, cat, fox) are natural hosts of *Heterophyes heterophyes*.

Pathogenicity.—At the point of attachment of the worm in the intestine inflammation occurs. Diarrhea is a common symptom of infection. It is possible that eggs of this form lodge in the myocardium, brain, and elsewhere and cause serious local pathology.

---

[7] Common synonyms: *Distomum heterophyes; Fasciola heterophyes.*

Diagnosis.—The determination of the presence of eggs in the feces is proof of infection with *Heterophyes* (Figure 16).

Specific therapy.—Tetrachlorethylene is effective for eliminating *Heterophyes* from man.

Prophylaxis.—If fish from endemic areas is thoroughly cooked before being eaten, infection with *Heterophyes heterophyes* will be prevented.

METAGONIMUS YOKOGAWAI

Metagonimus yokogawai [8] was first described from man by Katsurada in material sent from Formosa by Yokogawa in 1912. The parasite is common in the Far East (China, Japan, Siberia) and has been found in Palestine, the Balkan countries, and Spain.

Morphology and life cycle.—The adult is very similar to *Heterophyes heterophyes* in appearance. It differs in lacking a genital sucker, although the acetabulum is pulled toward the side of the body. The genital pore opens at the anterior margin of the displaced acetabulum. The eggs are nearly identical with those of *Heterophyes heterophyes,* although their greatest diameter is toward the end opposite the operculum. They are mature when laid and must be ingested by snails, chiefly of the genus *Melania,* for development. One sporocyst and two redia generations are developed in the snail. The lophocercous cercariae have two eye spots and a somewhat cone-shaped anterior end. They become encysted as metacercariae on the skin or in the flesh of various fresh-water fish. Man is infected by ingesting the infected fish.

Pathogenicity.—*Metagonimus yokogawai* may occur in tremendous numbers in the small intestine, where they cause extensive irritation and superficial erosion of cells. There is often a diarrhea, the severity of which depends on the number of worms present. Eggs of the parasite may reach the small blood vessels and be lodged in almost any tissue.

Diagnosis.—The finding of eggs in the feces establishes the diagnosis of the infection.

Specific therapy.—Tetrachlorethylene is used in the treatment of *Metagonimus* infection.

Prophylaxis.—By abstinence from eating raw fish, one can avoid infection with *Metagonimus yokogawai.*

[8] Common synonyms: *Heterophyes yokogawai; Loxotrema ovatum.*

AMPHISTOMATE INFECTIONS (FLUKES OF THE INTESTINE)

Only two amphistomate flukes have been found in man: *Gastrodiscoides hominis* and *Watsonius watsoni*. Neither species has great significance in medicine. The second form has been recovered from so few human hosts that it will not be discussed.

GASTRODISCOIDES HOMINIS

Gastrodiscoides hominis [9] was discovered in 1876 by Lewis and McConnell in the caecum of a patient in India, where the form has since been found to be somewhat common. The parasite is also found in Indo-China. It is a fluke of the amphistome group—that is, one having the ventral sucker at the posterior end of the body. It is a small form, measuring about one centimeter in its greatest dimension. The adult worm lives in the caecum and large intestine not only of man but also of the pig, where it produces rather large eggs which are immature when laid. The rest of the life cycle, however, is as yet unknown. The adult worm is best removed from man by soap-water enemas. Thymol, carbon tetrachloride, and tetrachlorethylene have also been used in treatment.

[9] Common synonyms: *Amphistomum hominis; Gastrodiscus hominis.*

Chapter XVI

THE CESTODE INFECTIONS

THE CESTODE PARASITES, or tapeworms, belong to the class Cestoda of the phylum Platyhelminthes. They differ from worms of the class Trematoda, in the adult stage of development, by having no alimentary canal and by being distinctly segmented. Adult tapeworms characteristically occur in the lumen of the intestine of carnivorous hosts; larval stages characteristically occur in the somatic tissues of herbivorous hosts.

The tapeworms which infect man can be placed in either of two orders: Pseudophyllidea or Cyclophyllidea. These groups are rather easily differentiated by the following characters. The pseudophyllidean tapeworms have an unarmed scolex bearing two opposing bothria (slitlike sucking organs). Those found in man have genital organs which persist in the gravid proglottid, a uterine pore, an operculated egg with a single shell, and a ciliated mature embryo. The cyclophyllidean cestodes have four cuplike muscular suckers and, usually, one or more rows of hooks on the rostellum; the genital organs largely degenerate in the gravid proglottid; eggs are nonoperculate and have two enveloping membranes; the mature embryo is not ciliated; mature proglottids have the vitellaria collected to a single mass along the posterior margin. Some representatives of each order occur in the human intestine attached to the wall; other species of each order invade the somatic tissue. The medically important species of the two cestode orders are as follows:

Order	*Representatives*
Pseudophyllidea	Diphyllobothrium latum
	Diphyllobothrium mansoni

Order	*Representatives*
Cyclophyllidea	Taenia solium
	Taenia saginata
	Echinococcus granulosus
	Hymenolepis nana
	Hymenolepis diminuta
	Dipylidium caninum

THE PSEUDOPHYLLIDEAN TAPEWORMS

Two pseudophyllidean tapeworms are significant in medicine as parasites of man. These are *Diphyllobothrium latum,* an adult form which occurs in the intestine, and *Diphyllobothrium mansoni,* the larval stage (plerocercoid or sparganum) of which occurs in the somatic tissues.

DIPHYLLOBOTHRIUM LATUM

Diphyllobothrium latum, [1] the fish or broad tapeworm, has for centuries been known as a parasite of man. Linnaeus classified the organism in 1758, although it was a well-known form long before 1758.

Geographical distribution.—Endemic foci of human infection with *Diphyllobothrium latum* are found in much of central and, especially northern Europe, in Russia, Siberia, Palestine, Japan, Manchuria, Canada, and north-central United States (Michigan, Minnesota).

Morphology and life cycle.—*Diphyllobothrium latum* is a large parasite, sometimes reaching a length of twenty-five to thirty feet. (See Plate X, A, facing page 174.) The scolex is typical of the group: it measures two millimeters in length and bears a sucking groove on each side. The mature segment is usually broader than long. (See Plate XI, A, facing page 175.) A bilobed ovary is present toward the posterior part of each segment, and testes are disposed through the dorsal plane of the lateral fields. The coiled uterus lies in about the center of the proglottid. The vitellaria are disposed in the ventral plane of the lateral fields. In gravid segments, many oval, operculated, immature eggs are enclosed in the uterus. (See Plate XI, B, facing page 175, and Figure 16.) These are regularly extruded from the uterine pore. The gravid proglottids do not break off from the distal end of the worm but disintegrate after expelling their eggs.

---

[1] Common synonym: *Dibothriocephalus latus.*

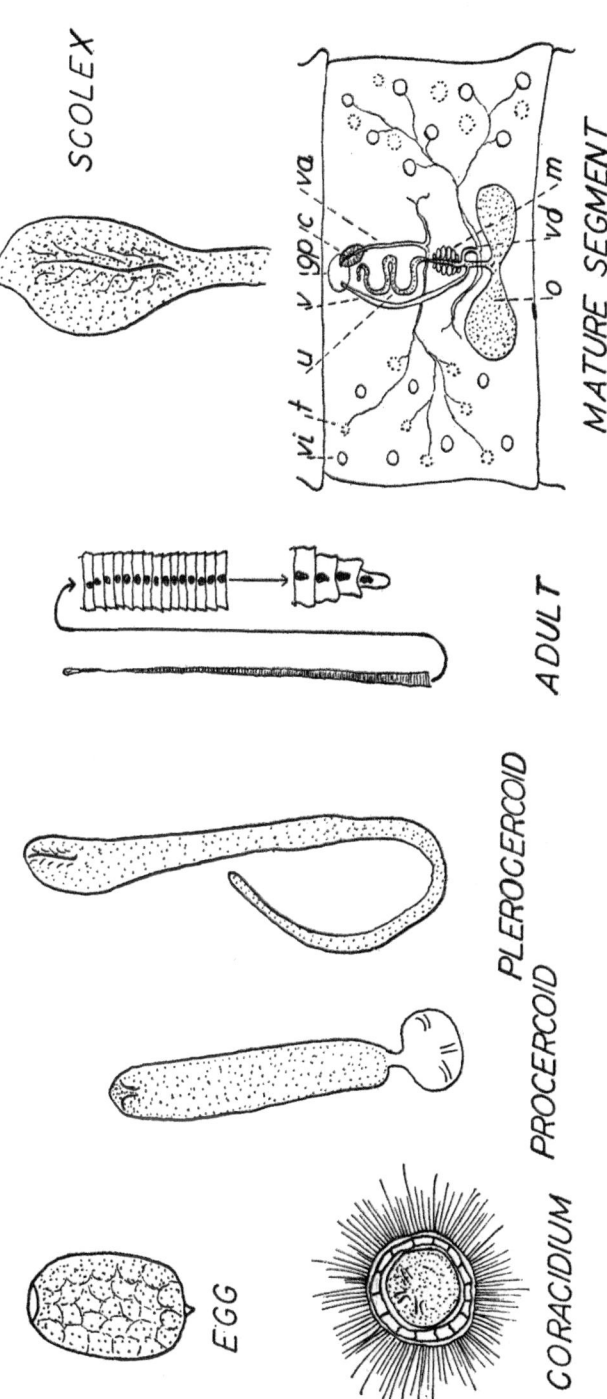

SCOLEX

MATURE SEGMENT

ADULT

PLEROCERCOID

PROCERCOID

CORACIDIUM

EGG

Figure 10. Stages in life cycle of typical pseudophyllidean cestode. c = cirrus; gp = genital pore; m = Mehlis's gland; o = ovary; t = testis; u = uterus; v = vagina; va = vas deferens; vd = vitelline duct; and vi = vitelline gland.

The eggs hatch in water after about three weeks to yield a ciliated hexacanth embryo. This free-swimming embryo must be ingested by a copepod (*Cyclops* spp.; *Diaptomus* spp.) within a few hours. In the copepod, the ciliated envelope is lost and, within another three weeks, the embryo bores to the body cavity of the crustacean and grows to the procercoid larva. When the copepod is swallowed by any of many species of fresh-water fish (perch, pike, trout, etc.) the procercoid makes its way into the fish muscle, where it grows to the plerocercoid or sparganum larval stage, which measures one or two centimeters in length. When man, or certain other fish-eating mammals, feeds upon the uncooked flesh of the fish, infection results, the worm developing to the adult stage attached to the wall of the mammalian intestine (Figure 10).

Epidemiology.—Not only man, but also dogs, foxes, cats, bears, pigs, mongooses, walruses, and seals, are responsible for the dissemination of *Diphyllobothrium latum*. Feces of these animals containing eggs of the parasite must reach water in which copepods occur, and the infected copepod must be devoured by a suitable fish. Man, or other susceptible mammal, is infected only by swallowing uncooked infected fish flesh. Usually, only a single worm occupies the intestine, although multiple infection is known. Infection may continue for twenty years or more in the absence of treatment.

Pathogenicity.—The presence of *Diphyllobothrium latum* in man often gives rise to no symptoms, although an intestinal catarrh is sometimes noted. A pernicious type of anemia ("bothriocephalus anemia") was formerly believed related to infection with this parasite, but at present such a relationship is questioned. An eosinophilia is often developed, and a toxic condition is revealed by those infected.

Diagnosis.—The finding of the characteristic eggs of the parasite in the feces of the patient proves infection with this tapeworm.

Specific therapy.—Oleoresin of *Aspidium* in capsule form is administered for the elimination of *Diphyllobothrium latum*. Carbon tetrachloride has also been used successfully.

Prophylaxis.—If fish be thoroughly cooked prior to its ingestion, infection with this tapeworm is prevented. Freezing the fish also is effective in killing the plerocercoids. The enactment and enforcement of legislation to prevent the shipping of susceptible species of fish from endemic areas is strongly advised, especially since the incidence of infection with this parasite seems gradually to be increasing.

DIPHYLLOBOTHRIUM MANSONI

Man is infected with the plerocercoid larva (sparganum) of *Diphyllobothrium mansoni*,[2] a parasite of the intestine of carnivores. The larval stage was first found by Manson in 1882 in a Chinese in Amoy. Many human cases have since been reported, these centering chiefly in the Far East, especially the East Indies, Malaya, Indo-China, China, and Japan. The procercoid is formed in *Cyclops*, but the plerocercoid or sparganum usually develops in frogs and snakes, and this grows to the adult stage in the intestine of canine or feline hosts. Human infection is never with the adult parasite, but regularly involves the sparganum or plerocercoid stage. Many of the human infections are accounted for through primitive customs in endemic areas where natives apply splitfrog poultices (containing a living sparganum) to open wounds or inflamed areas. The larva migrates from the frog toward and into the warmer tissues of man. It is possible that human infection also follows the ingestion of infected *Cyclops*. (See Plate XI, C, facing page 175.)

Any tissue of an infected person through which the sparganum migrates becomes inflamed and edematous. Many times the larval worm is killed in the tissue, and it subsequently degenerates, with the most intense local inflammation. When the tissues about the eye are invaded, continued lachrymation generally occurs from the irritation. Often the eye is partially closed, and sight may be lost if the eyeball is entered.

The infection is best diagnosed by recovering the larval worm from the lesions. The removal of the worm is possible only through surgical procedures. Prophylaxis in endemic areas involves the boiling of all drinking water and the avoidance of frogs or snakes which might transmit the plerocercoid stage.

THE CYCLOPHYLLIDEAN TAPEWORMS

Six cyclophyllidean tapeworms are significant in human medicine. These are: *Taenia solium, Taenia saginata, Echinococcus granulosus, Hymenolepis nana, Hymenolepis diminuta,* and *Dipylidium caninum,*

[2] Common synonym: *Sparganum mansoni.*

Of these *Echinococcus granulosus* is exclusively a somatic-tissue parasite in man. The other forms are chiefly intestinal parasites, although *Taenia solium* may also invade the somatic tissues. *Hymenolepis nana* regularly enters the intestinal villi for its larval development in man, but soon thereafter establishes itself in the lumen of the human intestine.

TAENIA SOLIUM

Taenia solium, the pork tapeworm, has been known as a human parasite since ancient times. Linnaeus named the species in 1758.

Geographical distribution.—The distribution of *Taenia solium* is world-wide, the parasite occurring wherever pork, and especially raw or poorly cooked pork, is eaten. It is largely unknown among Jews, Mohammedans, and other peoples whose religion dictates abstinence from the consumption of pig meat. At the present time, its incidence is highest in the countries of central and southeast Europe. It is not common in the United States.

Morphology and life cycle.—The adult parasite is found in the intestine of man exclusively, so far as is known, where it sometimes measures from five to ten feet in length. The scolex has four suckers, and its rostellum is armed with two rows of alternating large and small hooks. (See Plate XI, F, facing page 175.) The mature proglottid presents, in the posterior portion, an ovary with two large and one small lobe, and along the central part of the posterior margin, a collection of vitelline glands. The uterus extends forward through the central axis to near the anterior margin. Testes are very numerous and are disposed throughout the tissue. On the lateral margin is the genital pore, to which the vas deferens carries the sperm cells which have been collected from the testes. The vagina leads in from the genital pore to the oötype, where the eggs from the ovary are fertilized, provided with nutriment from the vitellaria, and passed forward into the uterus. (See Plate XI, D, facing page 175.) In gravid segments, the genitalia are gradually replaced by the branching egg-filled uterus. Generally there are not over thirteen branches in the gravid uterus of this species.

The gravid segments break off from time to time and, usually after they are passed from the body, open to free their eggs. The eggs have two membranes, the inner one being very thick and shell-like, and

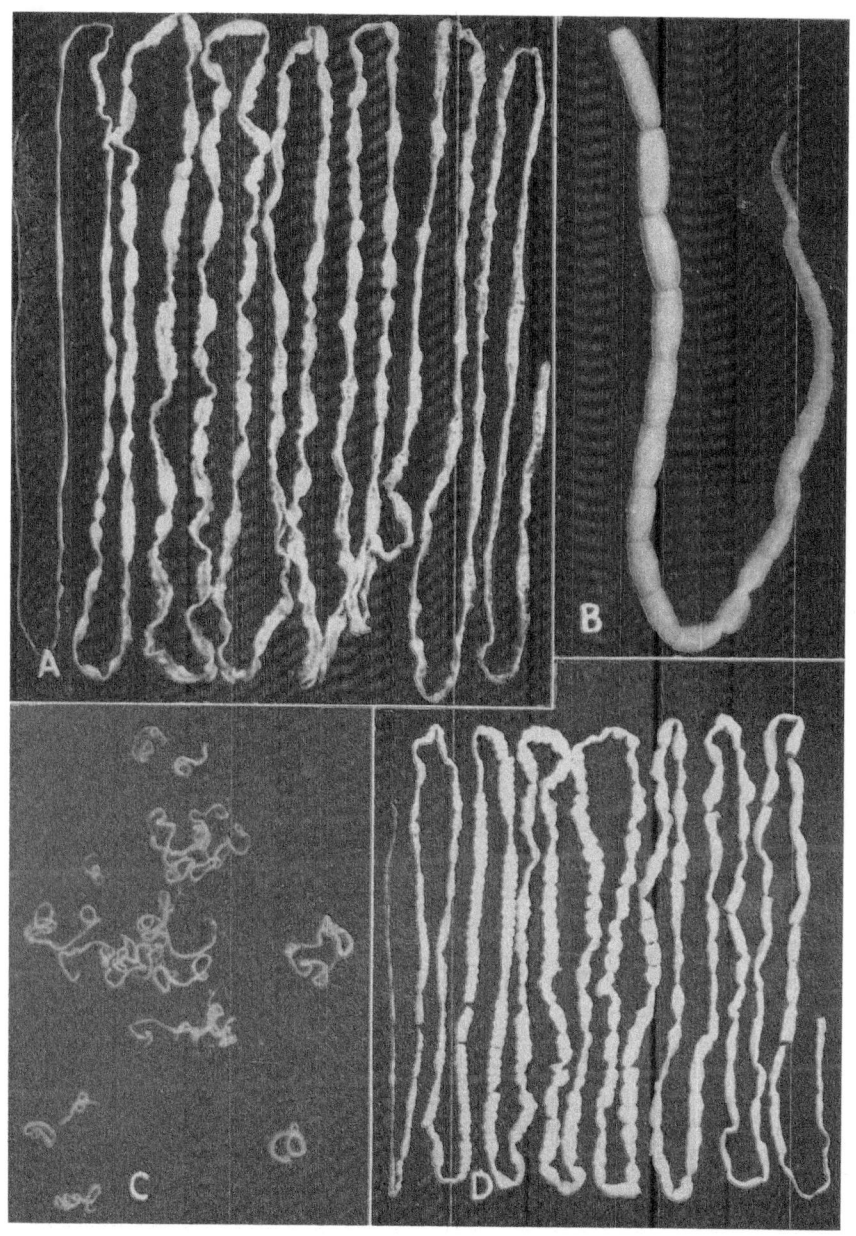

PLATE X

A. *Diphyllobothrium latum:* adult. (x¼)   B. *Dipylidium caninum:* adult. (x2)
C. *Hymenolepis nana:* adults. (x2)   D. *Taenia saginata:* adult. (x¼)

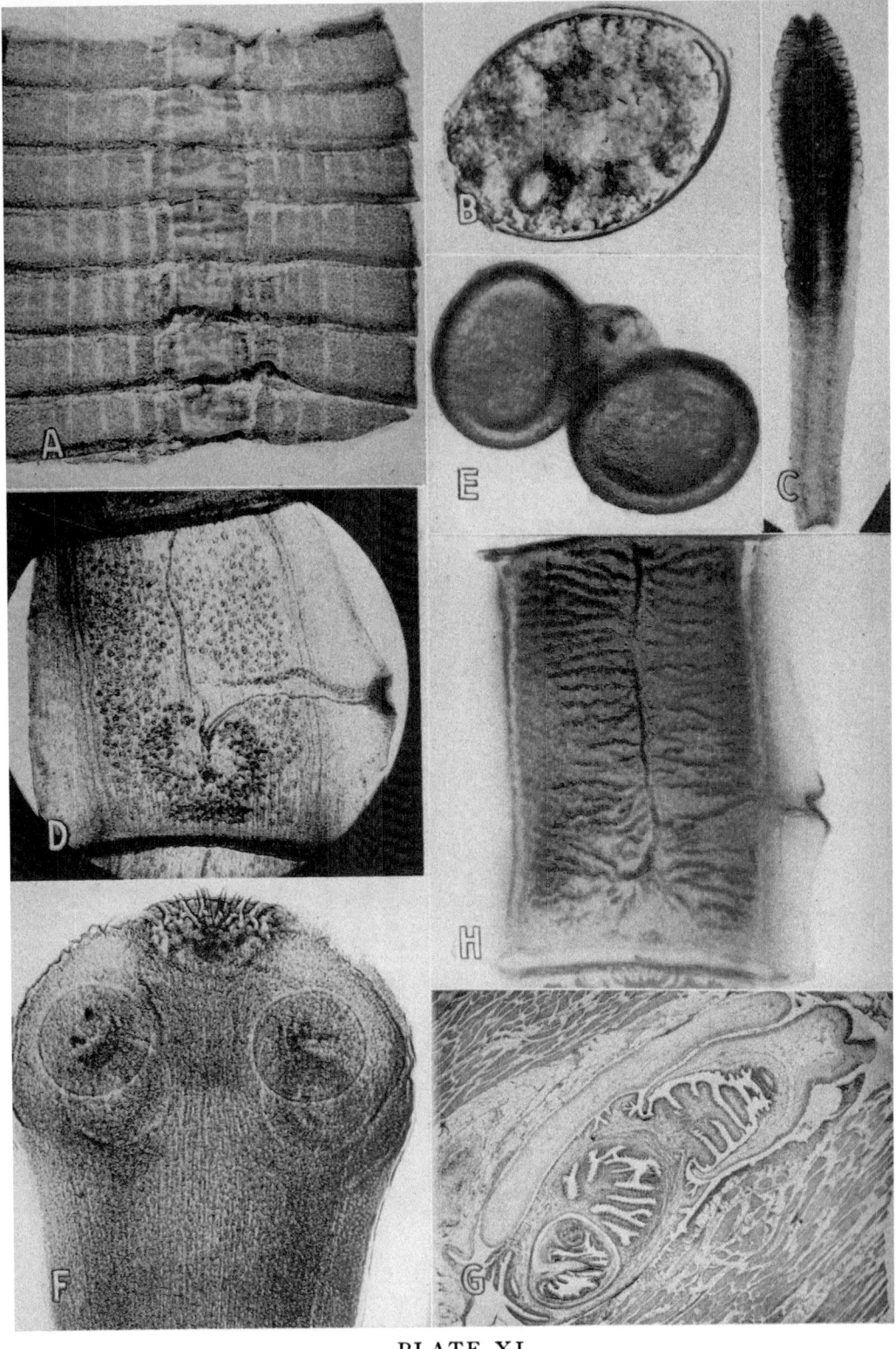

PLATE XI

A. *Diphyllobothrium latum:* mature segments. (x10) B. *Diphyllobothrium latum:* egg. (x600) C. *Diphyllobothrium mansoni:* plerocercoid. (x2) D. *Taenia solium:* mature proglottid. (x10) E. *Taenia saginata:* egg. (x500) F. *Taenia solium:* scolex. (x50) G. *Taenia solium:* cysticercus in section of pork muscle. (x8) H. *Taenia saginata:* gravid proglottid. (x8) the outer one quite thin and easily displaced. Within the inner shell is the hexacanth embryo. When the egg is swallowed by the pig, it hatches in the small intestine and the liberated embryo makes its way to the blood or lymph and thence to the muscles, connective tissue, brain, or elsewhere. Here an ovoidal fluid-filled bladder called a cysticercus is formed. The adult worm develops in man when he eats the uncooked pork which contains the cysticercus. When the cysticercus reaches the duodenum, the adventitial tissue of the bladder is digested away and the remaining head evaginates to become the typical scolex. This scolex attaches to the intestinal wall and gradually grows to the adult worm.

Epidemiology.—Man contracts the intestinal infection with *Taenia solium* by eating pork infected with the cysticercus. (See Plate XI, G, facing this page.) The pig becomes infected with cysticerci by swallowing eggs from human feces. Human infection with the cysticercus also can follow the ingestion of the eggs of the parasite. If eggs of the adult worm are carried forward in the intestine by reverse peristalsis, they hatch without leaving the patient, and the embryos then directly invade his tissue.

Pathogenicity.—Usually symptoms are mild in those persons who harbor the adult parasite. Evidence of toxemia is common, and an eosinophilia may be noted. Infection with the larval worm, the cysticercus, is more serious, and if the cyst lodges in a vital part, severe effects usually of a mechanical nature may ensue. Nearly all tissues are potentially subject to invasion by the larval worm. Cysts have been reported in such parts as the subcutaneous tissue, brain, skeletal muscle, orbit, heart, liver, and lung. There is, very early, a local reaction to the developing cyst in the host tissue, and soon the parasite becomes encased in a fibrous capsule. Very old cysts gradually become calcified. When the cyst develops in the brain, epileptiform symptoms are not uncommon.

Diagnosis.—The presence of the adult worm is determined by finding eggs or, more frequently, the gravid proglottids of the parasite in the feces of the host. The uterus of gravid proglottids generally has only about ten branches. If the scolex is examined, this is found to bear hooks.

The diagnosis of infection with the cysticercus has been carried out by performing a complement-fixation test on the serum of human patients or a precipitin test on the serum of pigs. The parasite itself can sometimes be excised and identified directly if it occupies a superficial site. Calcified cysts are revealed by X-ray photography.

Specific therapy.—Patients harboring the adult worm are treated with oleoresin of *Aspidium* or with carbon tetrachloride. These drugs cause the worm to release its hold on the wall of the intestine. A strong saline purgative is then administered, to flush the parasite from the intestine. It is especially important that the scolex be dislodged by the treatment. When the scolex is not dislodged, regrowth of the parasite soon occurs. The only known treatment for cysticercosis is the surgical removal of the parasite.

Cysticercosis of Brain, Case Report.—A female, forty years old, had experienced periodic convulsive seizures for one year before admission to hospital. The initial attacks had been relatively mild, consisting of uncontrolled jerking, preceded by paresthesias, in the left upper extremity, and lasting about one minute. Blood count showed an eosinophilia of eleven percent. Calcified cysticerci were revealed in thigh muscle by X-ray photography, and a tentative diagnosis of cysticercosis of the brain was made. Ten days before admission, the patient experienced a most severe attack involving all extremities and lasting for twenty minutes, without loss of consciousness. At operation, a mass two centimeters in diameter was removed from the cerebrum. This mass on section proved to be a cysticercus of *Taenia solium.* Symptoms were at once relieved, the eosinophilia disappeared, and during observations for four years subsequently no further symptoms were noted.[3]

Prophylaxis.—If meat is thoroughly cooked, or else frozen before cooking, any cysticercus which it contains will be killed. The parasites are not killed by salting methods or by liquid smoking.

TAENIA SAGINATA

Although the beef tapeworm, *Taenia saginata,* has been known since ancient times as a human parasite, the role of cysticercus-infected cattle in leading to human infection was not determined until 1862, when Leuckart demonstrated that the cattle cyst develops to the adult worm in man.

The parasite has cosmopolitan distribution but is especially frequent in Mohammedan countries and in Ethiopia, where raw beef is

[3] B. S. Ray, *Archives of Neurology and Psychiatry,* 45: 494 (1941).

commonly eaten. It occurs oftener than does *Taenia solium* in the United States.

Morphology and life cycle.—The adult *Taenia saginata* often measures from twenty to thirty feet in length. (See Plate X, D, facing page 174.) Its scolex differs sharply from that of *Taenia solium* in being unarmed. The mature proglottid is essentially identical with that of *Taenia solium*. The gravid proglottid differs from the corresponding stage of *Taenia solium* in having not less than fifteen, and usually more, branches of the uterus. (See Plate XI, H, facing page 175.) The egg is indistinguishable from that of *Taenia solium*. (See Plate XI, E, facing page 175.) The cysticercus, which develops in the muscles of cattle, measures about one centimeter in length and contains an invaginated scolex like that of the adult worm. After this is swallowed by man, the scolex evaginates and becomes attached to the intestinal wall where the worm develops to maturity in from eight to twelve weeks. Except for its residence as a larval form in cattle rather than the pig, *Taenia saginata* resembles *Taenia solium* in most respects in its life cycle.

Epidemiology.—*Taenia saginata* resides as an adult exclusively in the human intestine. Cattle are the only significant host of the larval stage, although sheep, llama, giraffe, and buffalo are said to be susceptible. Man is infected by consuming raw infected beef. Cattle are infected by food or drink contaminated with the eggs passed by man.

Pathogenicity.—Except for symptoms of hunger or loss of weight and a vague helminth toxemia, *Taenia saginata* is of small effect on man. An eosinophilia is usually developed. Human infection with the cysticercus only very rarely occurs.

Diagnosis.—Infection with *Taenia saginata* is established by finding eggs or proglottids of the worm in the feces of the patient. An effort is usually made to differentiate the form from *Taenia solium*, since persons with *Taenia saginata* need not fear somatic tissue infection with the larval stage. The eggs are identical with those of *Taenia solium*. The uterus of the gravid proglottids of *Taenia saginata* usually has more than sixteen branches.

Specific therapy.—The same methods are used for treating *Taenia saginata* infection as for *Taenia solium*. When the scolex of the parasite is not recovered, regrowth of the worm within two or three months can be expected.

Taenia Saginata Infection, Case Report.—A female fifty years old was admitted to hospital for removal of *Taenia saginata,* proglottids of this form having been recovered from the stool. A worm fourteen feet long was obtained after the administration of oleoresin of *Aspidium,* but the scolex was not found. Three months later, the patient returned and following *Aspidium* therapy a worm ten feet in length was recovered, again without the scolex. After another interval of three months the patient came back for a third treatment, and twelve feet of proglottids were removed, but once more the scolex could not be found. The patient did not return for further treatment, although probably she continued to harbor the worm.

Prophylaxis.—If all beef used as food is thoroughly cooked or frozen before ingestion, little danger of infection with *Taenia saginata* remains. If cattle are pastured on fields unpolluted with human feces, their meat will not contain the cysticercus.

ECHINOCOCCUS GRANULOSUS

Echinococcus disease is an old infection of man. Its occurrence was well known to the ancient medical writers, and its pathology was surprisingly well described in the first texts on pathology printed in the United States late in the eighteenth century. The disease is caused by the larval stage of a cestode named *Echinococcus granulosus.*[4]

Geographical distribution.—Although found over much of the world, echinococcus disease is a medical problem primarily in the great grazing areas. Its incidence is highest in the Argentine, and in South Africa, Australia, and New Zealand. It is common in the Mediterranean basin. It occurs also in much of Europe and the United States, although indigenous human cases in the United States seem rare. Most cases met in this country are among immigrants, chiefly from Mediterranean countries. In Iceland, the disease was once extremely common, as many as twenty percent of the entire population being infected. Fortunately, the condition in Iceland has been much improved in recent years, by reason of the institution of adequate public health measures.

Echinococcus Disease, Case Reports.—A female thirty-five years old was admitted to hospital for observation because of vague pains over the liver.

---

[4] Common synonyms: *Taenia echinococcus; Echinococcus hominis; Echinococcus alveolaris.*

She had been born in Turkey but had resided in New York city for ten years. Although previously hydatid disease was not suspected, at operation two unilocular hydatid cysts (one shown as Plate XII, B, facing page 190) were removed without rupture. There were no further symptoms during observation for three years, and recovery appeared complete.

A second patient was a male forty years old, born in California. About twenty years before admission to hospital he had worked as a seaman on cattle boats traveling to the Argentine and later on boats going to New Zealand and Australia. On admission to hospital he complained of extreme pain in the liver, and, during the first several days of residence, presented an eosinophilia up to ten percent. An X-ray photograph revealed what appeared to be a large cyst, and within this shadows suggestive of daughter cysts could be seen. A skin test with cestode antigen was positive; the complement fixation test for hydatid disease was also positive. At operation, a large alveolar cyst was found in the liver. It had ruptured and was infected with bacteria. As much as the cyst was removed as could be taken safely. After several weeks, the patient was able to leave the hospital, and eventually he resumed his employment which now was as a grocer's clerk. His prognosis was, however, bad. He continued to suffer with an intense urticaria and general malaise, which were caused doubtless by seepage of fluid from cysts still in the liver. Eventually, further operation for the removal of secondary cysts will probably be required, and little possibility exists for complete recovery.

Morphology and life cycle.—The adult form of *Echinococcus granulosus* (Plate XII, A, facing page 190) is found only in canines, particularly the dog, fox, wolf, jackal, and perhaps one or two others. The larval stage, which is known as a hydatid (Plate XII, B, C, D, and E, facing page 190) occurs in a broad range of hosts, such as sheep, cow, goat, horse, deer, moose, pig, kangaroo, elephant, camel, giraffe, squirrel, rabbit, mouse, and many others, besides man. Apparently only the canines harbor the adult worm because other mammals digest the larval stage after ingesting it. The adult worm is minute, measuring only two or three millimeters in length and possessing but four or five segments. Its armed scolex is like that of *Taenia solium,* although its few proglottids reveal a more abrupt progression of development than do those of the longer cestodes. The adult parasite produces onchospheres which cannot be distinguished from those of other Taenioid worms, the thin outer membrane generally being digested off while still in the dog intestine. After these onchospheres are passed in the dog feces, they are swallowed in food or drink by an animal susceptible to the larval parasite. In the anterior part of the small intestine, their thick shell is digested off, and the hexacanth embryo is freed. The embryo penetrates the intestinal wall, finally entering a capillary or mesenteric venule. It is carried by the blood to one of the several blood filters. This is usually the liver (sixty to seventy-five percent of all cases), but may be the lung (five to ten percent), muscles (five percent,) spleen (two percent), kidney (two percent), bones (one percent), brain (0.6 percent), or even other parts such as the orbit.[5] In any of these sites a fluid-filled bladderlike cyst containing usually very numerous brood capsules and scolices develops which, in man, may easily reach the size of a grapefruit, if it occupies a distensible organ. Usually from five to ten years or even more are required for the full development of the cyst in the human host. In the sheep the parasite reaches its full development more quickly, although its ultimate size is less than in man. Generally the cyst is gradually surrounded by a thick fibrous capsule which the host elaborates in response to the parasite. The larval parasite develops to an adult worm only if a susceptible canine host feeds on tissue containing the larval form.

Epidemiology.—Primary infection with the hydatid always occurs by swallowing eggs from the adult worm, generally along with food or drink. Man seldom contracts the disease except when living in close physical contact with dogs, and even then he is, more or less, an accidental host, being a substitute for the optimal hosts, the sheep, cow, or goat. Yet in grazing areas, where man and dog work together tending sheep or cattle, the parasite has ample opportunity to infect man. In Uruguay and the Argentine, for example, its incidence among some of the peons is about fifty percent. Generally, the world over, the dogs used to guard sheep and cattle harbor the adult parasite. In southern Australia, for example, at least forty percent of the dogs are infected.

Pathogenicity.—Echinococcus disease is a slowly developed condition, symptoms not appearing until years after infection. Its seriousness depends largely on the site occupied by the cyst. If the parasite develops normally, into a unilocular cyst, a cellular response is made by the host which finally walls it off more or less completely. Such persons may not even reveal an eosinophilia, and often the cyst dies and is calcified or even resorbed. If the cyst develops in cramped quar-

---

[5] F. Dévé, *Comptes rendus de la Société de biologie,* 74: 735 (1916).

ters, such as the canalicula of bones, it is inhibited in development and may remain sterile until it breaks out or erodes its way into tissue in which it can develop more freely. Alveolar cysts, however, are not uncommon. These have no well-described boundaries, and their metastasizing roots extend into neighboring tissue or may even be carried by the blood to distant sites. If a cyst is ruptured, as often happens at operation, bits of the germinative membrane may reëstablish themselves in the host. The sudden escape of the hydatid cyst fluid when a cyst ruptures may precipitate anaphylactic shock in the patient. Constant seepage of this fluid often causes serious and prolonged attacks of allergy, with urticaria, nausea, and asthmatic symptoms. Another complication is the infection of the cyst with other organisms, especially with blood-borne bacteria.

Immunity.—Probably some immunity is developed to reinfection with the hydatid by man, although certainly when a primary cyst ruptures reinfection occurs. Yet at such time the defensive facilities of the host are surely depressed, by reason of the anaphylactic reaction which the host has experienced as a result of cyst rupture. Antibodies appear in the serum of infected persons or animals, and these usually persist for at least several months after the cyst has been surgically removed.

The walling off of the parasite, which is accomplished through the collaboration of humoral and cellular defense agencies, as in a typical Arthus reaction, is also an evidence of an immune response. This resistance is magnified and accelerated in animals previously immunized artificially with killed antigens of the parasite. After such immunization, animals (sheep) are only slightly susceptible to infection.

Diagnosis.—The final proof of infection with hydatid disease is the demonstration of the parasite itself, but this is seldom possible directly with safety. In former times, fluid was routinely removed, if possible, by puncture of the suspected cyst, and examined for the presence of hydatid "sand," consisting of hooks and scolices. (See Plate XII, F, facing page 190.) It is now realized that this procedure must be discouraged, for it is attended with great danger from possible reinfection of the patient by material which escapes from the opened cyst. Several other suggestive or presumptive diagnostic procedures are available. X ray is helpful in revealing cysts of the lung, long bones, and some other sites. An eosinophilia of twenty-five percent or more may develop, which suggests infection. Antibody tests, however, are the most useful diagnostic procedures. Precipitin, complement-fixation, and skin tests all are used. The fixation and skin tests are most delicate, but of these the skin test is the simpler to perform. (See Plate XII, G, facing page 190.) Originally only the hydatid fluid was used for any of the antibody tests, but recently, at least for skin tests, extracts of related cestodes also have been shown to serve.

Therapy.—The only effective therapy for echinococcus disease is operation—surgical removal of the cyst. When the cyst is unilocular and can be perfectly enucleated, without rupture of its capsule, the patient is permanently rid of the infection. With alveolar cysts, operation is seldom successful in permanently curing the patient, although temporary relief from the extreme pressure pain generally experienced can thus be obtained. If a fertile cyst is ruptured at operation, multiple reinfection can be expected in five to ten years. As a precautionary measure at operation, cysts are generally injected with formaldehyde prior to their actual removal.

Prophylaxis.—Public health programs against echinococcus disease are designed to protect the human population from infection from the dog. The necessity of cleanly habits and the prevention of contaminating food or drink or one's person with dog feces, which contains the worm eggs, is stressed. However, before a community can be rendered free of the disease, other animals susceptible to the larval parasite must be similarly safeguarded. The dog population likewise must be protected, by preventing dogs from feeding on the raw tissue of animals infected with the larval parasite. In the endemic areas of South America, particularly, extensive educational programs are under way which doubtless, as earlier in Iceland, will reduce the incidence of the infection in those lands.

HYMENOLEPIS NANA

The dwarf tapeworm, *Hymenolepis nana*,[6] was discovered by Bilharz in 1851 in Cairo. It has essentially cosmopolitan distribution and is found with especial frequency in children. It is the commonest tapeworm in man in the United States.

[6] Common synonym: *Taenia nana*.

Morphology and life cycle.—The adult worm is a small form, seldom measuring over two or three centimeters long. (See Plate X, C, facing page 174.) The scolex has four suckers, and its rostellum is armed with a single row of hooks. Segments are broader than long, even when terminal. The eggs are distinct from those of cestodes of the genus *Taenia* in having two thin membranes about the hexacanth embryo. (See Plate IX, G, facing page 159.) Flagellalike strands arising from the poles of the inner membrane are seen especially in the living egg. No intermediate host is required, and when eggs passed by one person are swallowed by a second individual, the second becomes infected. The eggs hatch in the small intestine and the embryos penetrate the villi, where they develop to larvae called cercocysts. The cercocysts leave the villi in a few days and attach to the intestinal wall. In this position they grow to adults.

Epidemiology.—Not only man but also the gerbil and the rat and mouse are susceptible to infection by *Hymenolepis nana*. It is not proved, however, that man is infected from the rodent source or that rodents are infected from man. Among human beings, children are most commonly infected. Often the child, because of untidy habits, will continue to reinfect himself. If the eggs hatch in the intestine of patients without leaving the body, internal autoinfection will occur, the adult worms then lodging finally far toward the posterior end of the small intestine.

Pathogenicity.—Few or no symptoms are revealed by persons with light infections. Those with heavy infections, however, may manifest generalized toxicity and diarrhea or abdominal pain. Even epileptiform symptoms have been reported. An eosinophilia generally develops in those with heavy infections.

Diagnosis.—The presence of eggs in the feces establishes the diagnosis of infection with *Hymenolepis nana*.

Specific therapy.—Oleoresin of *Aspidium*, oil of chenopodium, and hexylresorcinol are administered in treating infections with *Hymenolepis nana*. Infections are difficult to cure because the larval stage occurs within the villus, and this may escape the effects of the administered drug and later return to the intestinal lumen to complete its development and reëstablish the infection.

Prophylaxis.—By avoiding contact with persons harboring *Hymeno-*

lepis nana and by abstaining from food or drink which may be contaminated with eggs of the parasite, individuals can protect themselves from infection with *Hymenolepis nana*.

HYMENOLEPIS DIMINUTA

Hymenolepis diminuta, the rat tapeworm, is a small cestode found naturally in the rat and mouse, as well as some other rodents, over much of the world. Cases of infection in man have occasionally been reported from many countries of South America and from Africa, Europe, the Far East, and various parts of the United States.

The adult worm may measure five or six centimeters in length. The scolex has four suckers, but, unlike *Hymenolepis nana*, it is unarmed. The lateral genital pores of the mature segments all open on the same side. (See Plate IX, E and F, facing page 159.) The egg has two thin membranes about the embryo, but, unlike that of *Hymenolepis nana*, no polar filaments come from the inner membrane. The eggs must be ingested by one of various insects, including larval lepidopterans, larval fleas, beetles, cockroaches, and earwigs. In the body cavity of the insect, the cysticercoid larval stage or cercocyst develops. The mammalian host, including man, becomes infected by swallowing the insect with food or drink, and the parasite develops to an adult worm in the intestine.

The human infection is determined by finding eggs of the parasite in the feces of the patient. Treatment is by the administration of oleoresin of *Aspidium*. Human infection is usually prevented by keeping foods, particularly grains and breakfast food, free of insects.

DIPYLIDIUM CANINUM

The double-pored dog tapeworm, *Dipylidium caninum*, has for several centuries been known as a parasite of man and was clearly identified by Linnaeus in 1758. It occurs over the entire world in dogs and cats, which often harbor many adult worms, as well as in other carnivores. Human infection is occasionally reported. The adult worm is comparatively small, usually measuring only about twelve to fifteen inches long. (See Plate X, B, facing page 174.) The scolex has four suckers and a protrusible rostellum armed with from three to seven rows of spines, which somewhat resemble carpet tacks whose points have been slightly bent. (See Plate IX, C, facing page 159.) The mature proglottids are supplied with two complete sets of genital organs, with a genital pore opening on each side of every segment. The gravid segments become filled with "nests" of eggs, which replace the genitalia. The hexacanth embryos are enclosed individually in one thin membrane, and a second thin membrane envelops the entire nest. (See Plate IX, D, facing page 159.) The gravid proglottids break off and either are expelled or else migrate from the anus of the infected animal. Once outside, they are ruptured and their egg nests are dispersed. In the case of the usual hosts, the dog and cat, larval fleas (*Ctenocephalides canis, Ctenocephalides felis*) ingest the eggs and serve as intermediate hosts for the cysticercoid larva of the worm. The parasite is retained in the body cavity of the fleas during their metamorphosis. If the adult flea is swallowed by the dog or cat, or by man, the parasite leaves the flea body in the vertebrate intestine and attaches to the intestinal wall to become an adult. Human infection is largely confined to children or those who have frequent and close contact with dogs and cats. Symptoms from the light infections usual in man are negligible.

The infection with *Dipylidium caninum* is diagnosed by finding the egg nests or proglottids in the feces of the patient. Oleoresin of *Aspidium* is an effective drug for treating patients with this parasite. Generally human infection is avoided by keeping house cats and dogs free of fleas, and by preventing children from close contact with animals which harbor fleas.

Chapter XVII

THE NEMATODE INFECTIONS

The THREADWORM PARASITES (class Nematoda, phylum Nemathelminthes) differ from all other helminths in having an alimentary canal complete with anus. They are slender forms, usually pointed at both ends. The sexes are separate. The posterior end of the male worm is often curved ventrad. The body of all forms is covered with a thick cuticula.

Many nematodes are free-living organisms throughout their development. Some species spend the early part of their life as free-living forms but later become parasitic. Others are obligate parasites during their entire life. A few forms experience complete development either as free-living or as parasitic worms depending on whether or not a suitable host is available.

TYPE MORPHOLOGY OF ADULT

The body wall of a nematode consists of an epithelial layer covered by cuticula. Motion is effected by the contraction of groups of longitudinal muscles beneath the body wall. The digestive canal is complete, with a mouth, oesophagus, intestine, rectum, and cloaca-anus. The mouth and oesophagus as well as the rectum and cloaca-anus are lined with cuticula. The excretory system may consist merely of cuticular glands, but in some species two longitudinal tubes, blind at their posterior ends, collect wastes and excrete them from the excretory pore on the mid-ventral line near the mouth. The nervous system consists of two commissures with ganglion cells. One commissure surrounds the oesophagus and innervates the head. The other surrounds the anus and sends nerve trunks to the tail. The commissures are connected by longitudinal trunks.

The reproductive system in the male consists of a single coiled testis, which opens into the seminal vesicle and thence into the cloaca-anus. A pair of spicules, protrusible from the spicule sheath through the cloaca-anus, aid in transferring sperm cells into the vagina of the female. Often there is a bursa copulatrix which helps attach the male to the female body.

The female reproductive system consists of two ovaries, two oviducts, two seminal receptacles, two uteri, a vagina, and a vulva. Eggs

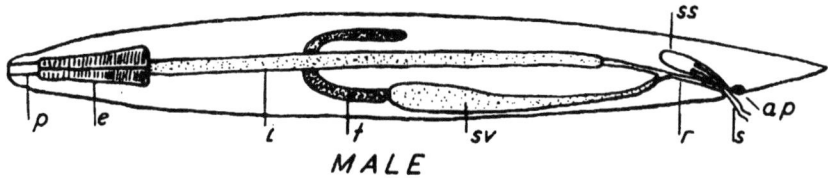

MALE

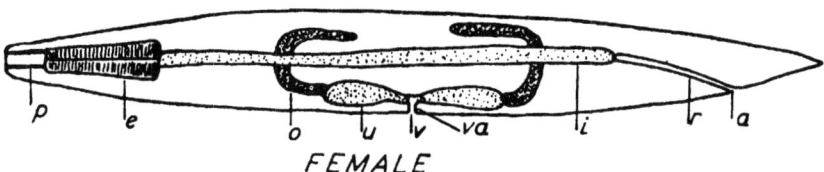

FEMALE

Figure 11. Diagram of typical male and female nematodes. a = anus; ap = accessory piece; e = oesophagus; i = intestine; o = ovarian tubule; p = pharynx; r = rectum; s = spicule; ss = spicule sheath; sv = seminal vesical; t = testis; u = uterus; v = vulva; va = vagina.

pass from each ovary through the oviduct and the seminal receptacle, where they are fertilized, to the uterus, where they are supplied with food and a shell of characteristic shape. They are stored in the uterus until they are ejected through the vagina and vulva. (See Figure 11.)

TYPE LIFE HISTORY

Nematode life histories are of such diverse character that the selection of a type is entailed with no small difficulty. Yet certain basic similarities run through many forms. For example, the adult worm is usually an intestinal parasite. The nematode egg is endolecithal and is generally passed in the host's feces. There are typically four larval stages in development. The first stage is that which emerges from the egg; the second stage is a free-living form; the third stage is the one infective for vertebrates, generally reaching the somatic tissues of the host; the fourth stage is the one which returns to the intestine where the adult development follows.

CLASSIFICATION

The nematode parasites of significance in human medicine are found in two orders: Trichosyringata and Myosyringata. The order Trichosyringata includes one superfamily, Trichinelloidea. The order Myosyringata includes six superfamilies: Rhabditoidea, Strongyloidea, Oxyuroidea, Ascaroidea, Filarioidea, and Dracunculoidea. These superfamilies can be differentiated by the following key:

A. Oesophagus a simple nonmuscular tube; anterior end of worm elongate and tapered; phasmids (caudal chemoreceptors) absent—Trichinelloidea
B. Oesophagus muscular; anterior end of worm not elongate; phasmids present
    I. Males bursate, buccal capsule present—Strongyloidea
   II. Males nonbursate; no buccal capsule
      1. Intermediate host required
        a. Intermediate development in bloodsucking insects—Filarioidea
        b. Intermediate development in Copepods—Dracunculoidea
      2. No intermediate host required
        a. Small (microscopic) forms; oesophagus with one or two bulbs; vagina transverse; many species free-living, with an alternating parasitic generation—Rhabditoidea
        b. Larger forms; oesophagus bulbed or cylindrical; vagina elongate; mouth with three to six lips
           (1) Large, stout worms; oesophagus muscular; tail of female not elongate—Ascaroidea
           (2) Medium-sized, transparent worms; oesophagus bulbed; tail of female usually elongate and sharply pointed—Oxyuroidea

The medically important species found in each of these superfamilies follow:

Superfamily	*Important Representatives*
Trichinelloidea	Trichinella spiralis, Trichuris trichiura
Rhabditoidea	Strongyloides stercoralis
Strongyloidea	Necator americanus, Ancylostoma duodenale

Oxyuroidea	Enterobius vermicularis
Ascaroidea	Ascaris lumbricoides
Filarioidea	Wuchereria bancrofti, Microfilaria malayi, Acanthocheilonema perstans, Mansonella ozzardi, Onchocerca volvulus, Loa loa
Dracunculoidea	Dracunculus medinensis

SUPERFAMILY TRICHINELLOIDEA

Two nematodes of the superfamily Trichinelloidea are important as human disease agents: *Trichinella spiralis*, the pork worm, and *Trichuris trichiura*, the whipworm.

TRICHINELLA SPIRALIS

The pork worm, *Trichinella spiralis*,[1] was first observed in human muscle in 1828 by Peacock in London, and in 1846 Leidy in Philadelphia observed cysts in the muscles of pigs. The life cycle was completed experimentally by Virchow in 1859. The adult worm was first seen in the human intestine in 1860 by Zenker.

Geographical distribution.—*Trichinella spiralis* has cosmopolitan distribution. It has its highest human incidence among peoples of Central Europe and the Western Hemisphere. Most of the recent studies suggest that at least fifteen percent of the general population of the United States harbor the parasite.[2]

Morphology and life cycle.—The adult male worm measures about one and one-half millimeters long. The body is slender and tapered gradually toward the anterior end. At the posterior tip are two papillae or "wings." The adult female worm is about twice the length of the male. The female genital opening lies relatively near the anterior end of the body. Females have but one ovary. No papillae occur at the posterior tip of the female body. (See Plate XIII, B, facing page 191.)

The embryos are about 0.1 millimeter long when born. The mature larva is approximately one millimeter long at the time of encystment. Sexual differentiation occurs in the larval stage.

During the first several days after meat containing encysted larvae is swallowed, the larval parasites which have been digested from their cysts reside in the superficial tissue of the intestinal wall, where they

---

[1] Common synonym: *Trichina spiralis*.

[2] K. B. Kerr, L. Jacobs, and E. Cuvillier, *Public Health Reports*, 56: 836 (1941).

experience several moults. They reach maturity within two or three days, and promptly mate in the gut lumen. Within a few days thereafter, the male worms are eliminated in the feces of the host. The female worms, however, penetrate the wall of the small intestine and pour forth embryos which reach the lymph or blood vessels of the hosts. These embryos remain briefly in the circulation but finally leave the blood and migrate into and through the striated muscles. Encystment of the larval worm occurs almost exclusively in skeletal muscle and is generally under way by the end of the fourth week following infection. The larval worm usually is coiled within the spindle-shaped cyst, and often some movement in the cyst can be detected. Leucocytes, and especially eosinophiles, can be seen around the cyst. (See Plate XIII, A, facing page 191.)

Epidemiology.—Infection with *Trichinella spiralis* is contracted by eating the muscle tissue of an animal containing the encysted larvae of this parasite. Human infection generally results from ingesting the meat of an infected pig. The pig in turn contracts its infection by feeding on uncooked scraps of infected pork, found usually in garbage, or on the tissue of an infected brown or black rat. The rat is the usual natural reservoir of the parasite. Many municipalities now require that garbage be cooked thoroughly before being fed to pigs, in order to prevent trichiniasis in the pigs. In 1942, the legislature of New York state passed a law to this effect.

Trichinella spiralis can infect a very broad range of animals, including representatives of all the mammalian orders. In herbivorous animals, however, natural infections do not often occur, even though these animals are potentially susceptible. Birds sometimes can be infected experimentally, but do not naturally harbor the parasite and certainly are insignificant in its transmission. Cold-blooded animals are insusceptible.

Pathogenicity.—Symptoms in very mild cases of trichiniasis are protean and often suggest various other diseases. In severe infections, there is usually an initial diarrhea with catarrhal inflammation, and sometimes blood and mucus appear in the stool. These symptoms follow irritation to the intestinal wall when the adult worms burrow through it. As larval worms begin to migrate through the muscle tissue, edema is often noted about the eyes and face. There is a gen-

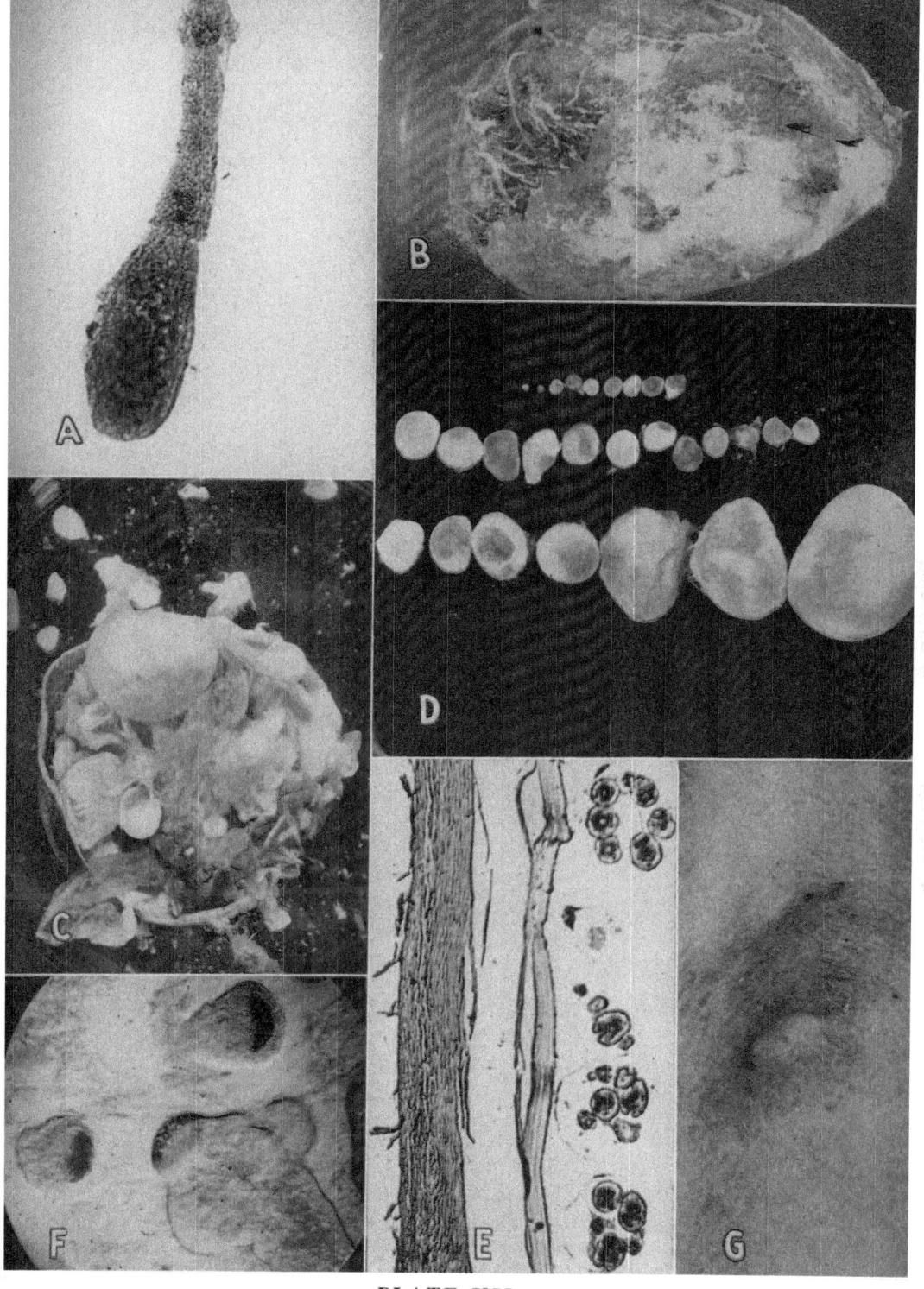

PLATE XII

A. *Echinococcus granulosus:* adult. (x25)   B. *Echinococcus granulosus:* hydatid cyst from liver. (x½)   C. *Echinococcus granulosus:* opened hydatid, showing daughter cysts. (x½) D. *Echinococcus granulosus:* daughter cysts. (x½)   E. *Echinococcus granulosus:* section of wall showing capsule, germinative membrane, and brood capsules. (x60)   F. *Echinococcus granulosus:* scolices of brood capsule. (x250)   G. Positive immediate skin test on volar surface of fore-arm of patient with hydatid disease.

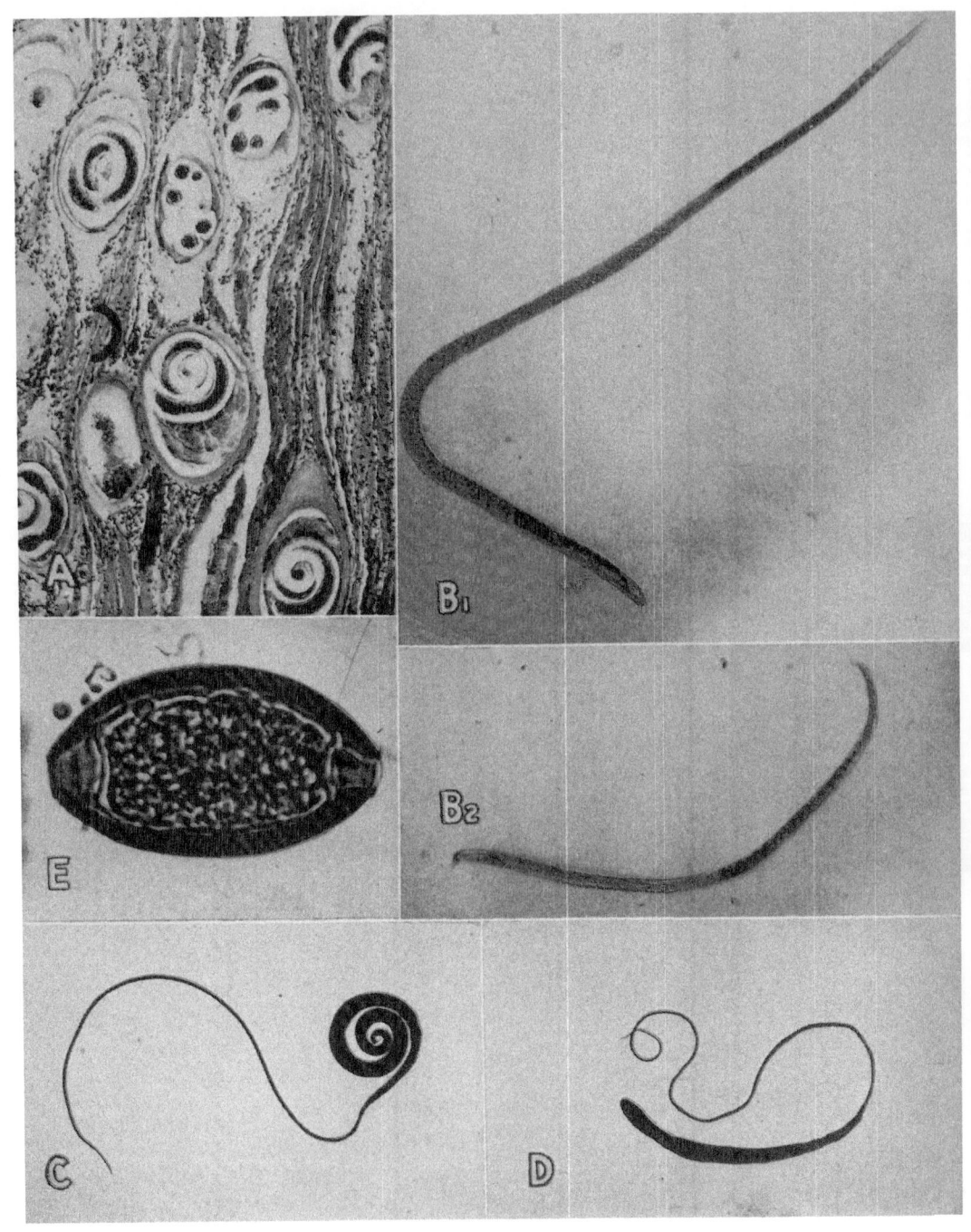

PLATE XIII

A. *Trichinella spiralis:* larvae encysted in skeletal muscle. (x75)   B. *Trichinella spiralis:* adults. 1, female; 2, male. (x75)   C. *Trichuris trichiura:* male. (x5)   D. *Trichuris trichiura:* female. (x5)   E. *Trichuris trichiura:* egg. (x750) eralized myositis, the muscles over the entire body becoming tender and aching when moved. The diaphragm is especially involved, and respiration is difficult and painful. Muscles of the legs and arms ache, and walking is sometimes impossible. The larynx is also involved so that speech is frequently lost or impaired. During the second week of the infection, an eosinophilia develops, eosinophiles often making up fifty percent or more of the leucocyte count. The most critical period of the infection is the third and fourth weeks, when encystment of the parasite is beginning and when tissue repair is initiated. Respiratory and circulatory disturbance then is often pronounced. Death may result from toxaemia, myocarditis, or secondary infection.

Diagnosis.—The detection of an eosinophilia is generally one of the first laboratory clues in the identification of trichiniasis. Somewhat earlier, adult worms—especially males—can be found in the feces, but usually symptoms are so poorly developed at the time that males are being eliminated that little reason is presented clinically to search the feces for the parasite. From the seventh day or so onward, embryos can be seen in the peripheral blood, although the procedure which must be followed to detect them is tedious. After the third week, larvae, either migrating through or encysted in the muscles, can be seen in biopsy material. It is chiefly through biopsy that absolute proof of infection is established. Positive immunological tests, especially precipitin and skin tests, also provide presumptive evidence of infection. In interpreting these tests, however, possible infection with other nematodes must be considered. Usually, unless a skin response is made to the antigen even after this has been used in a dilution of one thousand times or more, one cannot be certain the infection is not caused by a related species of nematode.

Specific therapy.—No specific therapeutic substance is available for treating trichiniasis. Sulfanilamide and butolan have been found by some authorities to be somewhat beneficial. An immune serum may also have slight therapeutic value. None of these materials, however, has seemed particularly useful for treating the disease.

Prophylaxis.—Pork can be eaten with safety from possible trichiniasis only if thoroughly cooked or refrigerated prior to ingestion. If the refrigerating temperature is −4° F., the meat is rendered innocuous by refrigeration for only twenty-four hours. Smoking, salting, and pickling procedures do not kill the parasite. Meat from large packing houses generally is rendered safe for use through refrigeration, and most epidemics or outbreaks of trichiniasis follow the use of meat from pigs killed at home or in small slaughterhouses. Hogs fed exclusively on corn are free from the parasite. The greatest incidence of infection occurs among garbage-fed hogs.

TRICHURIS TRICHIURA

The whipworm, *Trichuris trichiura*,[3] was first described by Morgagni in the late seventeenth century. Grassi completed the life cycle in 1887.

Geographical distribution.—*Trichuris trichiura* has a cosmopolitan distribution. Its incidence is highest in the warm parts of the world. Commonly, it is found in regions where *Ascaris lumbricoides* also occurs. In the United States it is known in the southern Appalachian mountains, in south-central Louisiana, and in Florida, near Tampa.

Morphology and life cycle.—The adult whipworm lives usually in the posterior small intestine, the caecum, or the appendix of man, its bulbous or fleshy posterior end protruding into the lumen and its long attenuated anterior portion being buried in the wall of the part occupied. The adult worms measure up to four or five centimeters in length. The males are generally very much coiled posteriorly, but the females are relatively straight. (See Plate XIII, C and D, facing page 191.) There is a single spicule in the male, which is often seen protruding from the extensible spine-covered penial sheath.

The eggs, which are immature when passed, are oval, with an extraordinarily thick shell with conspicuous mucous plugs at both ends. (See Plate XIII, E, facing page 191.) They develop within about two weeks outside the body, the formed embryo being then visible within. If the embryonated egg is swallowed, the embryo hatches from the egg and attaches to the wall of the small intestine. Later, it migrates posteriorly, where it grows to an adult worm. Eggs appear in the feces of the individual about three months after he became infected.

Epidemiology.—Man exclusively is infected with *Trichuris trichiura*. Infection occurs usually in children and results directly from polluted soil or by ingesting food or drink containing the embryonated

---

[3] Common synonym: *Trichocephalus trichiura.*

egg of the parasite. Soil in highly humid shaded areas which have heavy rainfall is most likely to harbor the organism.

Pathogenicity.—Infections of low intensity often reveal no symptoms, but persons infected with many worms become emaciated, have a severely reduced hemoglobin, and suffer a diarrhea, the stool usually containing mucus but rarely blood. Eosinophilia is generally said to be appreciable (twenty-five percent) in acute infections, although in chronic cases the blood picture is usually normal.

Diagnosis.—The identification of the distinctive egg of *Trichuris trichiura* establishes the diagnosis of infection with the parasite.

Specific therapy.—*Leche de higueron,* or its effective fraction, ficin, is specific for treating whipworm infection. The crude substance is the sap of trees of the genus *Ficus,* grown in Central and South America. The substance is not generally available, except in the tropics, and such materials as carbon tetrachloride, tetrachorethylene, and oil of chenopodium are usually employed in treating patients in temperate zones. These last drugs are effective in reducing the severity of heavy infections, although complete eradication of all parasites is seldom attained through their use.

Prophylaxis.—Prophylactic measures are usually directed to children, since they are more often infected with *Trichuris trichiura* than are adults. Children are advised not to play on ground likely to be polluted with the feces of infected children. Procedures which safeguard food and drink from such fecal contamination also are advised.

SUPERFAMILY RHABDITOIDEA

The superfamily Rhabditoidea includes but one species, found in man with sufficient frequency to deserve mention. This species is *Strongyloides stercoralis.*

STRONGYLOIDES STERCORALIS

Strongyloides stercoralis was first seen in 1876 by Normand in the feces of French colonial troops returned from Indo-China, some of which suffered a severe or even fatal diarrhea. Leuckart, in 1883, described the life cycle of the organism.

Geographical distribution.—*Strongyloides stercoralis* is rather widely distributed in the tropics, usually more or less coexistent with the human hookworm. In most areas, the infection rate is small, but occasionally it exceeds that of hookworm. In some parts of Panama, infection in as many as twenty percent of the population has been reported.

Morphology and life cycle.—*Strongyloides stercoralis* is unique among human parasites in being able to exist and reproduce indefinitely either as a parasite or as a free-living worm. Adults of the parasitic generation (at least the parasitic female) differ structurally from those of the free-living generation, although corresponding larval stages of the free-living and parasitic forms are the same in morphology. (See Figure 12.)

The parasitic female of *Strongyloides stercoralis* is a threadlike form, about two millimeters long. The oesophagus is cylindrical and extends through the anterior third of the body. The genital opening is at the mid-length. The thin-shelled eggs are partially embryonated when laid and hatch in the tissues. The parasitic male worm is very similar to the free-living male form, which will be described presently.

The free-living female worm is about one millimeter long and comparatively stouter than the parasitic female. It possesses an oesophagus of two portions: a slender anterior tube, and a posterior bulb which is set off from the anterior portion by a short constriction of the organ. The vulva is about mid-length, and partially embryonated eggs can usually be seen in the two-horned uterus. The free-living male is about 0.7 millimeter long. Its pointed posterior end is sharply curved ventrad. Two spicules generally are protruding from the anus of the male.

The rhabditiform larvae are slender forms with a distinctive oesophagus consisting of a slender anterior portion and a bulb situated immediately posteriorly. The filariform larvae are longer and comparatively more slender unsheathed forms whose simple oesophagus extends through almost half the body length and whose posterior tip is notched distinctively. It is sometimes necessary to distinguish these forms from the corresponding stages of hookworm larvae.

Since this form can survive and propagate itself as a free-living nonparasitic organism whenever necessary, the life cycle of *Strongyloides stercoralis* differs from that of other human parasites. When a suitable host is available, it can revert to the parasitic mode of life. The parasitic female dwells in the wall of the small intestine of man, and her eggs commonly hatch to the rhabditiform larvae before they leave the colon of the host. On reaching soil these forms moult to filariform larvae which enjoy the alternative possibilities of development into free-living males and females or infection of new vertebrate hosts. If the parasite develops to the free-living forms, these will mate, and first rhabditiform and then filariform larvae are produced. These

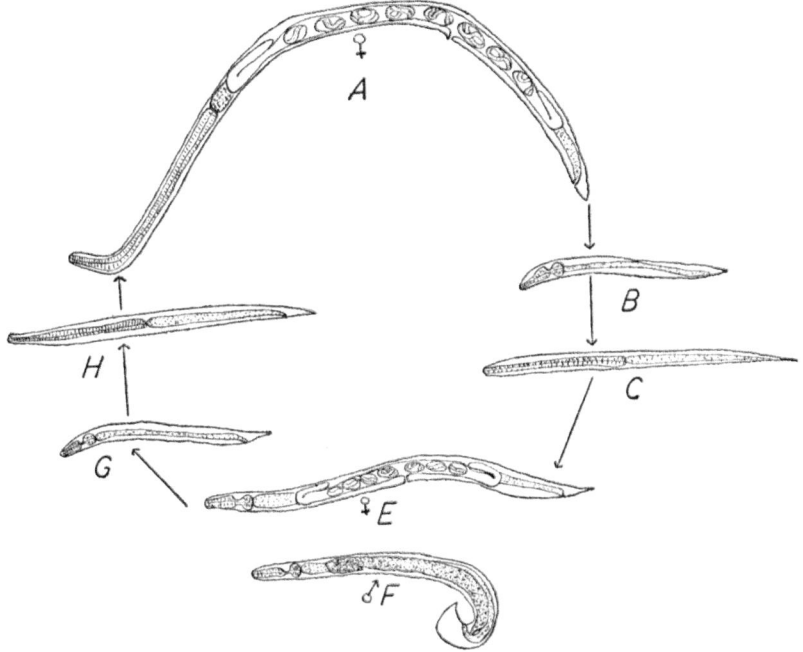

Figure 12. *Strongyloides stercoralis:* A, parasitic female; B and G, Rhabditiform larva; C and H, filariform larva; E, free-living female; F, free-living male.

filariform larvae, likewise, have the alternatives of growing to a new generation of free-living forms or, if a suitable vertebrate host is available, of taking up a parasitic existence. The vertebrate is usually invaded by way of the skin and venules. The larvae pass through the heart to the lungs, where they break out of the pulmonary veins into the alveoli. They then ascend the trachea and pass down the alimentary canal to the anterior small intestine. Here the parasitic female embeds herself in the intestinal wall and produces her eggs. The parasitic male presumably follows the same course as the female in its development, although it does not persist in the intestine. Fertilization of the female worm evidently occurs usually in the trachea or bronchi. It is possible that the female gives rise to young parthenogenetically.

Epidemiology.—Man and probably also dog, cat, and certain apes can be infected with *Strongyloides stercoralis.* Man is, however, decidedly the preferred host, since the parasite soon dies out in lower animals. Human infection usually results from contact with moist soil harboring filariform larvae but may occur after the ingestion of food or drink contaminated with such forms.

Pathogenicity.—There is only little local reaction to the skin penetration by filariform larvae, but symptoms suggestive of bronchopneumonia may be noted when infections are heavy and large numbers of worms break out of the pulmonary blood vessels into the aveoli. Hemorrhage into the aveoli and consolidation of parts of the lung are sometimes noted. Often the adult female worm lodges in the wall of the bronchi or trachea and leads to chronic bronchial inflammation. Perhaps the most serious effects, however, occur in the intestine, for here, because of the migration not only of the adult females but also of the newly hatched larvae, the intestinal epithelium and mucosa are badly eroded. A watery diarrhea without blood is usual. Not infrequently, especially in constipated individuals, infections are prolonged and internal reinfection may occur. This is a serious complication which, unless soon overcome, may lead to chronic invalidism.

Diagnosis.—Infection with *Strongyloides stercoralis* is diagnosed by finding rhabditiform larvae in the feces of the patient. The feces can also be cultivated, and within four or five days, the free-living adults appear. The sputum of those with bronchial infections sometimes contains larval forms. Usually, infected persons reveal a comparatively intense eosinophilia.

Specific therapy.—Gentian violet, sometimes given intravenously but much more commonly by mouth, is the only available drug which is effective in strongyloidiasis.

Prophylaxis.—Usually, infection with *Strongyloides* can be prevented by avoiding contact with soil or feces which contains the parasite.

SUPERFAMILY STRONGYLOIDEA

The superfamily Strongyloidea contains the important human hookworms, *Necator americanus* and *Ancylostoma duodenale*, as well as certain animal hookworms which sometimes cause disease in man.

NECATOR AMERICANUS

The species of hookworm which is found in man in the southern United States is *Necator americanus*.[4] It was described by Stiles in 1902 although observed earlier by Ashford and others.

Geographical distribution.—*Necator americanus* is found in the southern United States, in Mexico, through much of Central America, in the Caribbean Islands, and in northern South America, as well as in Central and South Africa and southern Asia.

Morphology and life cycle.—All hookworms possess an armed mouth capsule. *Necator americanus* has at the opening of this capsule one ventral and one dorsal pair of cutting plates (rather than "teeth," as in *Ancylostoma*). The anterior end of the worm is reflexed sharply dorsad. Females of this form are usually about one centimeter long, and males approximately 0.8 centimeter in length. The females are pointed at the posterior end, but males have a bursa copulatrix. This consists of a skirtlike extension of the chitinous body covering. It is supported by fleshy rays. In the female, the vulva opens somewhat anterior to mid-length.

The ovoidal egg which is passed in the feces of the infected person is enclosed by a thin hyaline shell. Usually, when passed, it is in the four-celled stage. The egg hatches in twenty-four hours or so after leaving the body to yield the first-stage rhabditiform larva, a free-living form about 250 microns long. After three days, this form moults to become a second-stage larva, in which the oesophagus gradually becomes (by the fifth day) filariform. This form, which also is free-living and measures about 300 microns long, moults on the sixth day to the third-stage larva, the old cuticle being retained by the third-stage larva as a sheath. The ensheathed third-stage form, which is about 600 microns long, is the infective stage for man. Its oesophagus is about one fourth the body length, and the posterior end of the larva is not notched (differences from filariform larva of *Strongyloides stercoralis*).

---

[4] Common synonym: *Uncinaria americana.*

Man is usually infected percutaneously, entrance being made through the skin of the toes or feet. The larva makes its way into small venules and is carried by the blood to the lung where it breaks out from the blood vessels into the aveoli. The larva then ascends the trachea and passes down the oesophagus to the anterior small intestine. Here it moults to the fourth-stage larva, which is like the adult except that it lacks sex organs. Within two or three days, this fourth-stage larva moults in the intestine to the fifth stage, which is the young adult form. This form matures during the ensuing three or four weeks, mates, and female worms produce the characteristic eggs found in the host's feces.

Epidemiology.—Hookworm infection is widespread in many parts of the tropics. In some rural areas of Puerto Rico, for example, eighty percent of the native population harbor the worm. Man usually becomes infected with *Necator americanus* by having contact with soil or water in which the third-stage filariform (infective) larvae are present. Man is probably the only significant vertebrate host, although certain apes, dog, cat, rhinoceros, pangolin, and possibly even the pig also are sometimes susceptible. Infection *per os* without the usual systemic development by the parasite probably can occur.

Pathogenicity.—In general, the pathology and symptoms in hookworm disease depend largely on the intensity of infections. When few worms are present, symptoms may be absent or negligible. With many worms, an acute or chronic wasting fatal disease may ensue. The disease involves chiefly the effects of the parasite in the skin, the lungs, and the intestine.

Most persons react rather severely to skin penetration by the larval stage. A dermatitis known as "ground itch" commonly develops. In this, papular or vesicular lesions occur chiefly in the skin between the toes. Pulmonary symptoms also are noted after intense infections and are caused by the larval worms breaking from the blood into the alveolar spaces of the lung.

The most severe damage caused by hookworms occurs when the adult worms are in the small intestine. When many worms are present, anemia and digestive disturbances may be manifest. The anemia usually results from the blood loss from the numerous sites where the worms are attached. The stools of such persons may contain much half-digested blood. Sometimes the anemia is profound, for not only does each worm itself withdraw constantly a significant volume of blood, but also hemorrhage continues from each bite wound long after the worm has detached itself and moved elsewhere. The worm evidently introduces an anticoagulant to the tissue of the intestinal wall which prevents the clotting of the host's blood. Blood formation also may be interfered with.

In children, physical growth as well as mental development may be seriously retarded by hookworm disease. Indeed, the skilled clinician in the tropics can diagnose, presumptively, many cases from the facial expression or manner which characterizes those who are infected. Such individuals seem lazy or shiftless and appear undernourished. They may show such symptoms as nervousness, potbelly, edema of the face, fever, bloody stool, and epigastric pain. Some patients have ravenous appetites, since food checks the pain in the epigastrium. Certain individuals are "dirt eaters," the desire to swallow soil coming from a need to fill the stomach and intestine with bulky materials. In fatal cases, there is fatty degeneration of the heart, liver, and kidneys and failure in heart action. Death generally occurs only after infection for several years.

Often, despite the presence of many worms in their intestine, individuals suffer little from hookworm disease. Their relative resistance seems to result from their having an adequate diet. If the diet is poor, the resistance is proportionately cut down.

Diagnosis.—The presence of the characteristic eggs in the feces is conclusive proof of infection with *Necator americanus*. (See Plate XIV, D, facing page 202.) The egg cannot be distinguished from that of the Old World hookworm, *Ancylostoma duodenale*. The presence of ground itch serves as a good point in clinical diagnosis of hookworm disease, although some other parasites cause similar skin reactions. An eosinophilia is usually noted.

Specific therapy.—Carbon tetrachloride and tetrachlorethylene are the two drugs used with best success in treating *Necator* infection. Often the administration first of iron compounds is advised, in order to overcome the patient's anemia and hemoglobin deficiency. When this condition has improved, specific treatment for the elimination of the parasite is then begun.

Prophylaxis.—The hookworm infection in any community is dependent upon pollution of the soil and the direct contact of the population with such polluted soil. Mass treatment of the population with drugs is often advised to reduce the possibility of soil infection. Educational programs, for both the individual and the community, are resorted to in an effort to inform the populace of the route of infection by hookworm and of methods to prevent infection. The installation of proper methods of sewage and feces disposal is always urged.

ANCYLOSTOMA DUODENALE

Ancylostoma duodenale [5] was first described by Dubini in 1843. Its relationship to miner's anemia, a disease of those engaged in digging the St. Gotthard railroad tunnel in the Alps, was first pointed out in 1878 by Grassi. The life cycle was experimentally completed by Looss in 1897.

Geographical distribution.—*Ancylostoma duodenale* is widely distributed, occurring in southern Europe, northern Africa, India, southeastern Asia, the East Indies, Australia, and South America.

Morphology and life cycle.—The life cycle of *Ancylostoma duodenale* is like that of *Necator americanus*, and most of the corresponding stages of the two parasites are very similar structurally. The adult worms, however, are easily differentiated. *Ancylostoma duodenale* is the larger, females of this species averaging twelve millimeters and males ten millimeters in length. The buccal capsule of *Ancylostoma duodenale* is oval rather than round in longitudinal section, and has on its ventral surface two pairs of teeth, of which the median pair is notched. There is no dorsal flexure of the head, as in *Necator americanus*. The vulva of the female is posterior, being about two thirds of the length from the head. The skirtlike bursa copulatrix of the male is supported by fleshy rays, from the pattern of which the species can be identified. (See Plate XIV, C, facing page 202.)

Epidemiology.—Man is infected with *Ancylostoma duodenale* by contact with soil or water contaminated with human feces from which the filariform larva of the parasite has developed. Although man himself is the probable source of essentially all human infections, the parasite will occasionally infect certain apes, pig, dog, and cat.

Pathogenicity.—Except for the fact that ground itch seldom is noted in infections with *Ancylostoma duodenale*, symptoms and pathology after infections with *Ancylostoma duodenale* and *Nector americanus*

---

[5] Common synonyms: *Anchylostoma duodenale; Agchylostoma duodenale.*

are the same, although more severe effects generally are seen with *Ancylostoma duodenale*. A few worms are of little significance but many lead to the typical hookworm disease—severe anemia, hemoglobin deficiency, and digestive disturbance.

Diagnosis.—The detection of eggs in the feces proves infection with hookworms. Often concentration procedures (salt or sugar flotation methods) must be resorted to for diagnosis, especially in old cases. Charcot-Leyden crystals sometimes occur in the feces. After a vermifuge, adult worms will be recovered.

Specific therapy.—The treatment of infection with *Ancylostoma duodenale* is the same as that with *Necator americanus*. Generally steps are taken first to overcome the anemia, then the hookworm itself is dislodged by carbon tetrachloride or tetrachlorethylene.

Prophylaxis.—Infection with *Ancylostoma duodenale* can be prevented in the same way as can that with *Necator americanus*—namely, by avoiding contact with soil or water in which filariform larvae occur. Proper disposal of infected human feces and the treatment of infected persons is advised.

ANCYLOSTOMA BRAZILIENSE AND ANCYLOSTOMA CANINUM

Two species of hookworms, found naturally in the dog and cat, sometimes cause disease in man. They are *Ancylostoma braziliense* and *Ancylostoma caninum*. They resemble *Ancylostoma duodenale* in most respects but differ in the "teeth" which guard the buccal capsule (Figure 13). *Ancylostoma braziliense* has two pairs of teeth, the median pair (which are unnotched) smaller than the lateral pair. *Ancylostoma caninum* possesses three pairs of buccal teeth. The life

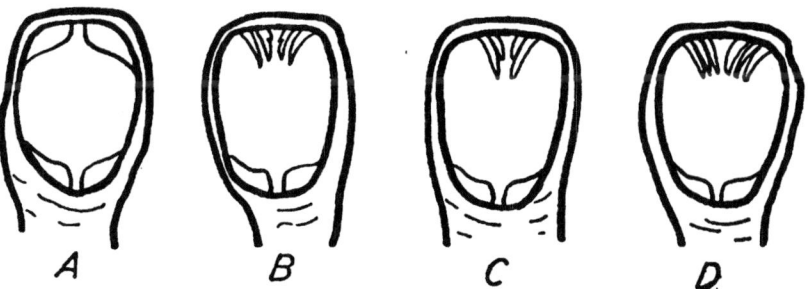

Figure 13. Mouth openings of adult hookworms: A, *Necator americanus;* B, *Ancylostoma duodenale;* C, *Ancylostoma braziliense;* D, *Ancylostoma caninum.*

cycles of these worms are essentially like that of *Ancylostoma duodenale*. The forms exist as adults in the intestine of the dog and cat and have only rarely been reported as adults from man.

In man, the larvae of these parasites cause a form of "creeping eruption," which has been observed especially in bathers on beaches of Florida. (See Plate XV, facing page 203.) Serpigenous tunnels are formed in the superficial layers of the skin of the patient, the larval parasite often going forward several centimeters during each day. Itching is severe, and inflammation marked. The parasites seldom get into the blood and do not develop beyond the filariform larva stage that penetrated the skin, even though present for months. The larvae can be killed in their tunnels by applying directly ethyl chloride or carbon dioxide snow. Prophylaxis involves avoiding soil contaminated with dog or cat feces. Infected dogs and cats should be treated to eliminate their adult worms.

SUPERFAMILY OXYUROIDEA

Only one species of this group is significant as a human parasite. This form is *Enterobius vermicularis*.

ENTEROBIUS VERMICULARIS

The human pinworm or seatworm, *Enterobius vermicularis*,[6] has been known since ancient times. The life cycle was experimentally completed by Leuckart in 1865.

Geographical distribution.—The pinworm has cosmopolitan distribution. Persons of untidy habits are especially likely to contract infection.

Morphology and life cycle.—The adult female *Enterobius vermicularis* is approximately one centimeter long (see Plate XIV, E, facing this page), and the adult male about half that length. Both are pointed terminally, the posterior end in the female particularly being greatly drawn out. The adults have a distinctive double-bulbed oesophagus, no "neck" occurring between the bulbs. The cuticle at the head end of the worm is inflated, and that along the body wall is extended as a "wing." The eggs are thick-shelled asymmetrical bodies which contain a tadpolelike larva (Plate XIV, F, facing this page). They are usually not laid by the gravid female until she has migrated through

---

[6] Common synonym: *Oxyuris vermicularis*.

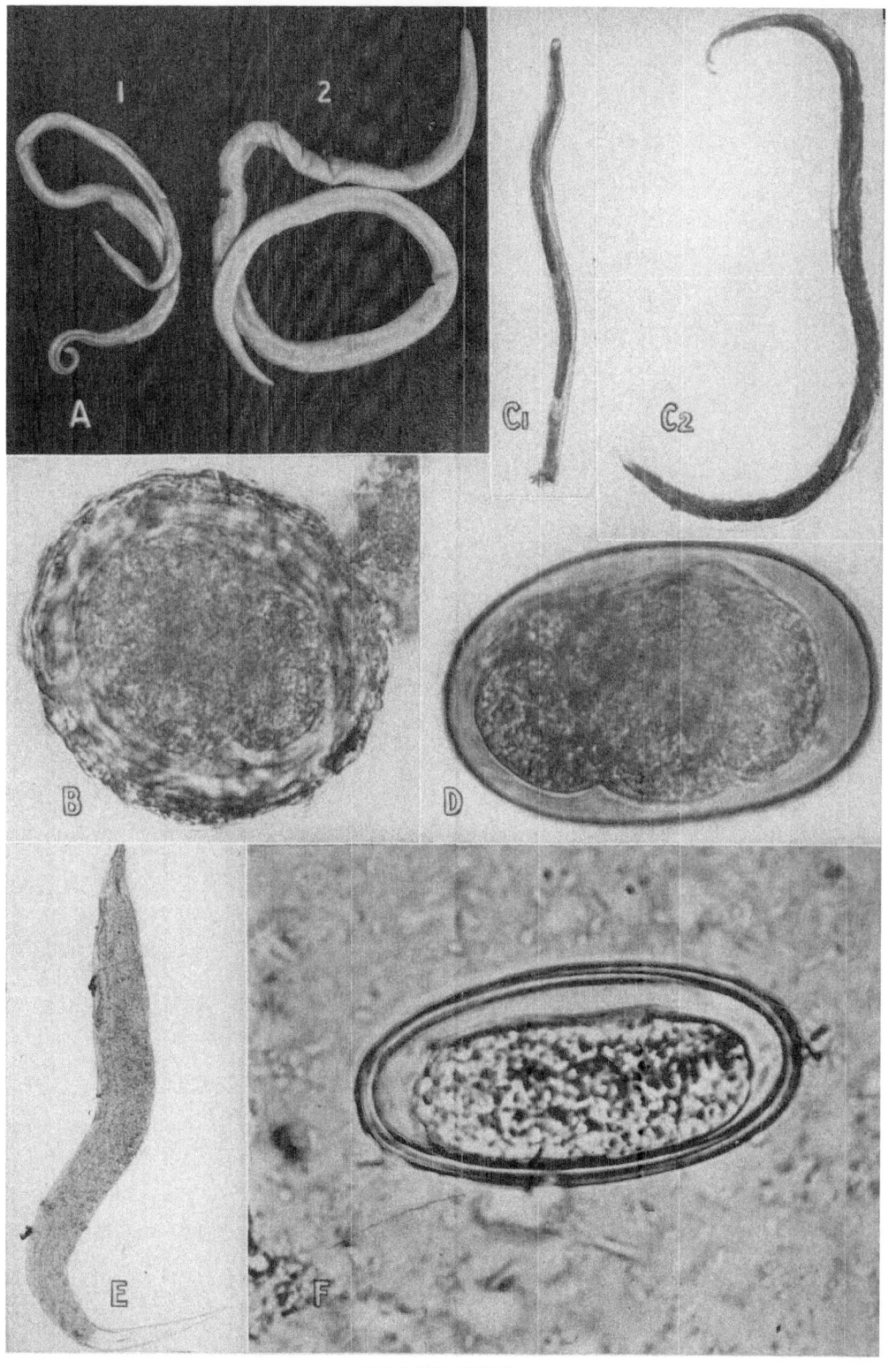

PLATE XIV

A. *Ascaris lumbricoides:* 1, male; 2, female. (x⅔) B. *Ascaris lumbricoides:* egg. (x750)
C. *Ancylostoma duodenale:* adults. 1, male; 2, female. (x10) D. Hookworm egg. (x750)
E. *Enterobius vermicularis:* gravid female. (x25) F. *Enterobius vermicularis:* egg. (x600)

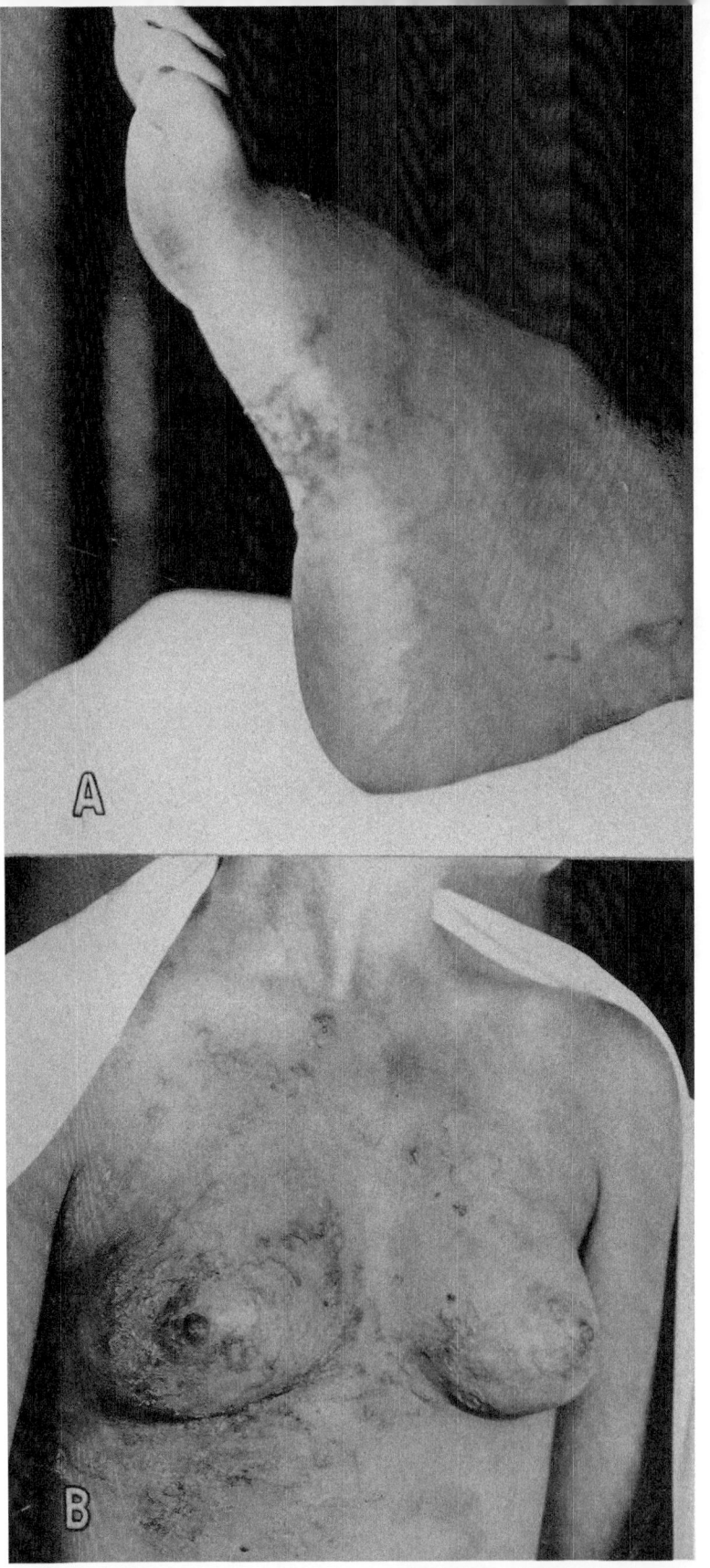

PLATE XV

A. Creeping eruption of the foot. Note tunnel of larval worm. B. Creeping eruption of the breast.

the large intestine and out of the anus. As she crawls over the perianal skin, she causes the infected person to scratch or rub the part. The gravid female body is ruptured during the scratching, and her eggs are sprayed over the surrounding clothing, and the hands and fingers. The egg must eventually reach the mouth of the same or of another person, if it is to develop. After the egg is swallowed, the rhabditiform larva is freed in the duodenum. It moults twice and grows to the adult stage which resides in the small intestine. After mating, the adult worms move to the large intestine, the caecum, or the appendix.

Epidemiology.—Pinworm infection is largely a familial disease, and if any in the family harbor the parasite, others are likely to become infected. The incidence of infection is particularly high in institutions, such as children's homes, in which many are crowded together, often with defective hygienic facilities. Man alone harbors the human species of pinworm. Children of school age are more commonly infected than adult persons.

Pathogenicity.—Nervous symptoms are frequently noted in infected persons if there is sufficient erosion of the intestinal mucosa to expose sympathetic nerves. Insomnia is common, and even epileptiform symptoms may develop. An intense and aggravating pruritis ani is usual, especially at night after the person has retired. Occasionally the worms cause vaginitis in women.

Diagnosis.—The embryonated eggs of the parasite as well as the adult worms may be recovered from the skin about the anus of infected persons, usually appearing in this site soon after the individual has retired. The eggs may also be observed in scrapings from beneath the fingernails. The adults can be recovered by enemas. Skin tests with extracts of *Enterobius* as well as of a rabbit pinworm have given promising results experimentally in diagnosis.

Specific therapy.—The administration of gentian violet is recommended for the elimination of the pinworm. Tetrachlorethylene also has been successfully used for the purpose. Repeated warm-water or soap enemas also are advised. Every member of a family should be examined, and all those infected given appropriate treatment. Great care must be exercised to prevent reinfection during the course of treatment.

Prophylaxis.—Infection can usually be prevented by avoiding contact with infected persons, their underclothing, their sleeping garments, and their bedclothes. Children should sleep in closed garments which prevent their scratching about the anus. Reinfection can thus be largely eliminated.

ASCARIS LUMBRICOIDES

Only one species of the superfamily Ascaroidea is significant as a human parasite. This is *Ascaris lumbricoides,* the large intestinal roundworm of man. It has been known since ancient times, but its complete life cycle was elucidated only in 1917. The worm has cosmopolitan distribution.

Morphology and life cycle.—*Ascaris lumbricoides* is a large worm, the females often measuring up to thirty centimeters in length and the males up to twenty-five centimeters. The ends of the worms taper to a point, and the posterior end of the male is coiled (Plate XIV, A, facing page 202). The head end has three lips, one dorsal and two ventrolateral. The vulva of the female worm is one third the body length from the head.

The eggs, which are immature when laid, are of oval shape. (See Plate XIV, B, facing page 202.) They are enclosed by a very thick shell, which is usually covered with an albuminous layer stained by the host's bile. After some weeks in the open, the eggs become embryonated and finally, after two moults, a third-stage larva is developed within the egg shell. This is the infective stage. Infection follows ingestion of the embryonated egg. The shell is digested off in the small intestine, and about three days later the larva appears in the liver. On the sixth or seventh day, it reaches the lung. It soon breaks out of the blood vessels to the alveoli, and then, after ascending the trachea, passes down the oesophagus to the small intestine, which it reaches about ten days after the embryonated egg was first ingested. In the intestine, it moults once more and grows to the adult stage.

Epidemiology.—Man is infected with *Ascaris lumbricoides* by swallowing the embryonated eggs of the parasite, generally directly from polluted soil, or as contaminants of food or drink. Children are chiefly infected and are chiefly responsible for the spread of the parasite.

Apparently man is alone the source of human infections, although morphologically identical parasites occur in the pig.

Pathogenicity.—Severe effects commonly follow heavy infections with the larval stage of *Ascaris lumbricoides*. Pneumonic symptoms develop as a result of the parasite breaking into the alveoli from the pulmonary vessels. Consolidations occur through the lung from the hemorrhage and trauma. The adult worm seldom causes great harm, although many worms may cause intestinal obstruction. When the adult worm migrates into the common bile duct or the appendix, acute and severe inflammation may result. Often the parasite migrates into the mouth or nose of a child or is vomited by him.

Diagnosis.—The recovery of the usually numerous eggs of *Ascaris lumbricoides* from the feces of patients is sufficient to prove infection with the parasite. Generally eosinophile counts do not rise greatly during this infection. Immunological tests are seldom used for diagnosis, although infected persons as well as some others manifest sensitivity to the antigens of the parasite.

Specific therapy.—Hexylresorcinol "crystoids" or a mixture of tetrachlorethylene and oil of chenopodium serve for eliminating *Ascaris lumbricoides*.

Prophylaxis.—Since infection with *Ascaris lumbricoides* generally occurs from soil polluted with infected feces, the treatment of all known cases is advised in prophylaxis. Children should be instructed not to defecate in the dooryard but to use sanitary privies. The infection of other children with whom they play and the reinfection of themselves will then be less probable. The use of human feces as fertilizer should, furthermore, be discouraged, for *Ascaris* eggs from such feces may persist on vegetables for months and retain their infectivity.

SUPERFAMILY FILARIOIDEA

Six species in the superfamily Filarioidea are of importance in human medicine. These are *Wuchereria bancrofti*, *Microfilaria malayi*, *Acanthocheilonema perstans*, *Mansonella ozzardi*, *Onchocerca volvulus*, and *Loa loa*. All are very specific parasites, the adult worms occurring, so far as known, only (or almost exclusively) in the human host. All are transmitted by bloodsucking insects.

WUCHERERIA BANCROFTI

The microfilariae of *Wuchereria bancrofti* [7] were first seen in 1863 by Demarquay in hydrocoele fluid. In 1866, Wucherer in Brazil observed them in chylous urine. The adult female worm was first recovered by Bancroft in Australia in 1876. In 1878, Manson passed the parasite through *Culex fatigans* and showed this insect to be an intermediate host, but transmission from the insect back to man was not accomplished until 1900.

Geographical distribution.—*Wuchereria bancrofti* is found in southeastern Asia and the East Indies, in India, Arabia, and the Near East, in Africa, and in northern South America and the Caribbean Islands. It occurs but little in Europe, being reported only from Barcelona in Spain and from Turkey and Hungary. In the United States it occurs only in the vicinity of Charleston, South Carolina.

Morphology and life cycle.—The threadlike adult worms occur in connective tissue. The female worms measure from five to ten centimeters long, the males about half this size. They are bluntly rounded at either end. No buccal capsule is present. The oesophagus is a single muscular bulb. The vulva of the female is located on the ventral side at about the mid-length of the oesophagus. The eggs become embryonated while still within the body of the adult female worm. After the embryos leave the female, the egg shell persists as a sheath. These so-called microfilariae, which measure from 150 to 300 microns in length, reach the lymph and blood vessels. Blood films of infected persons, if stained appropriately, reveal little internal structure for the microfilariae, although a column of nuclei is seen (Plate XVI, A, facing page 210). The microfilariae of different species of filarioid worms can be distinguished by the spacing of these nuclei. In *Wuchereria bancrofti*, the nuclei are absent from the tail end of the embryos. Typically, the embryos of this species are in the peripheral blood only at night, appearing at about seven or eight o'clock. They reach their greatest density between ten and two o'clock and are largely gone from the blood by six o'clock the following morning. In the Fijis and some other Pacific islands, no such periodicity is observed.

Wuchereria bancrofti is transmitted among human beings by the bite of certain mosquitoes. *Culex pipiens* and, in the warmer regions,

---

[7] Common synonym: *Filaria bancrofti.*

Culex fatigans are most widely implicated as natural transmitters. Many other species, including some of the genera *Aëdes* and *Anopheles* have been proved by experiment to be capable of transmitting the parasite. Within a few hours after the mosquito has bitten the infected person, the filarial embryo, which meanwhile has lost its sheath, migrates from the intestine into the thoracic muscles of the insect. Here it remains for some days, developing as a sausage-shaped larva generally lying parallel with the muscle fibers. After two moults during the course of ten days or so, a third-stage filariform larva is formed. This is the infective stage for man. It migrates into the head capsule of the mosquito and down to the labellae of the mouth parts. When next the mosquito bites a susceptible person, the larva migrates to his skin, which it actively penetrates, usually through the bite wound. The larvae probably pass through the blood vessels and the lympathics to lymph nodes. Here they grow to adults and mate and the females produce their embryos.

Epidemiology.—Man is the only vertebrate known to be infected with *Wuchereria bancrofti*. He becomes infected only through the bite of a mosquito carrying the larva of the parasite. Human blood containing microfilariae injected directly into another person will not lead to the infection of that person, since the parasite must develop to the infective larval stage in the body of the mosquito. As many as sixty percent or more of the native population in some endemic centers of the tropics will harbor the parasite.

Pathogenicity.—Symptoms are not manifested by most persons infected with *Wuchereria bancrofti*. No tissue reaction has been described against the circulating microfilariae, although the host tissue may hypertrophy about the adult worms. When the worms have been in the tissue for some time, leucocytic infiltration becomes marked. The parasites may become encapsulated and then are soon killed (Plate XVI, B and C, facing page 210). The microfilariae disappear from the peripheral blood after the adult worm dies. If the lymph flow is completely blocked by the tissue reaction to the adult parasites, an elephantoid condition of the part normally drained by the lymph vessel follows. This elephantiasis, as it is called, is noted most often in the legs but also in the scrotum, the vulva, the mammary glands, the arms, and other parts (Plate XVII, A and B, facing page 211). In the beginning the swelling may be temporary and accompanied by pain and fever. The affected region seldom recedes to its original size, however, and with subsequent attacks, grows even larger, with less recession subsequently. Bacterial infection may develop, and some authorities believe toxins of these bacteria, particularly streptococci, are responsible for the elephantiasis.

Diagnosis.—Infection with *Wuchereria bancrofti* is diagnosed by finding microfilariae in blood films of the patient (Figure 14). Calcified adults in lymph vessels can often be detected by X-ray photography. An extract of the dog heart worm, *Dirofilaria immitis*, will elicit a skin reaction or serve as antigen for the complement fixation test in filariasis.

Specific therapy.—No drug is effective upon the adult worms in *Wuchereria* infection, although various arsenicals may temporarily eliminate microfilariae from the peripheral blood. Surgical removal of elephantoid tissue or of calcified adult worms in or near lymph nodes may give temporary relief. Pressure bandaging of the swollen part is used with considerable success in some cases of elephantiasis.

Prophylaxis.—The avoidance of endemic areas is the best means of escaping *Wuchereria* infection. Where possible, steps should be taken to curb the multiplication of potential mosquito vectors.

MICROFILARIA MALAYI

Microfilaria malayi was first observed by Lichtenstein in 1927 in the peripheral blood of Celebes natives. It is now known to occur widely among the peoples of the East Indies and southeastern Asia. The adult parasite has not as yet been described. The ensheathed microfilariae are distinctive in possessing two discrete nuclei near the pointed posterior end of the body. (See Figure 14.) The parasite is transmitted by mosquitoes chiefly of the genera *Mansonella* and *Anopheles*, complete development to larvae occurring in about six days. Elephantiasis is rather frequently associated with this infection.

ACANTHOCHEILONEMA PERSTANS

The "persistent filaria," *Acanthocheilonema perstans,* was found by Daniels in British Guiana and was described by Manson in 1891. It is a widely distributed form, occurring in tropical and North Africa, in eastern South America, and in New Guinea. It is found in man and possibly in certain monkeys. It is transmitted by certain flies of the genus *Culicoides*. The adult worms dwell in the body cavity. Females, of which the posterior tip is bifurcated, are about seventy-five millimeters long, and males about half that size. The unsheathed microfilariae occur in the blood throughout the twenty-four-hour day, although they are more abundant during night hours. Nuclei are seen in the microfilariae all the way to the posterior tip. (See Figure 14.)

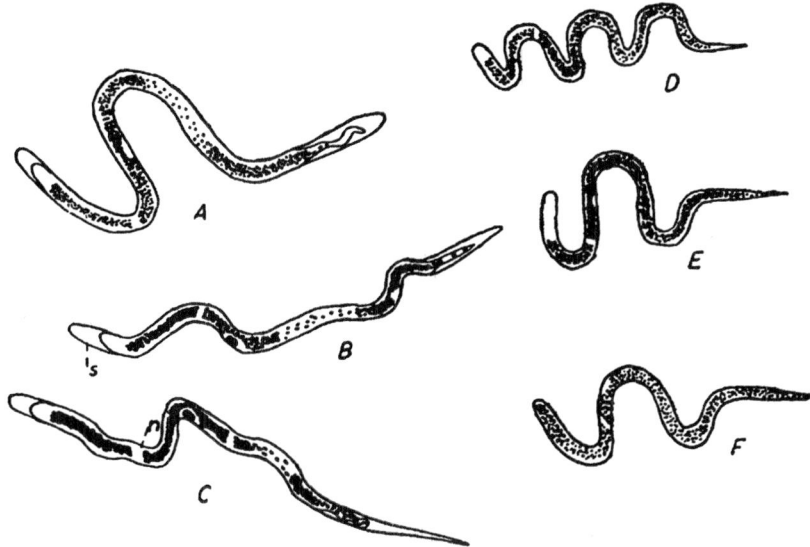

Figure 14. Diagram of microfilariae of man: A, *Wuchereria bancrofti;* B, *Filaria malayi;* C, *Loa loa;* D, *Onchocerca volvulus;* E, *Mansonella ozzardi;* F, *Acanthocheilonema perstans.* n = nerve ring; s = sheath. (Original)

No clinical condition is known to result from infection with this parasite. Its presence is diagnosed by finding the microfilariae in the peripheral blood. No specific treatment is known. Infection is prevented by avoiding the bite of species of *Culicoides* in endemic areas. The insects bite only in rather complete darkness.

MANSONELLA OZZARDI

Ozzard's filaria, *Mansonella ozzardi,* is a New World species, confined to certain Caribbean islands, Yucatan, Panama, northern South America, and Argentina. It was found by Ozzard and first described by Manson in 1897.

The adult worms live in the body cavity. Female worms, which are from seventy to eighty millimeters long, are identified by a pair of flaplike processes at the posterior end of the body. The microfilariae have no sheath, and appear in the peripheral blood with no periodicity. Unlike those of *Acanthocheilonema perstans*, the microfilariae of *Mansonella ozzardi* have no nuclei at their posterior ends. (See Figure 14.) The parasite is spread by *Culicoides furens*, developing in the thoracic muscles of this insect in about seven days.

Infected persons reveal no symptoms. The infection is diagnosed by finding the microfilariae in the peripheral blood. No treatment is known. Infection is prevented by avoiding the bites of *Culicoides furens* in endemic areas.

ONCHOCERCA VOLVULUS

Onchocerca volvulus [8] from an African source was first described by Leuckart in 1893. In 1915, the parasite was found in the New World—on the western slope of Guatemala. In 1926, Blacklock showed black flies to be intermediate hosts of the worm.

Geographical distribution.—*Onchocerca volvulus* occurs throughout Central Africa as well as in southern Mexico and Guatemala.[9]

Morphology and life cycle.—Adult female worms are often from forty to fifty centimeters long; male worms are about one tenth this size. Usually the adults are found fixed in nodules or cysts, from the tissue of which they can be extricated only with extreme difficulty. The microfilariae have no sheaths and are sharply pointed posteriorly. They are unique among the microfilariae of human filarioid worms in seldom entering the blood and in dwelling in cutaneous tissue especially near the parent worm, and in the tissue of the eye. The microfilariae have no nuclei either in their anterior or their posterior ends. (See Figure 14.) The parasite is transmitted by the black fly (e.g., *Eusimulium damnosum*) following its development during about six days in the thoracic muscles of that insect.

Epidemiology.—Man may be the only vertebrate host of *Onchocerca volvulus*, although similar worms occur in such animals as horse, deer, and cow. Man is infected by the bite of an infected black fly, insects which bite only during the day time. The flies occur only near well-

---

[8] Common synonym: *Onchocerca caecutiens*.

[9] R. P. Strong and associates, *Onchocerciasis in Africa and Central America*, *American Journal Tropical Medicine*, Supplement to Vol. 18 (1938).

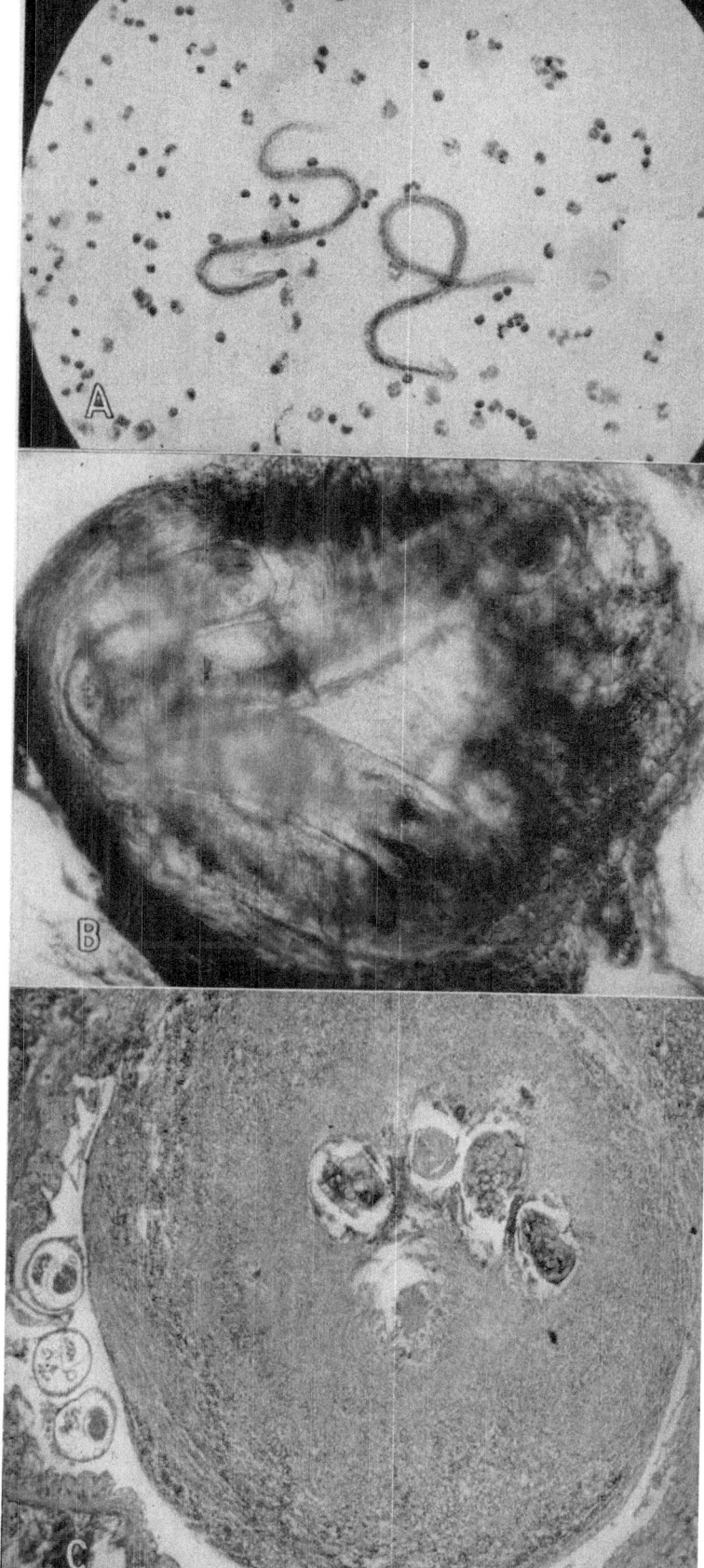

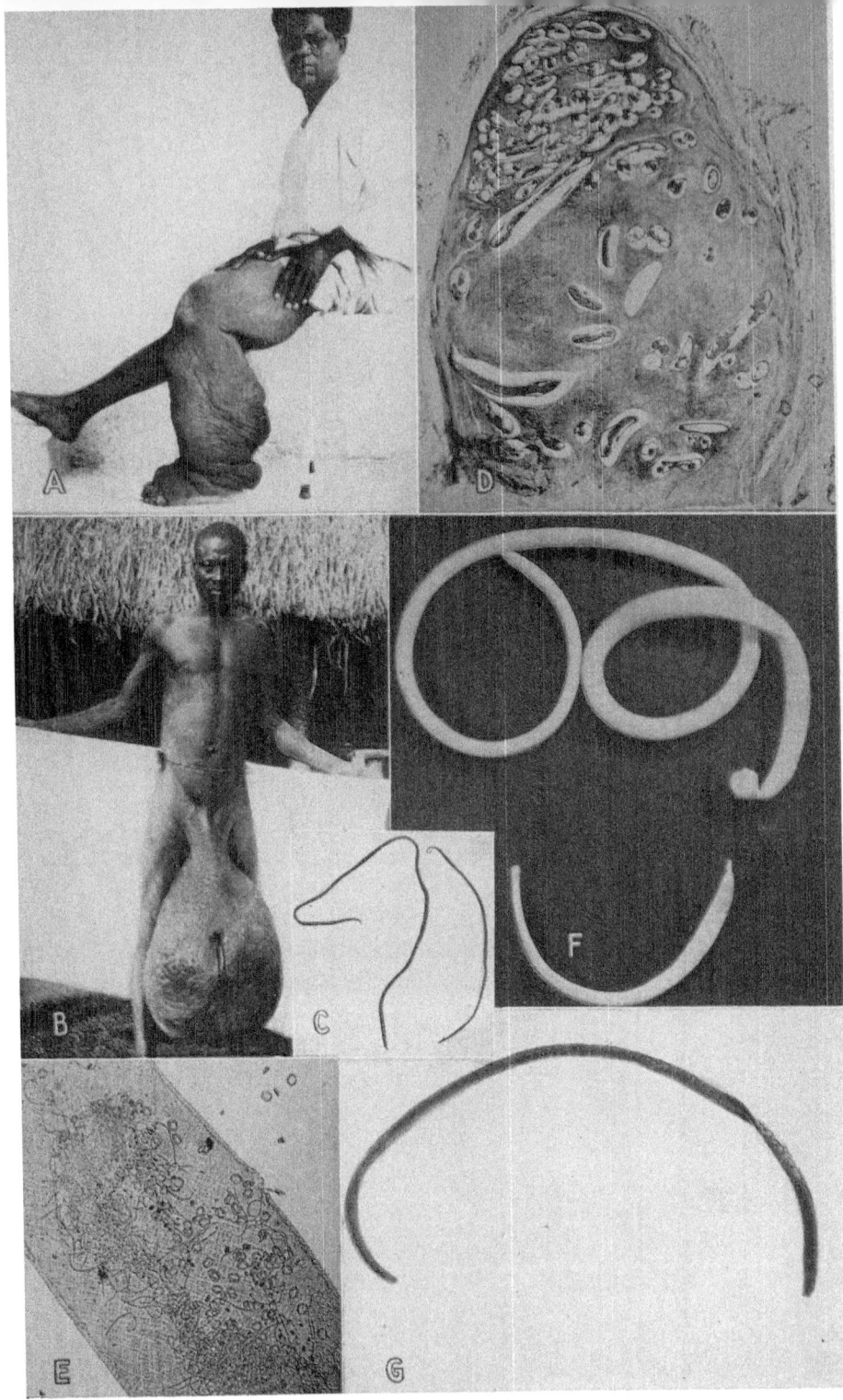

PLATE XVII

A. Elephantiasis of leg. B. Elephantiasis of scrotum. C. *Loa loa:* adults. (x1) D. *Onchocerca volvulus:* section of nodule showing portions of coiled adults. (x15) E. *Dracunculus medinensis:* embryos in strip of uterus of adult worm. (x750) F. *Macracanthorhynchus hirudinaceus:* adults. (x1) G. *Moniliformis moniliformis:* adult. (x3) aerated water, such as that of splashing, turbulent mountain streams, since their larvae require such water for development.

Pathogenicity.—Usually onchocerciasis is characterized by the formation of fibrous nodules about the parent worms (Plate XVII, D, facing this page). In the African disease, the nodules generally occur on the trunk, arms, or legs. In the New World cases, most nodules occur on the head. Usually the nodule is somewhat removed from but near the site where the fly has bitten the individual. Frequently many nodules occur on the same person. When nodules occur near the eye, blindness sometimes develops. This follows because the microfilariae invade the tissue of the eye and cause vascularization of the cornea, with resulting keratitis. When they migrate in tissue near the optic nerve, vision is disturbed, and if the optic nerve itself is invaded, complete blindness results. It is possible that "toxins" from the worms likewise disturb vision.

Diagnosis.—Onchocerciasis is diagnosed by finding microfilariae in the fluid from the nodules or by sectioning an excised nodule. In ocular infections, the microfilariae may be found in tissue obtained by biopsy from the conjunctiva. An eosinophilia is noted in persons whose blood contains microfilariae. The complement fixation or the skin test also is useful in diagnosis, antigen from the dog heart worm (*Dirofilaria immitis*) serving for the test.

Specific therapy.—The treatment of onchocerciasis is best carried on, when possible, by surgical removal of the superficial nodules enclosing the worms. Sometimes gentian violet or other anthelmintic, injected directly into cysts, kills the parasites. Plasmochin and fuadin seem to destroy the microfilariae, and their use is advised to avert blindness.

Prophylaxis.—Infection with *Onchocerca volvulus* is contracted only by persons who enter endemic areas and expose themselves to the bites of black flies. If all infected natives were treated surgically, or otherwise, the black fly population would probably soon lose its infection, since lower animals are not reservoirs of this parasite. Measures directed against the black flies themselves also are useful.

LOA LOA

The "eye worm," *Loa loa*, was evidently first removed from the eye of a Negress in Santo Domingo by Mongin in 1770. The life cycle was experimentally completed by the Connals in West Africa in 1922.

Geographical distribution.—The parasite occurs almost exclusively in Central and West Africa, where often the majority of persons in small villages will be infected.

Morphology and life cycle.—The adult female worm measures from five to seven centimeters long, and the male about half the size (Plate XVII, C, facing page 211). The cuticle bears small "warts" or bosses, which in the males are absent toward the ends of the body. The microfilariae which occur in the blood during the daytime are ensheathed, but, unlike those of other ensheathed forms, their nuclei are continuous to the posterior tip of the body. (See Figure 14.) Larval development occurs in the thoracic muscles of tabanid flies (*Chrysops dimidiata* and *Chrysops silacea*), the third-stage larva being the infective one for man.

Epidemiology.—Man and, possibly, the baboon are the only vertebrates known to harbor *Loa loa*. Infection occurs only through the bite of tabanid flies.

Pathogenicity.—As the adult worms migrate through subcutaneous tissue, temporary swellings (calabar swellings) are commonly noted. These are painless, and presumably result from prior sensitization of the patient to the excretions or "toxins" of the worm. They occur near the elbow or hip joint with considerable frequency but also are found about the eyes. The worm sometimes migrates across the bridge of the nose or the eyeball, and at this time can be removed surgically. It can be brought to the eyeball surface by applying hot compresses to the eye.

Diagnosis.—The presence of the characteristic microfilariae in the day blood proves infection with *Loa loa*. Skin tests or complement fixation tests also are useful in diagnosis, the antigen usually coming from the dog heart worm.

Specific therapy.—No drug is available for treating loaiasis. Surgical removal of the adult worms is practiced, if these appear on the eyeball or bridge of the nose.

Prophylaxis.—Infection is prevented by avoiding the bites of tabanid flies in endemic areas.

SUPERFAMILY DRACUNCULOIDEA

The only species of the superfamily Dracunculoidea infective for man is *Dracunculus medinensis*,[10] the guinea worm or the "fiery serpent" of ancient times. The infection with this worm is called dracunculiasis or dracontiasis.

DRACUNCULUS MEDINENSIS

The guinea worm has been known since biblical times. Its life cycle was first completed in a monkey by Leiper in 1907.

Geographical distribution.—Even today the guinea worm has about the same Old World distribution which it had in ancient times. It occurs in Egypt, Central and West Africa, the Near East, Russia, and India, as well as in the Dutch East Indies. In the Western Hemisphere, it is known in the islands of the Caribbean Sea, Brazil, and the Guianas.

Morphology and life cycle.—The gravid female is a large form, measuring up to about four feet in length. The adult male, at least as seen in experimentally infected dogs, is relatively minute, seldom measuring as much as three centimeters long. The female generally is seen deep in the subcutaneous tissue. When about to deliver her young embryos, the anterior end of the worm moves to the superficial tissues and the worm then secretes from this end a toxic fluid which causes the overlying skin to blister and break down, leaving an open ulcer. When water is poured repeatedly over the ulcer, the worm ejects some of the milky fluid with which the entire body is filled. This fluid contains many embryos (Plate XVII, E, facing page 211) which for development must infect copepods usually of the genus *Cyclops*. After all the embryos have been ejected, the parent worm is resorbed by the host. These embryos which succeed in entering *Cyclops* go on into the body cavity where they moult twice to become the third-stage (infective) larvae. When *Cyclops* containing this third-stage larva is swallowed by man (at least, as suggested in experiments with the dog), the vertebrate host becomes infected. The development in man has not been studied.

Epidemiology.—Man is infected presumably by swallowing, with raw water, *Cyclops* harboring larval worms. *Cyclops* is infected when per-

[10] Common synonym: *Fuellebornius medinensis*.

sons bearing the gravid female in their subcutaneous tissues enter streams or pools—the female at such times ejecting the embryos from the ulcer in the skin of the host.

Pathogenicity.—At the time the female worm secretes her toxin to form the cutaneous blister, patients generally suffer their first symptoms, which include such various anaphylaxislike effects as nausea, urticaria, asthma, diarrhea, and fainting. Later symptoms usually are the effects not of the guinea worm but of bacterial infection of the open ulcer, and these often are severe and sometimes are fatal.

Diagnosis.—The living adult worm itself can be seen in the subcutaneous tissue of patients, and dead calcified forms can be revealed by X-ray photography. Skin tests also are helpful in diagnosis, an extract of the specific parasite or of the dog heart worm being used as antigen in the test.

Specific therapy.—No specific drug is available for treating dracontiasis. Usually worms are removed mechanically a little at a time by intermittent traction.

Prophylaxis.—If water in endemic areas is boiled before being swallowed, infection with the guinea worm will be prevented. As a means of protecting others, infected persons must be prohibited from using wells or other open water supplies in which *Cyclops* might occur, in order not to infect the crustacean vector.

Chapter XVIII

THE ACANTHOCEPHALAN INFECTIONS

THE CLASS ACANTHOCEPHALA [1] includes those roundworms (phylum Nemathelminthes) which possess a retractile proboscis armed with recurved hooks. The bodies of the worms are cylindrical or flattened. There are no digestive organs. The sexes are separate, male worms being much smaller than females. The worms are parasitic in all stages. Transmission is through the dissemination of eggs, which, in the species which infect man, are mature when they leave the host. The egg is ingested by insects in which larval development takes place. Vertebrates become infected by ingesting the insect host.

Only two species of acanthocephalan (spiny- or thorny-headed) helminths infect man: *Macracanthorhynchus hirudinaceus* and *Moniliformis moniliformis*. Both forms are primarily parasites of animals and are merely accidental or sporadic parasites of the human host. Many other acanthocephalans are known, but these are confined to lower animals, notably to fish and birds.

MACRACANTHORHYNCHUS HIRUDINACEUS

Although the parasite was discovered in the pig in 1781 by Pallas, *Macracanthorhynchus hirudinaceus* [2] has been known to infect man only since 1859, when it was found by a Russian investigator, Lambl, in a child. Its occurrence was said by Lindemann in 1865 to be common among peasants of the Volga region of Russia, where the natives ate beetle larvae or grubs in which the parasite experiences part of its development. In the pig and some of its close relatives, such as wild boar and peccary, the worm has practically cosmopolitan distribution. It also occurs in the dog and certain monkeys.

[1] See footnote 1, Chapter II, p. 17.
[2] Common synonyms: *Gigantorhynchus hirudinaceus; Echinorhynchus gigas.*

Morphology and life cycle.—Three stages occur in the development of *Macracanthorhynchus hirudinaceus:* egg, larva, and adult. The female worm is quite large, measuring twenty-five to sixty centimeters in length by one-half to one centimeter in breadth (Plate XVII, F, facing page 211). The males are smaller, being generally from five to ten centimeters long by 0.3 to 0.5 centimeter broad. The white or pinkish posteriorly tapered body is flattened dorsoventrally and has transverse annulations which suggest segmentation. At the anterior end is a very small protrusible proboscis armed with five or six rows of recurved thornlike spines. The posterior tip of the female is rounded bluntly, whereas that of the male bears a bursa copulatrix.

The oval brown-shelled egg measures eighty to one hundred microns in length by forty to fifty microns in breadth. They are embryonated when laid, the embryos bearing anteriorly two pairs of hooks and having a spine-covered body. There are three embryonic envelopes.

The embryonated eggs which are passed with the host feces are ingested by any of various coleopteran (beetle) grubs, such as those of the June bugs, certain dung beetles, and some water forms. They hatch in the grub intestine, penetrate into its body cavity, and there develop to mature larvae which become encysted. The vertebrate host becomes infected by swallowing the beetle grub, the larval parasites promptly developing to adults in the vertebrate intestine.

Epidemiology.—The infection with *Macracanthorhynchus hirudinaceus* is one primarily of pig, wild boar, peccary, and related vertebrates which root through earth and eat the grubs found in earth. Man is infected only when he accidentally ingests an infected beetle grub. The incidence of human infection is negligible, although that of pigs is considerable.

Pathogenicity.—The pathogenicity of *Macracanthorhynchus hirudinaceus* for man is not known. The pig, however, suffers considerably from local trauma and inflammation at the site where the adult parasite is attached to the intestinal wall. Occasionally the wall is perforated and serious complications or even death may then occur. In intense infections, the host suffers marked emaciation.

Diagnosis.—Infection with *Macracanthorhynchus hirudinaceus* can be diagnosed by observing eggs of the parasite in the feces of the vertebrate host.

Specific therapy.—No very effective drug is available for the elimination of *Macracanthorhynchus hirudinaceus*. Nicotine sulphate and carbon tetrachloride have proved to be the most effective of numerous materials tested.

Prophylaxis.—Prophylaxis against the pig acanthocephalan involves either of two procedures: (1) eliminating adult worms from vertebrates, so that beetle grubs cannot be infected, or (2) preventing the ingestion of beetle grubs by vertebrates.

MONILIFORMIS MONILIFORMIS

Moniliformis moniliformis [3] is found in rats over much of the world but has been reported only rarely in man.

Morphology and life cycle.—The female parasite measures from ten to thirty centimeters long by 0.3 to 0.5 centimeter broad. (See Plate XVII, G, facing page 211.) The male worms are about one third this size. The body, which falsely gives the impression of segmentation, has rather square ends and bears, at the anterior end, a protrusible proboscis with from twelve to fifteen rows of hooks. The ellipsoidal eggs, which measure one hundred microns long, are embryonated when laid. The spinose embryos carry two pairs of hooks. When the eggs are swallowed by any of several roaches or beetles, they hatch and larvae (acanthors) penetrate the intestinal wall of the insect, where they encyst. After four to six weeks, the mature larvae, then measuring up to 1.8 millimeters long, are found in the body cavity of the roach. The rat or, rarely, human beings become infected by swallowing the infected roach, the worms reaching maturity in the vertebrate intestine in about five weeks.

Pathogenicity.—Little is known of the pathogenicity of *Moniliformis moniliformis* although local trauma and inflammation at the point of attachment in the intestine could be expected. In one experimentally infected human case, gastrointestinal symptoms set in nineteen days after infection.[4]

Diagnosis.—The presence of *Moniliformis moniliformis* is established by finding the eggs of the parasite in the feces.

---

[3] Common synonyms: *Echinorhynchus moniliformis; Gigantorhynchus moniliformis.*
[4] B. Grassi and S. Calandruccio, *Centralblatt für Bakteriologie, Parasitenkunde, und Infektionskrankheiten, Originale,* 3: 521 (1888).

Specific therapy.—Little is known concerning specific therapy of *Moniliformis* infection. *Aspidium filix-mas* was said to have eliminated the parasite from the experimental human case referred to above. The trial of nicotine sulphate and of carbon tetrachloride seems indicated.

Prophylaxis.—Infection of man is prevented by safeguarding food and drink from contamination with the bodies of roaches or beetles infected with the larval stage of the parasite.

Chapter XIX

ARTHROPODA OF MEDICAL IMPORTANCE: HEXAPODA (INSECTA)

T HE PHYLUM ARTHROPODA includes most of the ectoparasites of man and some forms which dwell within human tissues. Many species of the phylum are important, not because they themselves cause disease, but because they transmit other organisms which are disease agents. The arthropods are bilaterally symmetrical, metamerically segmented forms which are encased in a chitinous exoskeleton. Most species are divided structurally into three parts: head, thorax, and abdomen, from some or all of which arise jointed appendages. Motion is effective by the contraction of striated muscles which pass from one body segment to the next. Respiration is by tracheal tubes in the terrestrial forms and by gills in the aquatic species. The nervous system consists of a pair of ganglia in each segment, the units of each pair being connected with those of the other segments to form two longitudinal nerve trunks. The ganglia in the head represent the brain. Reproduction is chiefly by sexual methods, the sexes being separate.

The arthropods of medical importance are found in the classes Hexapoda (or Insecta), Arachnida, Crustacea, and Myriapoda. The members of these classes are rather easily differentiated, as is indicated in Chapter II, by the number of their legs. In the present chapter, representatives of the class Hexapoda (the six-legged forms) are described and their significance in medicine is indicated. Those of the other classes are discussed in Chapter XX.

HEXAPODA

The hexapods or insects have bodies which are divided into segments grouped into three distinct regions: head, thorax, and abdomen.

A pair of antennae arise from the head, these serving as sense organs. A pair of compound eyes, as well as several simple eyes called ocelli, are usually present. The mouth parts may be suited for sucking blood or other fluids, for rasping tissue, or for chewing solid substance. There are three pairs of legs and usually two pairs of wings attached to the thorax. The abdomen of insects has no appendages.

The insect food canal consists of a fore-intestine, of which the salivary glands represent a diverticulum, the mid-intestine, and the hind-intestine. The blood is a colorless fluid which fills the "body cavity" or hemocele. The excretory system consists of the Malpighian tubules, which arise where the mid- and hind-intestine join and float in the blood of the hemocele. Respiration is chiefly through long tracheal tubes which arise from spiracles on the sides of the body and float in the hemocele.

The sexes are separate. Females have paired ovaries, made up of ovarioles. The ovarioles open into oviducts which unite to form a vagina which opens just ventrad of the anus. A spermatheca, which is a diverticulum of the vagina, receives and stores sperm cells. Males have a pair of testes, each with a vas deferens swollen at one point along its length to form a seminal vesical. The two vas deferens unite posteriorly to form an ejaculatory duct which is partially enclosed in a chitinous invagination adapted for intromission.

The metamorphosis of insects is either gradual or complete. In gradual metamorphosis, the egg hatches to a young form (nymph) which resembles in general appearance the adult insect which it eventually becomes. In complete metamorphosis, the egg hatches to a young form (larva) which after growth passes through a quiescent stage (pupa) in which profound changes in structure and appearance take place. The adult—which appears strikingly different from the earlier stages—emerges from the pupa.

The insects of significance in medicine occur in seven orders of the class Hexapoda: Anoplura, Hemiptera, Coleoptera, Lepidoptera, Diptera, Siphonaptera, and Hymenoptera. These orders can be differentiated by the following key:

A. Typically wingless forms; mouth parts for sucking
    I. Body compressed dorsoventrally; hind legs not for jumping; tarsi with single large claw; metamorphosis incomplete—Anoplura (lice)

II. Body compressed laterally; hind legs for jumping; tarsi without large claw; metamorphosis complete—Siphonaptera (fleas)

B. Typically winged forms; mouth parts for sucking or chewing

    I. One pair of wings only; second pair of wings replaced by halteres (balancing organs)—Diptera (flies, mosquitoes)

    II. Two pairs of wings

        1. All wings membranous, sometimes with scales

            a. Wings without scales; female abdomen often terminating in sting—Hymenoptera (bees, wasps, ants)

            b. Wings covered with scales; female without sting—Lepidoptera (moths)

        2. Some wings not membranous

            a. Anterior wings thickened (leathery) basally; mouth parts for sucking; metamorphosis incomplete—Hemiptera (true bugs)

            b. Anterior wings thickened throughout to form protective covering or elytra; mouth parts for chewing; metamorphosis complete—Coleoptera (beetles)

The different insect orders vary much in relative importance. Some include but few forms with little medical significance, whereas others include species responsible either directly or indirectly for some of the greatest scourges of mankind. The mode of causing harm to man also varies much. Some species attack man and suck his blood, inoculate him with their venom, or actually invade his tissues. Other species are themselves relatively harmless but transmit disease agents to man. Table 6 presents information for some of the more significant insects.

THE ANOPLURA (LICE)

GENERAL MORPHOLOGY

The Anoplura or lice are wingless insects which live on the skin or in the hair of mammals. Their extensible mouth parts are adapted for piercing the skin and sucking the blood of their hosts. Their bodies are flattened dorsoventrally, with the head free and horizontal. Their compound eyes are vestigial or absent, and ocelli are always lacking. Their antennae have from three to five joints.

LIFE CYCLE

Lice eggs or nits, which are cemented to the hairs of the host or to the fibers of clothing, hatch several days after being laid to yield a

TABLE 6

REPRESENTATIVE INSECTS IMPORTANT IN MEDICINE

Order	Scientific Name	Common Name	Importance
Anoplura	Pediculus humanus	human louse	irritating bite; vector of rickettsiae of typhus and trench fever; vector of spirochetes of relapsing fever
Hemiptera	Cimex lectularius	bedbug	irritating bite
	Triatoma megista	kissing bug	vector of *Trypanosoma cruzi*
Lepidoptera	Euproctis phaeorrhoea	brown-tail moth	hairs of caterpillars contain venom causing urticaria
Diptera	Phlebotomus argentipes	Sand fly	probably transmits *Leishmania donovani*
	Phlebotomus papatasii	Sand fly	probably transmits *Leishmania tropica;* vector of virus of Pappataci fever and bartonella of Verruga peruana
	Culex pipiens and Culex fatigans	mosquito	transmit *Wuchereria bancrofti*
	Aëdes aegypti	mosquito	vector of yellow fever and dengue fever
	Aëdes sollicitans	mosquito	fierce biter
	Anopheles quadrimaculatus	mosquito	vector of malaria (in United States)
	Eusimulium damnosum	black fly	vector of *Onchocerca volvulus*
	Culicoides austeni	gnat	probable vector of *Acanthocheilonema perstans*
	Chrysops dimidiata	mangrove fly	vector of *Loa loa*
	Chrysops discalis	deer fly	vector of tularemia
	Tabanus striatus	horsefly	vector of anthrax
	Stomoxys calcitrans	biting stable fly	irritating bite
	Glossina palpalis	tsetse fly	vector of *Trypanosoma gambiense*
	Glossina morsitans	tsetse fly	vector of *Trypanosoma rhodesiense*
	Musca domestica	housefly	vector of cysts and eggs of intestinal parasites and of enteric bacilli
	Cochliomyia macellaria	screwworm fly	eggs laid in open wounds
	Cordylobia anthropophaga	tumbu fly	larvae penetrate skin of feet of children
	Dermatobia hominis	human warble fly	larvae cause boil-like lesion in man
Siphonaptera	Tunga penetrans	sand flea	fertile female enters soft skin (e.g., between toes) for egg development

Order	Scientific Name	Common Name	Importance
Siphonaptera	Pulex irritans	human flea	irritating bite; potential vector of bubonic plague
	Xenopsylla cheopis	tropical rat flea	important vector of bubonic plague; vector of endemic typhus fever
Hymenoptera	Apis mellifica	honeybee	irritating sting

nymphal form morphologically similar to the adult louse. The nymphs develop through two subsequent nymphal stages and within a month after the eggs are produced become sexually mature adults. The lice are wholly dependent upon their hosts for food and usually do not leave the host for more than a few hours at any time. They readily transfer to other hosts of the same species on the slightest contact, although they do not generally live for long on other species of vertebrates.

SPECIES IMPORTANT IN MEDICINE

Two species of human lice are important in medicine: *Pediculus humanus*, the body or head louse and *Phthirus pubis*, the crab louse. Two distinct types or varieties of *Pediculus humanus* are recognized, *Pediculus humanus* variety *capitis*, found on the head, and *Pediculus humanus* variety *corporis*, found in the clothing or in the hair of the chest. Several lice of animals also are important in the transmission among animals of disease agents responsible for potential infections of man. (See Plate XVIII, A, B, and C, facing page 228.)

Pediculus humanus.—A characteristic roughness and pigmentation of the skin of frequently bitten areas (vagabond's disease) is noted in persons who harbor lice more or less continuously. Even a single bite is irritating to most people, and frequent bites cause nervousness, loss of sleep, and general irritability. Some individuals, however, seem immune to the bites of lice.

The two types of *Pediculus humanus* cause disease in man not only through their bites but also through transmitting other disease agents. The head louse and the body louse are both responsible for the spread of the rickettsial infections, European epidemic typhus fever and trench fever, as well as for the transmission of the spirochetal disease, relapsing fever, in India and parts of Africa. Infection with the rickettsiae may result from the insect bite or by contamination of the bite wound with the louse feces or the crushed louse tissue which contains rickettsiae. Infection with the relapsing fever spirochete evidently occurs when the louse body is crushed on the skin or between the fingernails. The spirochetes penetrate either through the skin or through the membrane under the nails.

Phthirus pubis.—The crab louse is most commonly found on the pubic hair but may attach itself to hair elsewhere on the body. Sometimes it is found on the chest hair and also on eyelashes. The local irritation in those bitten by the crab louse is the chief effect, this irritation sometimes being extremely annoying. Relapsing fever is said to be transmitted by the crab louse, although typhus fever is not.

Lice of lower animals.—*Polyplax spinulosa*, the common louse of the rat, is the vector among rats of the rickettsia of endemic typhus (murine typhus) in southeastern United States. (See Plate XVIII, D, facing page 228.) The rabbit louse, *Haemodipsus ventricosus*, is a natural vector of tularemia among rabbits. Neither of these lice, however, carries the disease named to man.

CONTROL MEASURES

Measures for the control of lice are directed either against the infested individual or against the infested community. The infested individual should be segregated, then thoroughly cleansed with soap and water, his hair shaven if necessary, and his scalp and other hairy parts treated with larkspur, phenol, kerosene, or other pediculicide. His clothing should be sterilized, especially by steam under pressure. Mass treatment must be used in heavily infested communities, and the general population instructed in or given facilities for the elements of personal cleanliness.

THE HEMIPTERA (TRUE BUGS)

GENERAL MORPHOLOGY

The members of the order Hemiptera typically have four wings, the first pair of which are thick and leathery at the base but thin and membranous terminally. The mouth parts of all are fitted for piercing and sucking, the beak arising from the front of the head. The forms experience gradual metamorphosis.

The hemipterans or true bugs which have importance in medicine are confined to two families: The bedbugs of the family Cimicidae, and the assassin or cone-nosed bugs of the family Reduviidae.

Bedbugs.—Two species, *Cimex lectularius* in the temperate zone and *Cimex hemiptera* in the tropics, are the most important bedbugs of man (Plate XVIII, E, facing page 228.) These forms both feed naturally on human blood, and some individuals suffer much from their bites. Nervous symptoms or even symptoms of digestive upset are manifested by some persons following frequent bites. Children suffer most. Neither of these species, despite the close association of both with man, has been shown naturally to transmit any disease agent among human beings, although both forms can be infected experimentally with such human disease agents as the plague bacillus (*Pasteurella pestis*), the leishmanias of kala azar (*Leishmania donovani*) and Oriental sore (*Leishmania tropica*), the spirochetes of relapsing fever (*Borrelia recurrentis*), the trypanosome of Chagas's disease (*Trypanosoma cruzi*), and the filtrable virus of yellow fever.

The eradication of bedbugs from houses is not an easy task but is generally possible. The bugs are killed by any of various fumigants, such as sulphur dioxide, hydrocyanic acid, or "cyanogas" (calcium cyanide). Steam or hot air also is effective in killing the bugs. Various sprays, often consisting largely of kerosene, also are used. Generally, unless the premises are thereafter kept clean, the insects will soon return.

The assassin bugs.—A number of assassin bugs are domesticated forms known to act as bloodsuckers upon man or animals. These are found mostly in the Reduviid genera *Triatoma, Rhodnius, Melanolestes, Erathyrus,* and *Rasahus.* They are capable of inflicting painful wounds, although usually there is comparatively little discomfort, and individuals bitten at night are seldom awakened by the injury. Since they often insert their proboscis in their sleeping victim near or at the edge of the lips, they are sometimes called "kissing bugs."

A few assassin bugs are natural vectors of *Trypanosoma cruzi*, which causes Chagas's disease. The species most important in transmitting this parasite to man are *Triatoma megista, Rhodnius prolixus,* and *Rhodnius pictipes.*

The Coleoptera (Beetles)

GENERAL MORPHOLOGY AND LIFE CYCLE

Most beetles have four wings, the anterior pair being greatly thickened to form an elytron which affords protection to the membranous posterior wings and the insect body. The mouth parts are suited to chewing rather than piercing. The metamorphosis is complete. Eggs are produced which hatch to grubs commonly found in soil, wood or plant tissue, food stores, or decaying matter. After pupation, adult beetles appear.

SPECIES IMPORTANT IN MEDICINE

Beetles of two families, the Meloidae or blister beetles and the Staphylinidae or rove beetles, are of occasional significance in medicine because of the urticating or vesicating properties of certain representatives. The blister beetles (e.g., *Meloe* spp.) contain cantharidin in their body fluids. This drug is active externally as a blistering agent and internally as a stimulant of the urinary and reproductive systems. A dermatitis may be produced by handling the forms and especially by crushing them against the skin. The rove beetles which have vesicating properties are found in the genus *Paederus*.

The larvae (grub) of some beetles serve as the intermediate hosts of helminth parasites. The pig acanthocephalan, *Macrocanthorhynchus hirudinaceus*, is found in the grubs of June bugs (*Phyllophaga* spp.).

The Lepidoptera (Moths and Butterflies)

GENERAL MORPHOLOGY AND LIFE HISTORY

Lepidopterans have four membranous wings covered with overlapping scales. They have mouth parts fitted for sucking the nectar of plants, although not for piercing the skin of animals for blood. Their metamorphosis is complete. The egg hatches to a caterpillar which pupates in a cocoon or a chrysalis from which the insect emerges as an adult moth or butterfly.

SPECIES IMPORTANT IN MEDICINE

A considerable number of species of the order Lepidoptera have larvae (caterpillars) of which certain modified body hairs cause more or less severe urticaria in man. Their effect stems from the presence within these special hairs of a poisonous fluid. When these hairs are broken, the contained fluid pours from them. When the fluid either penetrates the human skin or flows over it, a severe urticaria follows. People vary much in their susceptibility to the urticating effect. When a species to which many persons are susceptible, such as caterpillars of the flannel moth (*Megalopyge opercularis*), occurs in great abundance, as this form sometimes does, an epidemic of dermatitis follows in a community. Many persons also are susceptible to the poison from hairs of the brown-tail moth caterpillar, *Euproctis phaeorrhoea*. The poison is apparently of the character of a true venom.

THE DIPTERA (FLIES AND MOSQUITOES)

GENERAL MORPHOLOGY AND LIFE CYCLE

The dipterans have but two wings, which are borne by the mesothorax. Nearly all forms have, in place of the second pair of wings, knobbed halteres. Mouth parts are adapted for sucking. The metamorphosis is complete. Eggs hatch to larvae known as maggots, which pupate and then emerge as adults.

SPECIES OF MEDICAL IMPORTANCE

The dipterans of medical importance are found in the families Psychodidae (moth flies or sand flies), Culicidae (mosquitoes), Simuliidae (black flies), Chironomidae (gnats), Tabanidae (horseflies), Muscidae (houseflies, tsetse flies, blowflies, etc.), Anthomyidae (lesser houseflies and latrine flies), Oestridae (warble and bot flies), and Syrphidae (hover flies). In some of these families, especially in the Culicidae, numerous species of great importance are included. The most significant representatives of each family will be briefly discussed.

PSYCHODIDAE (MOTH FLIES, SAND FLIES)

Moth flies or sand flies are small insects, seldom over 0.5 centimeter in length. Their bodies are covered with hair. They have oval wings of simple venation and long antennae with sixteen segments, each of which bears numerous short hairs. Some have mouth parts fitted for sucking blood.

The bloodsucking members of the family Psychodidae are contained in the single genus *Phlebotomus*. Certain species of this genus are important as the vectors of various diseases. Doerr proved in 1908 that a sand fly, *Phlebotomus papatasii*, could transmit the filtrable virus of three-day fever (also called Pappataci fever and phlebotomus fever). Sand flies, *Phlebotomus verrucarum* and *Phlebotomus noguchii*, have also been known since 1912 to transmit the bartonella (*Bartonella bacilliformis*) of Oroya fever (also called Verruga peruana and Carrion's disease) in South America. The transmission of leishmania infections by sand flies has also long been suspected, although proof of such transmission is till now lacking. The parasites of kala azar and Oriental sore are known to develop in sand flies, and macerated infected flies injected into human beings cause the corresponding diseases, but infection naturally by the sand fly bite or by natural contamination of the bite wound by feces of the sand fly does not occur. *Phlebotomus argentipes*, *Phlebotomus chinensis*, and *Phlebotomus sergenti* are all suspected of transmitting *Leishmania donovani* of kala azar, *Phlebotomus papatasii* is probably the vector of *Leishmania tropica* of Oriental sore, and *Phlebotomus intermedius* is the suspected vector of *Leishmania braziliensis* of espundia.

CULICIDAE (MOSQUITOES)

Mosquitoes are identified by the characteristic venation of their wings and by the presence of scales on the veins and the posterior border of the wings. The antennae are long, and each segment bears a whorl of hairs. In males, these hairs often give a bushy appearance to the antennae.

The metamorphosis of mosquitoes is complete. Eggs are laid on or very near water. The larvae, known as wigglers or wrigglers, are aquatic but breathe air through a breathing tube which extends from the posterior end of the body. This tube is protruded through the surface film of water to the air, for respiratory purposes. Pupation goes on in water, and adults emerge from the pupae directly to the air.

The mosquitoes of medical importance occur in the two tribes, Culicini and Anophelini. These tribes include the transmitters of such important diseases as yellow fever, dengue fever, malaria, and filariasis. Furthermore, some species, although not known to transmit any

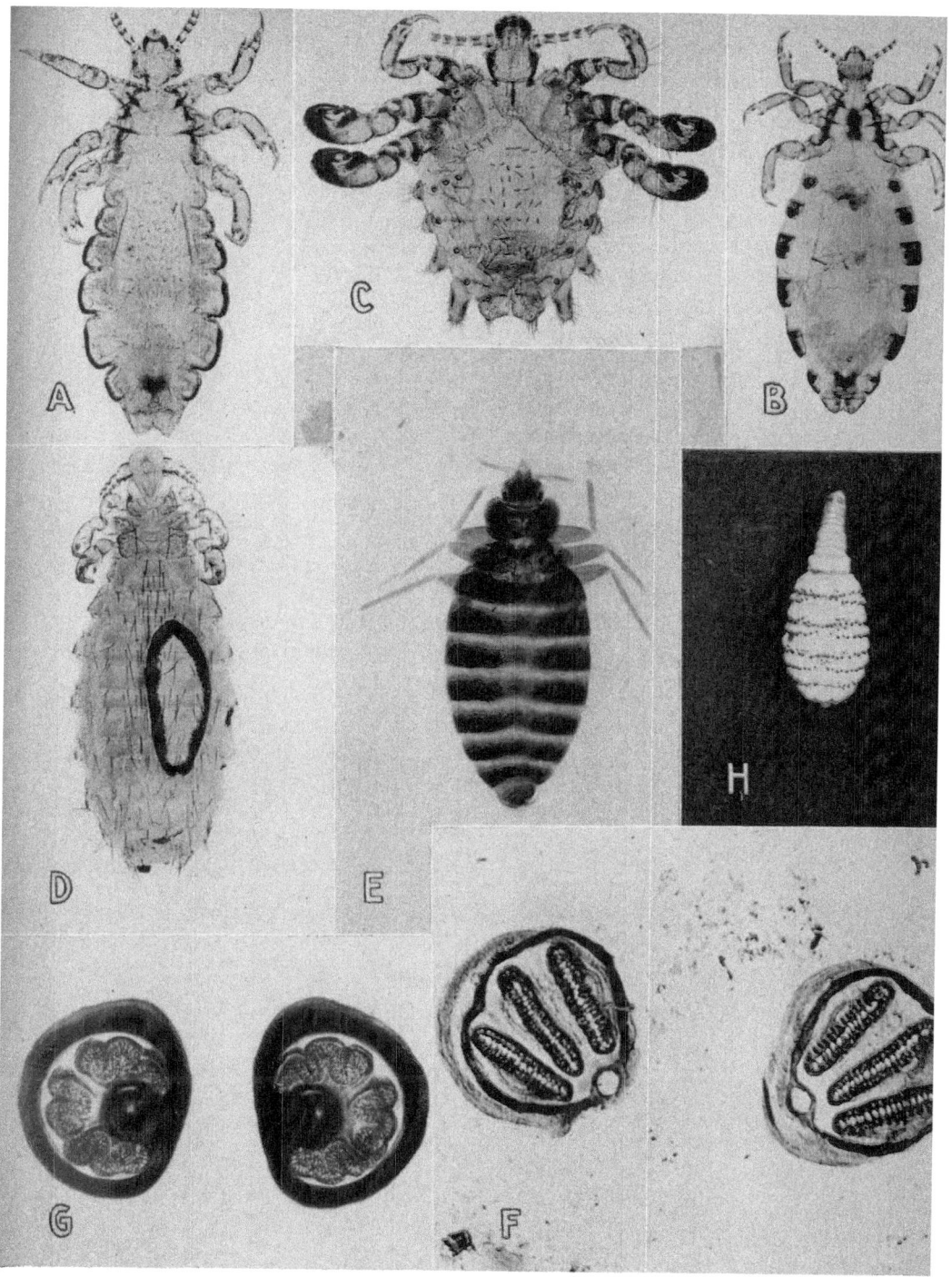

PLATE XVIII

A. *Pediculus humanus*, var. *capitis:* head louse. (x15)   B. *Pediculus humanus*, var. *corporis:* body louse. (x15)   C. *Phthirus pubis:* crab louse. (x15)   D. *Polyplax spinulosa:* rat louse. (x15)   E. *Cimex lectularius:* bedbug. (x10)   F. *Lucilia sericata:* spiracles of larva. (x125) G. *Musca domestica:* spiracles of larva. (x125)   H. *Dermatobia hominis:* larva. (x1)

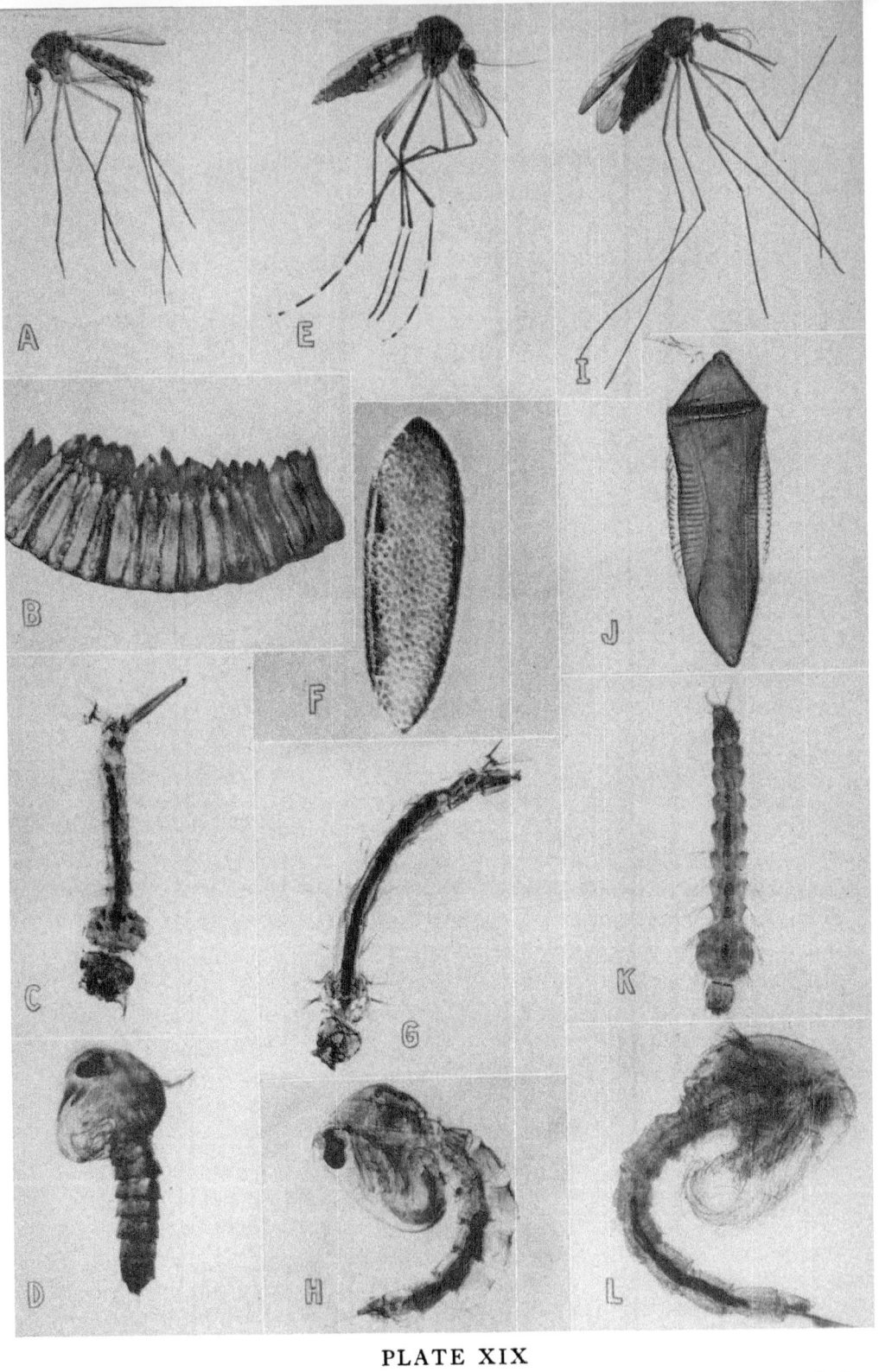

PLATE XIX

Culex fatigans: A. female. (x5)   B. raft of eggs. (x15)   C. larva. (x5)   D. pupa. (x5).
Aëdes aegypti: E. female. (x5)   F. egg. (x50)   G. larva. (x5)   H. pupa. (x5). *Anopheles quadrimaculatus:* I. female (x5)   J. egg, showing floats. (x50)   K. larva. (x5)   L. pupa. (x5)

given disease, often occur in such tremendous hordes and can bite human beings with such voracity and fierceness that human residence in areas infested by them is impossible. The females alone are able to suck blood.

CULICINI

The mosquitoes of the tribe Culicini which have medical importance are found in the genera *Culex* and *Aëdes*. The most significant species of these genera are *Culex pipiens, Culex fatigans, Aëdes aegypti, Aëdes albopictus, Aëdes taeniorhynchus, Aëdes vexans,* and *Aëdes sollicitans.*

Culex pipiens and *Culex fatigans.*—*Culex pipiens* is one of the most widely distributed species in the temperate zone and, because of its usual residence in or very near human dwellings, is one of the forms most annoying to man. In the tropics and subtropics, *Culex pipiens* is replaced by a closely related and almost indistinguishable species, *Culex fatigans.* Both forms are known transmitters of *Wuchereria bancrofti.* They are both night-biters and become infected with this helminth by biting patients with filariasis, whose blood contains the infective microfilariae only during night hours. (See Plate XIX, A, B, C, and D, facing this page.)

Aëdes aegypti.—*Aëdes aegypti* is probably the most completely domesticated of all mosquitoes. It does not exist except within or near human dwellings. It breeds almost exclusively in artificial containers, such as wells, rain barrels, flower vases, tin cans, and gutters of roofs, although also in holes in tree stumps. The adult form of this insect can be rather easily recognized by the lyre-shaped silvery lines on the dorsum of the thorax and by the silvery banding of the tarsi. (See Plate XIX, E, F, G, and H, facing this page.)

Aëdes aegypti is the known vector of the filtrable viruses of yellow fever and dengue fever (also called breakbone fever). The yellow fever virus must be taken up within three or four days after the patient exhibits symptoms. From nine to fourteen days thereafter, the infected mosquito becomes capable of passing the virus to a next person. Once the capacity to infect is developed, it is retained by the mosquito for at least several months.

In order to transmit dengue fever, *Aëdes aegypti* must bite a patient during the first three days of fever. From eight to eleven days later, the mosquito becomes infective for a next person, and it remains so for life.

Aëdes albopictus, Aëdes stokesi, etc.—Until a few years ago, *Aëdes aegypti* was considered the only vector of yellow fever and dengue fever. Several other forms have now been proved potential transmitters. One of the most important is *Aëdes albopictus*, which is widely distributed in the Orient. In West Africa *Aëdes stokesi* and in Ethiopia *Aëdes luteocephalus* have been shown capable of transmitting the yellow fever virus. The vector of "jungle fever," the form of yellow fever in the South American jungle, is not yet established. *Aëdes aegypti* is completely absent from the endemic area, but other forms (*Aëdes leucolaenus*) have been found naturally infected in Brazil. Certain species of *Aëdes* transmit equine encephalomyelitis to man.

Other species of Aëdes.—Many species of *Aëdes* mosquitoes are known vectors of no disease agent but are annoying to man through their fierce and frequent bites. In some regions they occur in such abundance that human residence is impossible. *Aëdes sollicitans* is the common salt marsh New Jersey mosquito, of which everyone in the East has heard. Actually, it occurs along the entire Atlantic and Gulf coast of the United States. Along the Pacific coast, it is replaced by *Aëdes squamiger*, which similarly is a vicious biter. *Aëdes taeniorhynchus* occurs in salt marshes along both the Atlantic and Pacific coasts of both North and South America, extending on the Atlantic as far north as Connecticut, and on the Pacific to California. In the northern woodlands of the United States, *Aëdes stimulans* and *Aëdes excrucians* are well known. One of the most widely distributed of all mosquitoes is *Aëdes vexans*.

ANOPHELINI

The mosquitoes of the tribe Anophelini (the anophelines) as a group are somewhat easily identified at any stage of development. The eggs are equipped with lateral floats and are laid singly. The larvae, which bear no siphon or air tube, feed and rest parallel to the surface of the water in which they occur. The body of the adult is usually held at a distinct angle (30° to 90°) to the surface on which the insect is resting, the head and proboscis being in the same plane as the body. With mosquitoes of the genus Culex, on the other hand, eggs are laid commonly in "rafts," without special floats. The larvae have an air siphon and rest with the head end suspended downwards. The adult body is held parallel to the surface on which the insect rests, with the head and proboscis in a plane different from that of the body. (See Plate XIX, I, J, K, and L, facing page 229.)

Altogether about one hundred and fifty species are found in the single genus, *Anopheles*, of the tribe Anophelini. Of these, thirty-two species are known to be good vectors of malarial parasites, and some others are known to be susceptible to experimental infection and thereafter capable of transmitting the organisms. Often a good vector in one community will not be a significant transmitter in another. The most important transmitters in the United States are *Anopheles quadrimaculatus* and *Anopheles maculipennis*.

Anopheles quadrimaculatus.—*Anopheles quadrimaculatus* is found in southern Canada, in much of eastern and southern United States, and in Mexico, where it is the most important vector of malaria. It is chiefly a night-biting form, although, sometimes, it will bite persons in darkened rooms during the daytime. Usually in the lighted hours it remains in dark, secluded areas.

Anopheles maculipennis.—*Anopheles maculipennis* is the most widely distributed species of anopheline mosquito. It occurs in Europe, North Africa, Asia Minor, the Orient, Alaska, western Canada, and northwestern United States. In all these areas it is a dangerous transmitter of malarial organisms. It bites by day as well as by night.

Anopheles pseudopunctipennis.—*Anopheles pseudopunctipennis* is an important vector of malaria in the Argentine and elsewhere in South America, where it is widely distributed. It is said, on the other hand, not to be a carrier in the United States, where it occurs in the valleys and coastal areas of the Southwest.

Other species of Anopheles.—Many other species of *Anopheles* are known to be important vectors in certain parts of the world. In the West Indies *Anopheles albimanus*, in North Africa *Anopheles algeriensis*, in tropical Africa *Anopheles gambiae*, and in Malaya and the Far East *Anopheles maculatus*, *Anopheles ludlowi*, and *Anopheles stephensi* are significant transmitters. *Anopheles gambiae* has recently been introduced from Africa to Brazil.

The eradication and control of mosquitoes is a problem of the greatest concern to public health officials. Generally the problem is attacked through the drainage of swamps or the spraying of oil or Paris green over waters which cannot be drained. When even this is not practicable, perhaps because of its great cost, such measures are resorted to as the stocking of the waters with fish (*Gambusia* sp.) which feed on the mosquito larvae, or with plants such as *Chara* spp. which presumably repel adult mosquitoes and thus prevent their egg-laying. An intensive inspection of the grounds about houses, as well as of the rooms inside, is also essential, for some species of mosquito are more or less completely domesticated and will not be affected by more obvious community measures. Individuals also can be protected from mosquito bites. The screening of houses provides effective protection to those indoors. Citronella oil, pennyroyal oil, and some other substances rubbed on the skin of those who must go out-of-doors, and especially into wooded areas, are often considered to act as mosquito repellants.

THE SIMULIIDAE (BLACK FLIES, BUFFALO GNATS)

GENERAL MORPHOLOGY

Black flies are small insects, one to several millimeters long, with humpbacked bodies and short legs. The antennae have eleven joints. The mouth parts of both sexes are suited for piercing and sucking, although only females are known to suck blood.

Eggs are laid near the surface of water, and hatch in from four to twelve days, depending on the temperature. The larvae, which pass through six moults during several weeks, are generally found attached to rocks in swift streams, especially mountain brooks splashing over stones. Pupation occurs in the same type of environment and lasts from two days to a week.

SPECIES IMPORTANT IN MEDICINE

Black flies are important both directly through their bites and indirectly through transmitting disease agents. The bites are peculiarly severe, considering the small size of the insect. During the bite, saliva is injected, and the anticoagulin which it contains prevents the healing of the bite wound. Consequently, blood will stream from the wounds of those bitten and when many bites are suffered this blood loss is serious. Many regions are uninhabitable during the black fly season, and persons who unwisely visit such areas run grave risks. Outbreaks approaching epidemic character have been reported in Central Europe and the United States. Animals as well as man are attacked. In man, the relatively painless bite is followed by prolonged hemorrhage. In a few hours, a papular lesion develops, often with extensive edema. Intense itching and inflammation are then noted. Lymphatic gland involvement may follow, tenderness and pain being noted on pressure. Generally symptoms subside so long as no further bites are experienced. Many persons who have long resided in black fly areas develop an immunity to the effects of the bite.

Eusimulium damnosum and *Eusimulium caecutiens.—Eusimulium damnosum* occurs widely in tropical Africa, where it transmits the filarial worm, *Onchocerca volvulus. Eusimulium caecutiens,* which occurs in the mountains of Guatemala, transmits the same filarial worm in Central America. Nodular swellings occur on the head, shoulder blades, ribs, and elsewhere of the bitten person, and these contain the adult worms as well as many microfilariae. Blindness is a not-infrequent sequel of this infection, the microfilariae often invading the eyeball. The parasite will also develop in some other species of black fly.

CONTROL MEASURES

Protection of the exposed individual against black flies is generally attempted through applying various repellants to his skin. These usually involve essentially the same materials employed as repellants of mosquitoes. Measures directed against the breeding habits of the fly are seldom effectual. The fact that it develops in splashing rather than still water adds to the difficulty of its control.

THE CHIRONOMIDAE (GNATS; PUNKIES; NO-SEE-UMS)

The bloodsucking chironomid flies are small insects having wings ornamented with dark spots, and antennae with thirteen to fifteen segments. The larvae are aquatic.

Nearly all the chironomid flies of medical importance belong to the genus *Culicoides*. Several species, including *Culicoides furens*, *Culicoides guttipennis*, *Culicoides obsoletus*, and *Culicoides mississippiensis* occur more or less widely over the United States and bite man and other animals with avidity. Usually some redness and swelling follow, with intense itching. No serious effects generally ensue.

Culicoides austeni, Culicoides grahami, and Culicoides furens.—Culicoides austeni and *Culicoides grahami* are believed to be the transmitters of *Acanthocheilonema perstans*, a filarial worm widely distributed in Africa and found in some parts of South America. In northern South America, *Culicoides furens* is believed to transmit another filarial worm, *Mansonella ozzardi*.

THE TABANIDAE (HORSEFLIES; DEER FLIES)

GENERAL MORPHOLOGY

The tabanid flies are stout, strong-looking, brilliantly colored flies with few bristles and large, prominent eyes. The costal vein extends around the entire wing. The third joint of the antenna is annulated but bears no style. Some species are no larger than the common housefly, but others have a wing expanse of more than two inches. The mouth parts are adapted for piercing. The female flies alone suck blood, males taking only more available liquids such as plant juices and other fluids.

LIFE HISTORY

Horseflies are usually encountered near streams or other bodies of water. Eggs are laid in masses on objects over water, such as foliage or the stems of plants. The larvae live in water and are usually actively carnivorous or even cannibalistic. Growth is comparatively slow, often requiring nearly a year. Pupation, lasting but a few weeks, occurs in dry, compact soil.

SPECIES IMPORTANT IN MEDICINE

Many tabanid flies (e.g., *Tabanus* spp., *Chrysops* spp.) are extremely annoying not only to man but also to animals by reason of their persistence in obtaining blood as food. They are particularly active on sunny, hot, humid days. Their bite is painful, and even horses which many forms attack, are sensitive of their presence. The loss of blood itself is serious, for, in proportion to their weight, these insects ingest large amounts of blood. In addition, some forms are important as vectors of disease agents.

Chrysops dimidiata.—The mangrove fly, *Chrysops dimidiata,* is the natural transmitter of the filarial worm *Loa loa* in Africa. It is a day-biting insect, and the microfilariae of this parasite occur in man's peripheral blood in the daytime. Biologic development of the parasite goes on in the fly, and ten to twelve days must elapse following an infective feeding before a fly can transmit the disease agent. Within a week, usually, unless it becomes reinfected, the fly loses its capacity to transmit the organism.

Chrysops discalis.—*Chrysops discalis* is a mechanical transmitter of *Pasteurella tularense,* the bacillus of tularemia or rabbit fever. The disease can be carried by the fly not only among wild rodents but also from rodents to man.

Tabanus striatus; other tabanids.—*Tabanus striatus* is a potential mechanical vector of the bacillus of anthrax (*Bacillus anthracis*). Human as well as animal infections by fly bite have been reported. A number of tabanid flies, including *Tabanus nemoralis,* are believed capable of transmitting mechanically the trypanosomes of surra (*Trypanosoma evansi*) and of dourine (*Trypanosoma equiperdum*).

THE MUSCIDAE (BITING STABLE FLIES; TSETSE FLIES; HOUSEFLIES; BLOWFLIES)

In the family Muscidae are grouped a number of species of biting flies as well as many forms which are not adapted for bloodsucking. Those of medical importance will be described individually. With the exception of the tsetse flies, none of the forms is known to act as the biologic transmitter of any disease agent. The classification of the group is not as yet well worked out.

Stomoxys calcitrans.—The biting stable fly, *Stomoxys calcitrans,* resembles the common housefly but has a proboscis for piercing, distinct wing venation, and rounded spots on its abdomen. It frequents stables and dwellings in late summer and autumn, and both males and females bite cattle, horses, and man, as well as many other animals. Larval development goes on in the dung of many barnyard animals. Although extremely annoying because of its bite, the insect is not otherwise harmful. It is not the biologic vector of any human disease, although it is known to be able to transmit mechanically several trypanosomes among animals, notably *Trypanosoma evansi* of surra.

Glossina spp.—The tsetse flies (*Glossina* spp.) are all confined to tropical Africa, where they have great importance as the biologic vectors of trypanosomes of man and other animals. They are very distinctive forms in appearance. They have a proboscis for piercing, their wing venation is distinctive, and their wings when at rest are folded scissorslike over the abdomen. *Glossina palpalis* is the vector of *Trypanosoma gambiense* of man in Central and West Africa, and *Glossina morsitans* transmits *Trypanosoma rhodesiense* in man and *Trypanosoma brucei* in animals in Rhodesia. In tsetse fly belts of Africa, the flies are often controlled by removing underbrush, or even by the more direct methods of killing individual flies or especially their larvae and pupae. Reproduction in these flies is slow, and each female produces but few eggs per year. The eggs are not deposited as are those of most insects, but are developed one at a time and retained within the uterus. The larva obtains its nourishment from the mother fly through sucking upon milk glands which open into the uterus. After three months, the larva leaves the uterus of the mother fly and pupates on sand or other suitable substance. Direct methods of destruction, because of the slow development, are of considerable effect in keeping down the total fly population.

Musca domestica.—The housefly (or typhoid fly) is found in and about dwellings over the entire world. The body is of grey color, with four black lines running the length of the thorax. The wing venation is rather distinctive, the fourth longitudinal vein turning forward near the margin so as nearly to meet the vein next in front.

Larval development of the housefly goes on rapidly in manure, and the entire life cycle is usually completed in from eight to sixteen days. In the tropics, breeding is continuous. (See Plate XVIII, G, facing page 228.)

Because of its habits of visiting fecal deposits of man as well as human food, the housefly is an admirable potential transporter of many types of human intestinal disease agents. It is known to carry on its hairy body or in its own intestine many intestinal bacteria, such as typhoid and dysentery bacilli, and the cysts of protozoans. Even the eggs of tapeworms can be carried in this way. None of the human pathogens, however, is known to experience development in the body of houseflies.

The control of houseflies is a difficult problem. Community measures are helpful, and cleanliness must be observed by any community which hopes to keep down the housefly menace. The incineration of garbage and the covering of manure dumps is absolutely essential in the control of the housefly. Individual homes can be protected by screens and by such added instruments as fly traps and poisons.

Blowflies.—The blowflies are important in medicine because the habit of their larvae is to bore through fresh or decaying animal tissue. Two of the important species will be mentioned.

Cochliomyia macellaria (the screwworm fly) is medically the most significant blowfly. It is a widely distributed form, being found from Canada to Patagonia. In the tropics it is a particularly troublesome pest. The females oviposit in wounds or in infected or decaying tissue of animals including man. Often eggs are laid in the nostrils or in the vagina. Within three to five days, the eggs hatch and the larvae begin migrating about, often carrying with them serious pathogens or boring into and destroying vital parts. Solutions of chloroform are often helpful in ridding an infested site of the larvae. *Chrysomyia bezziana* is confined to Africa, Asia, and the Philippines, where it causes infections much like those of *Cochliomyia macellaria*.

Bottle flies.—Several species of bluebottle flies (*Calliphora* spp.) and green-bottle flies (*Lucilia* spp.) are known to infect wounds in animals and, occasionally, man. The black-bottle fly, *Phormia regina*, also has been reported from man. All are widely distributed. (See Plate XVIII, F, facing page 228.)

Cordylobia anthropophaga.—The tumbu fly, *Cordylobia anthropophaga*, occurs widely in tropical Africa. Larvae penetrate the skin of the feet of children and reside therein for nine or ten days, after which they fall to the ground and pupate.

Auchmeromyia luteola.—The "Congo floor maggot" is the larva of *Auchmeromyia luteola*. It is a bloodsucker and feeds at night usually upon persons sleeping on earthen floors. After feeding, it retires to the soil.

THE ANTHOMYIDAE (LESSER HOUSEFLY; LATRINE FLY)

The lesser housefly (*Fannia canicularis*) and the latrine fly (*Fannia scalaris*) are two very similar forms, most easily differentiated in the larval stage, which in both species possesses featherlike or spinelike appendages on each segment. The larvae are sometimes recovered from the stomach, intestines, or urethra of both male and female persons. Infection occurs probably by anus or by urethra when the person is sitting in a crudely constructed privy.

THE OESTRIDAE (WARBLE FLIES)

All members of the family Oestridae are, in the larval stage, parasitic on mammals. The adult female fly visits the mammal only for egg deposition.

Dermatobia hominis.—The human warble fly, *Dermatobia hominis*, occurs widely in Mexico and Central and South America. The female flies oviposit on the abdomen of mosquitoes, usually of the genus *Psorophora*. The mature eggs hatch at once when the mosquitoes bite man, the fly larvae within the eggs evidently being stimulated by the warm temperature of the vertebrate host. The larvae transfer to the human host at this time and penetrate his skin, forming a boil or warble. They migrate in the tissue of the mammal for from six to eight weeks, then emerge for pupation. The lesion often persists for some weeks after the larva has emerged. (See Plate XVIII, H, facing page 228.)

Oestrus ovis.—The sheep nasal botfly, *Oestrus ovis*, oviposits in the nose or eyes of sheep. Oviposition has been reported also in the eyes of man.

Other oestrid flies.—The larvae of some other oestrid flies are occasionally reported from man, particularly *Hypoderma lineata* and *Gastrophilus intestinalis*. The second of these forms causes, in its first and second stages, a form of "creeping eruption" of the skin.

SYRPHIDAE (HOVER FLIES)

The larvae of various hover flies, but especially *Eristalis tenax*, are recorded occasionally from the feces of man. The form of the *Eristalis tenax* larva is distinctive in having a lengthy "rat-tail." Infection of man is probably by swallowing the egg in water or food. It causes no known pathology.

PLATE XX

A. *Pulex irritans.* (x50) B. *Xenopsylla cheopis.* (x50) C. *Ceratophyllus fasciatus.* (x40) D. *Ceratophyllus fasciatus:* larva. (x75) E. *Ctenocephalides felis.* (x50)

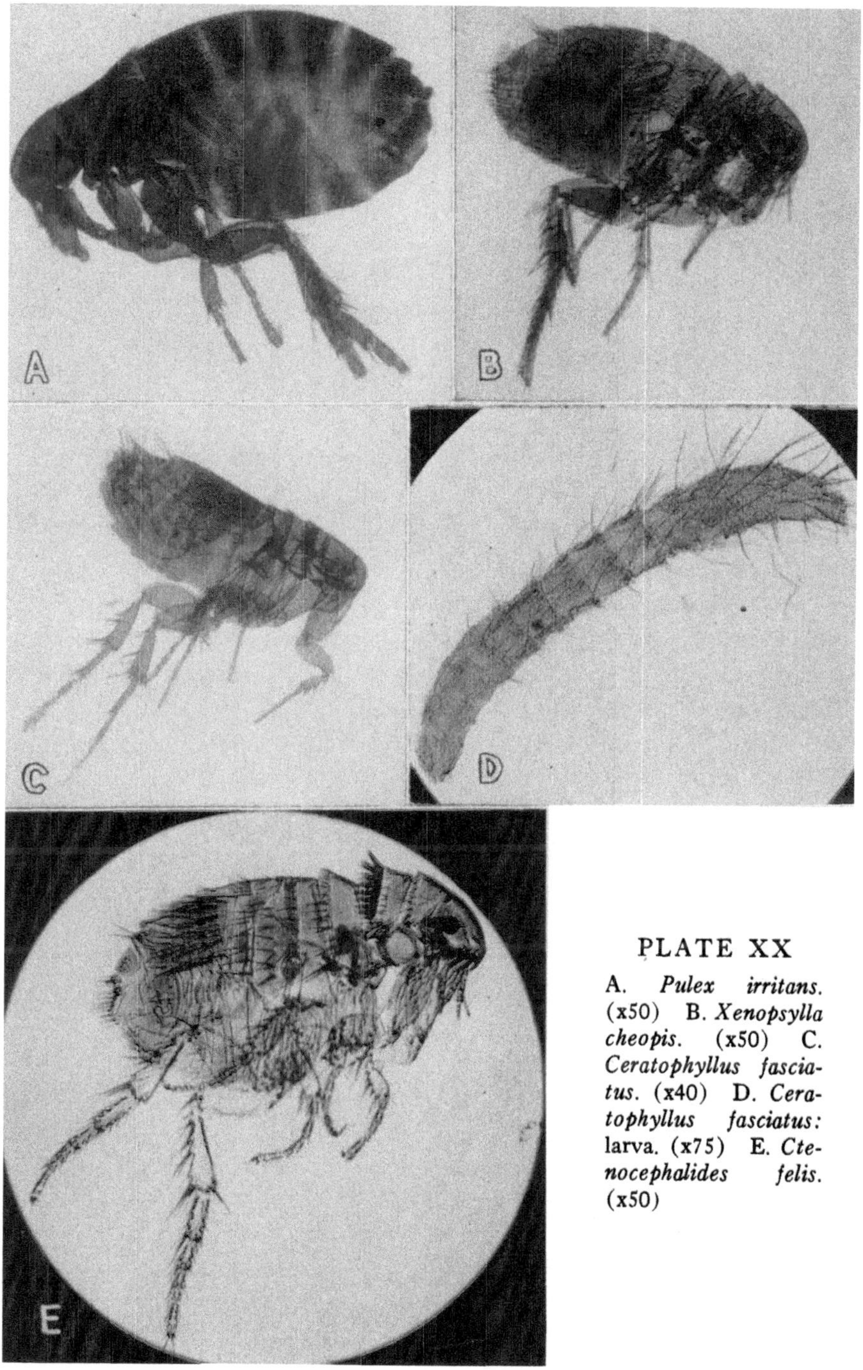

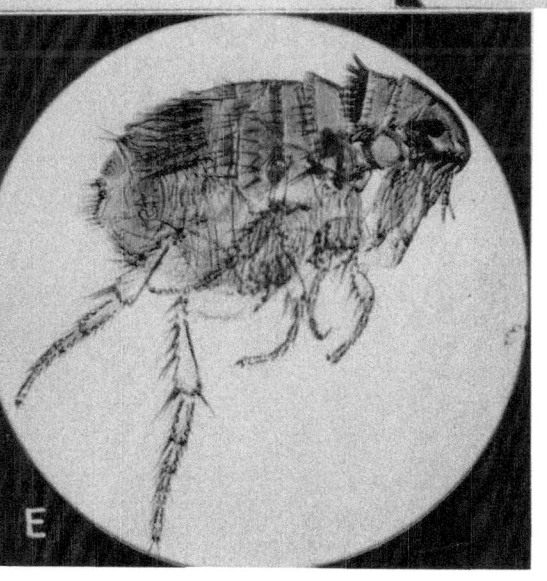

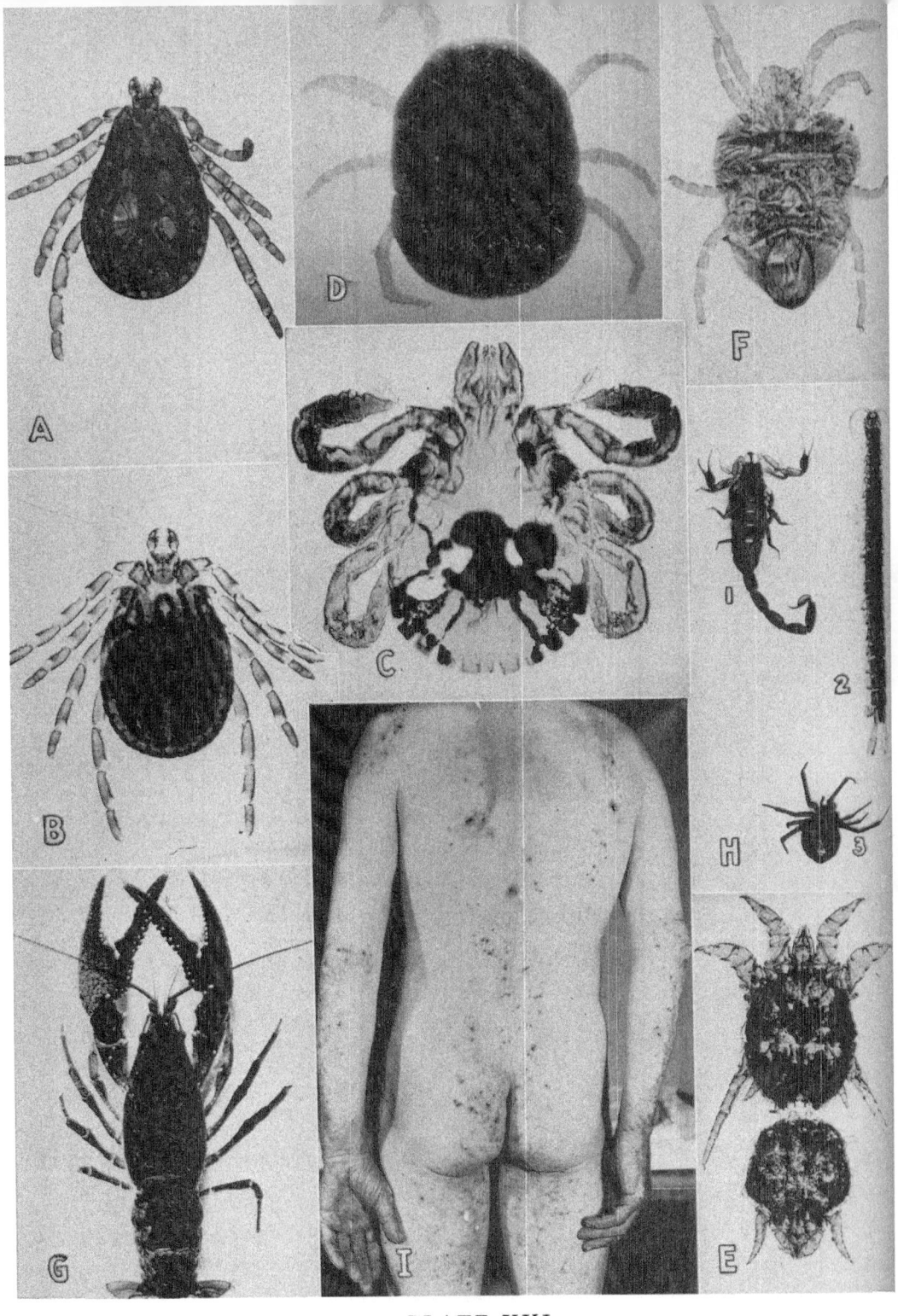

PLATE XXI

Dermacentor andersoni: A. male. (x3)   B. female. (x3)   C. larva. (x75)   D. *Ornithodorus moubata:* adult. (x5)   E. *Psoroptes communis:* in copulation. (x75)   F. *Trombicula irritans:* adult. (x10)   G. *Astacus* sp.: crayfish. (x½)   H. Venomous arthropods: 1, centipede; 2, scorpion; 3, *Lactrodectes mactans* (hourglass or black widow spider) (All, x½)   I. Human scabies.

The Siphonaptera (Fleas)

GENERAL MORPHOLOGY

Fleas are small wingless insects of which the body is compressed laterally. Mouth parts are suited for piercing and bloodsucking.

LIFE HISTORY

Flea eggs are usually deposited in the nests or on the fur of the host. They generally hatch in from two to twelve days. The larvae live in the nest or the fur for from seven to thirty days or so. They pupate in cocoons spun by the larvae. The adults are periodic bloodsucking parasites. They are not generally absolutely specific as to host, although they do reveal strong preferences. They may live for long periods. The human flea, *Pulex irritans,* survives up to about 500 days.

SPECIES IMPORTANT IN MEDICINE

Fleas are important not only because they annoy man by their bite but also because they transmit disease agents to man.

Pulex irritans.—The human flea, *Pulex irritans* (Plate XX, A, facing page 238), attacks skunks, dogs, squirrels, and even other animals besides man. It lives in bedding or in the crevices of houses and bites man chiefly at night. The bites are rather annoying to many persons. "Flea vaccines" have been injected with some success in the hope of artificially immunizing persons against attack by these creatures. The human flea also may serve as a transmitter of the bacillus of bubonic plague.

Tunga penetrans.—The jigger flea, sand flea, or chigoe, *Tunga penetrans,* occurs widely in many tropical and subtropical countries. It is one of the few forms of interest in parasitology which are known to have originated in the New World and to have spread to the Old World. Since late in the nineteenth century it has spread through Africa to India and the Far East. It is the smallest species of flea known. The fertilized female flea penetrates the skin usually between the toes and remains there while her eggs are being formed. During this time, her abdomen becomes swollen to the size of a pea. Itching and inflammation in the host is severe. Finally eggs are expelled usually to the soil by the flea, and the female herself then shrivels and drops out of the skin, her departure often being hastened by ulceration of the tissue. Many vertebrates, but man and the pig especially, serve as host.

Xenopsylla cheopis.—The Indian rat flea, *Xenopsylla cheopis* (Plate XX, B, facing page 238), is the most important vector of bubonic plague. It bites rats chiefly, but in the absence of rats it bites man about as readily. It transmits bubonic plague from the rat to man. In the United States, this species occurs along the east, south, and west coast. It is in part responsible in the southeastern United States for the transmission of endemic typhus from rat to man.

Ceratophyllus fasciatus.—The European rat flea, *Ceratophyllus fasciatus* (Plate XX, C and D, facing page 238), is widely distributed in all temperate climates. It bites rats, squirrels, or man and transmits plague bacilli among these hosts. It is responsible for the transmission of endemic typhus in the southeastern United States from rat to man.

Ctenocephalides canis; Ctenocephalides felis.—The dog and cat fleas (Plate XX, E, facing page 238) are important in disease chiefly by reason of the irritation which accompanies their bite. These fleas also serve as host for the cysticercoid stage of *Dipylidium caninum,* a cestode found as an adult in the intestine of the dog or cat and occasionally in children. The child is infected by swallowing an infected flea.

THE HYMENOPTERA (BEES, WASPS, AND ANTS)

GENERAL MORPHOLOGY AND LIFE HISTORY

Winged members of the order Hymenoptera have two pairs of membranous wings, the posterior pair being considerably smaller than the anterior pair. The wing venation is generally reduced. The mouth parts are suited for chewing or for both chewing and sucking. The abdomen of the females usually bears a modified ovipositor capable of functioning as a sting. The metamorphosis is complete.

SPECIES IMPORTANT IN MEDICINE

The order Hymenoptera owes its importance in medicine to those insects which are provided with a sting. Indeed, all the stinging insects are found in this order. They are the honeybees (family Apidae), bumblebees (family Bombidae), wasps and hornets (Vespidae), digger wasps (Sphecidae), velvet ants (Mutillidae), and stinging ants (Formicidae). A true venom is injected during the sting, and when many stings occur simultaneously the effect may be serious. In the case of the worker honeybee, *Apis mellifica,* the sting cannot be withdrawn after insertion and the whole tip of its abdomen is usually torn from the body by the bee as it struggles to get away. The sting and poison glands are left in the wound. The bee dies, therefore, as the result of stinging. Persons such as beekeepers, who may be stung many times through the course of a single season, develop an immunity not only to the bee venom but to the mechanical injury from the sting as well.

Chapter XX

ARTHROPODA OF MEDICAL IMPORTANCE: ARACHNIDA, CRUSTACEA, AND MYRIAPODA

THE ARTHROPODS, besides insects (which are discussed in Chapter XIX above), which have medical importance are found in the classes Arachnida, Crustacea, and Myriapoda of the phylum Arthropoda. These groups can usually be distinguished by any of several characters (see Chapter II), but most easily by the number of their legs. The arachnids possess four pairs, the crustaceans five pairs, and the myriapods still greater numbers of legs. Insects, on the other hand, have but three pairs of legs. Those species of arachnids, crustaceans, and myriapods of medical importance are mentioned in Table 7.

THE ARACHNIDA

The arachnids of significance in medicine are found in three orders, Acarina (ticks and mites), Araneida (spiders), and Scorpionida (scorpions), of which the first is decidedly the most important. These orders can be distinguished by the following key:

A. Abdomen segmented and armed with a sting—Scorpionida (scorpions)
B. Abdomen not segmented; sting absent
    I. Abdomen joined to fused head and thorax (cephalothorax) by a stalk—Araneida (spiders)
    II. Abdomen fused with cephalothorax, to form a saclike body—Acarina (ticks and mites)

THE ACARINA (TICKS AND MITES)

The species of the order Acarina are distinguished from other arachnids by the absence of segments in the abdomen and by the fusion of the abdomen with the cephalothorax. They vary much in size, some representatives being two centimeters or more in length while others are microscopic. Seven distinct groups (superfamilies) are generally considered as medically significant: Ixodoidea, Sarcoptoidea, Parasitoidea, Tyroglyphoidea, Trombidoidea, Tarsonemoidea, and Demodicoidea. These groups can be differentiated by the key which follows. An eighth group, the tongue worms of the family Linguatulidae, also is by many authorities included in the order Acarina.

Key to the Superfamilies of the Order Acarina (after Matheson [1]):

A. Body vermiform, distinctly segmented; legs rudimentary; parasites in hair follicles—Demodicoidea
B. Body not vermiform; not parasitic in hair follicles
    I. Trachea present; two spiracles opening through stigmal plates
        1. Hypostome large, with recurved teeth; skin leathery; large forms—Ixodoidea
        2. Hypostome small, without recurved teeth—Parasitoidea
    II. Trachea, if present, not opening through stigmal plates
        1. Trachea usually present, spiracle openings at base of chelicerae; larvae often parasites, adults free-living—Trombidoidea
        2. Trachea, if present, not opening at base of chelicerae
            a. Trachea present; body divided into cephalothorax and abdomen; abdomen showing segmentation—Tarsonemoidea
            b. Trachea absent; no division between cephalothorax and abdomen; abdomen without segmentation
                (1) Tarsi with stalked suckers; parasitic in all stages—Sarcoptoidea
                (2) Tarsi not with stalked suckers; not true parasites—Tyroglyphoidea

IXODOIDEA (TICKS)

The superfamily Ixodoidea includes all the large Acarina, which are commonly called ticks. These are distinguished from the other forms by their large size, their leathery skin, and, especially, their stigmal plates just behind and above the base of the fourth pair of legs. Many species of ticks occasionally bite man, although only one form, *Ornithodorus moubata*, is primarily an ectoparasite of the human host. Those species of medical importance are found in two families: Ixodidae (hard ticks) and Argasidae (soft ticks). The mouth

[1] R. Matheson, *Medical Entomology*, Springfield, Ill., C. C. Thomas, 1932.

parts of soft ticks (*Argas; Ornithodorus*) are concealed under the anterior margin of the body, whereas those of hard ticks (*Dermacentor; Haemaphysalis; Amblyomma*) are exposed. The bodies of the soft ticks are more flexible and leathery than those of hard ticks. The medically important forms of both families will be discussed.

Dermacentor andersoni.—*Dermacentor andersoni* [2] is commonly called the Rocky Mountain spotted fever tick, because it serves as vector of this disease. It is largely confined to the states of Washington, Oregon, Idaho, Montana, Wyoming, Nevada, Utah, and Colorado, although its presence is also recorded in states adjoining these.

The eggs of this species are laid on the ground in the spring. The six-legged larvae (Plate XXI, C, facing page 239), which hatch in a few weeks, feed on the blood of any of several rodents, such as ground squirrels, chipmunks, and rabbits. After feeding for a week or so, they drop to the ground and moult. The eight-legged nymphal ticks which are formed do not feed till the following spring, and then attach themselves to the same type of host (rodent) as was used by the larvae. After feeding, the nymphs drop to the ground and moult to the adult stage. The adult ticks (Plate XXI, A and B, facing page 239) do not feed till the spring of the next year, and then search for a larger mammal, such as horse, cattle, deer, coyote, bear, or man. On this host, mating occurs and the fertilized females engorge themselves with blood and drop to the ground for egg-laying.

Dermacentor andersoni is important in medicine for three reasons: (1) the direct effects of its bite, (2) its production of a generalized disease called "tick paralysis," and (3) its transmission of the rickettsia of Rocky Mountain spotted fever, *Rickettsia rickettsi.* Tick bites are often serious, for the capitulum which the tick inserts for drawing blood is dislodged only with difficulty and with considerable trauma. Because an anticoagulin is injected by the tick in biting, local hemorrhage commonly occurs. Fever is reported in many persons who are especially sensitive to tick bite.

The paralysis caused by *Dermacentor andersoni* is of an acute ascending type, sometimes fatal to children and to the smaller domesticated animals, such as sheep and dogs, if the tick is not removed. Presumably the disease results from the injection of a venom into the circulation by the tick, although the precise nature of the

[2] Common synonym: *Dermacentor venustus.*

inciting substance has not been proved. Recovery is complete soon after the tick is removed.

The transmission of the rickettsia of Rocky Mountain spotted fever by *Dermacentor andersoni* represents the activity of greatest medical significance carried on by this tick. The tick carries the rickettsia from the reservoir rodent host to man. The rickettsia can pass between male and female ticks in coitus and likewise can pass through the egg to the next generation from infected female ticks. The disease agent can, therefore, persist in the tick independently of the human host.

Dermacentor variabilis.—The dog tick, *Dermacentor variabilis*, occurs over the entire eastern and southern United States and on the western coast. It readily bites man and is believed to transmit among human beings the eastern variety of Rocky Mountain spotted fever, as well as tularemia.

Species of Ixodes.—Three species of the genus *Ixodes* are known to cause tick paralysis, *Ixodes ricinus*, *Ixodes pilosus*, and *Ixodes holocyclus*. These forms readily bite man, as well as many species of lower animals.

Haemaphysalis leporis-palustris.—The rabbit tick, *Haemaphysalis leporis-palustris*, is important because of its transmission of the rickettsia of Rocky Mountain spotted fever among rodent reservoirs. It does not bite man and therefore does not carry this infection to man.

Amblyomma cajennense and Amblyomma americanum.—*Amblyomma cajennense* occurs in Central and South America and in the West Indies. *Amblyomma americanum* is found in southern United States, Mexico, Central America, and parts of South America. Both species cause particularly painful bites which often become secondarily infected. Neither, however, is known to transmit any infectious agent.

Argas persicus.—*Argas persicus* is the common "soft" tick of fowls, which also readily bites man. It is said to transmit Miana fever among humans in Persia, although little is yet established concerning such transmission. Among fowls, it transmits a virulent spirochete, *Spirochaeta marchouxi*.

Ornithodorus moubata.—*Ornithodorus moubata* (Plate XXI, D, facing page 239) is a "soft" tick which prefers man as host but feeds on nearly all domesticated animals as well as other forms. It occurs widely in Africa. It is nocturnal in its habits and feeds on sleeping hosts, being sometimes called the "bedbug tick." It transmits the spirochete of African relapsing fever.

Other species of Ornithodorus.—Several species of *Ornithodorus* ticks which occur in Central and South America attack man. The most important are *Ornithodorus turicata, Ornithodorus talaje,* and *Ornithodorus venezuelensis.* The last two of these forms transmit the spirochete of South American relapsing fever. *Ornithodorus turicata* transmits the relapsing fever spirochete in southwestern United States.

SARCOPTOIDEA (ITCH OR MANGE MITES)

The superfamily Sarcoptoidea includes two species of mites of importance in human medicine: the itch mite of scabies, *Sarcoptes scabiei,* and the scab mite, *Notoedres* spp.

Sarcoptes scabiei.—The female itch mites burrow into and through the skin, particularly that of the fingers, wrists, axillae, groin, back of the knees, ankles, and toes. The burrow is serpigenous and eggs are laid along it. These hatch in three or four days and the six-legged larvae migrate to the surface and form vesicles in hair follicles. After two days or so, the larvae moult to eight-legged nymphs which form superficial burrows. Following two nymphal stages, adults are developed. After mating, the adult female then forms a new burrow and, at once, begins egg-laying. The entire cycle requires only from eight to fifteen days. (See Figure 15.)

The local irritation from the presence of sarcoptic mites is extreme,

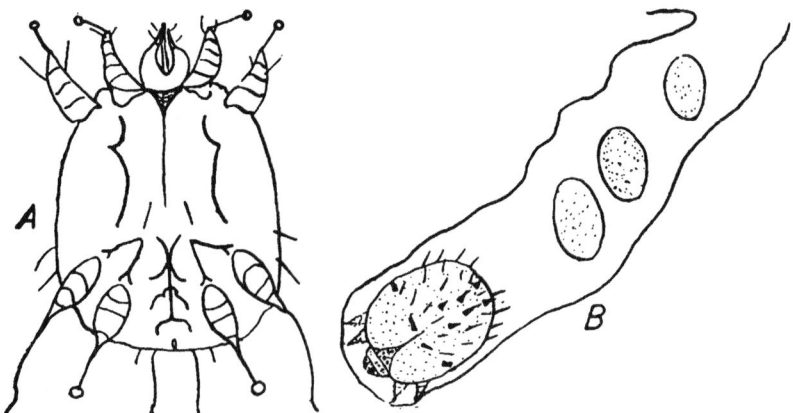

Figure 15. *Sarcoptes scabiei:* A, male; B, female laying eggs in tunnel in skin.

and bacterial infection of the irritated area often occurs from scratching. Unless treated, usually with sulphur ointment, lesions may become extensive. Particularly serious mite infections in Central Africa, known as craw-craw, and in northern and central Europe, known as Norwegian itch, are caused by this species. Transmission is through contact with infected persons or with their clothing. It is largely confined to armies and prisons. (See Plate XXI, I, facing page 239.)

Species of Notoedres.—The so-called psoroptic mites do not burrow but cause a most intense itching from superficial injury to the skin. Scabs develop characteristically, and hair falls out. Psoroptic mites infest many animals, but those of only one genus, *Notoedres*, attack man. The forms found on man are primarily ectoparasites of the cat. (Plate XXI, E, facing page 239.)

PARASITOIDEA (PARASITOID MITES)

In the large superfamily Parasitoidea are several mites that are found naturally on chickens and that sometimes infest handlers of these birds. The forms most significant are *Dermanyssus gallinae*, the common chicken mite, and *Liponyssus bursa* and *Liponyssus sylviarum*. The tropical rat mite, *Liponyssus bacoti*, also will infest man. All of these forms cause a dermatitis in man. The tropical rat mite also is capable of transmitting the rickettsia of endemic typhus. This mite passes the rickettsia to its offspring through the egg.

TROMBIDOIDEA (HARVEST MITES, CHIGGERS, REDBUGS)

Trombicula irritans and Trombicula autumnalis.—*Trombicula irritans*, the North American chigger mite (Plate XXI, F, facing page 239), occurs throughout eastern and middle-western United States. It is a small form, which attaches itself usually to the feet, ankles, and legs by its hooked chelicerae and armed palpi. It causes an intense itching and dermatitis. Many animals besides man, including rodents, birds, toads, and snakes, are infested. In Europe, a related species, *Trombicula autumnalis*, causes a similar infestation.

Trombicula akamushi.—*Trombicula akamushi* is found in parts of southeastern Asia, Japan, and Formosa where the six-legged larval stage readily attacks man, as well as field rodents. It is important as the vector of tsutsugamushi disease, which, presumably, is a rickettsial infection. The disease agent is retained by the mite during development, and adult mites, which feed only on plant juices or organic debris, can pass the agent congenitally to the next generation of larval mites.

TARSONEMOIDEA (PREDACIOUS MITES)

One species of the large superfamily Tarsonemoidea causes disease in man. This is *Pediculoides ventricosus,* the grain itch mite. Man is attacked while handling or otherwise having contact with infested grain. A vesicular or pustular rash spreads over the entire body of those attacked, and itching is extreme. Recovery occurs promptly when further contact is prevented or avoided.

TYROGLYPHOIDEA (CHEESE MITES, ETC.)

Mites of this superfamily abound in foodstuffs, and a dermatitis caused by them is often seen among those who handle food products. Workers in copra mills have copra itch, caused by *Tyroglyphus longior* var. *castellani;* vanilla workers have vanillism, caused probably by *Tyroglyphus siro;* and grocers have grocer's itch, caused by *Glyciphagus prunorum.* Many species of this superfamily have been recorded from the intestinal tract.

DEMODICOIDEA (FOLLICULAR MITES)

Mites of the superfamily Demodicoidea are parasitic in the hair follicles and sebaceous glands of mammals. They are very small, elongate forms with vestigial or stumpy legs. The form in man is *Demodex folliculorum,* which lives deep in the sebaceous glands and hair follicles. A related species, *Demodex canis,* causes follicular or red mange of dogs. The differentiation of many follicular mites of animals is difficult or impossible.

LINGUATULIDAE

The tongue worms or linguatulids are endoparasitic bloodsuckers, which are usually classed with the Acarina. They are wormlike forms without legs but with two conspicuous pairs of retractile fanglike hooks near the mouth. There are rather conspicuous annulations along the entire length, which falsely suggest segmentation. Development of all species, including *Linguatula serrata,* involves two hosts. Eggs of this form are eaten by rabbits, sheep, or by man. They hatch in the intestine, and larvae migrate to the liver and encyst while nymphal development occurs. If such liver is eaten by dogs or by man, nymphs may reach frontal sinuses and grow to adults. Eggs are then discharged in the mucus and waste from the sinus. Inflammation of the sinus tissue often occurs, with bleeding. Two species found in pythons are sometimes recovered from native peoples who eat python steaks. These are *Armillifer* (*Porocephalus*) *armillatus* in Africa and *Armillifer moniliformis* in the Orient. Human infection is known as porocephaliasis.

THE ARANEIDA (SPIDERS)

In all spiders, there is a fused cephalothorax to which an unsegmented abdomen is attached by a short pedicel. The mouth parts consist of a pair of chelicerae armed with a poison gland and a pair of pedipalps. Simple eyes may number from two to eight but may be absent.

All spiders possess two poison glands, the poison escaping from the saclike glands through ducts opening near the tip of the claw of each chelicera. With most species, including the tarantulas which so often induce dread, this poison is too mild for the bites of the forms to have medical importance.

Latrodectes mactans.—The only spider in the United States which can truly be called poisonous is *Latrodectes mactans*, the hourglass spider or black widow, which is found only in southern states. (See Plate XXI, H, facing page 239.) After persons are bitten by this form, their heartbeat may be slowed and local pain may be considerable. Usually symptoms persist for only a few hours.

THE SCORPIONIDA (SCORPIONS)

Scorpions are the only Arachnids which have a segmented abdomen, of which the posterior tip is armed with a sting. They also have large pedipalps bearing chelate claws. They are nocturnal animals, confined to warm countries. (See Plate XXI, H, facing page 239.)

The venom expressed during the stings of scorpions is fatal to small animals and even to children and, if several stings are experienced simultaneously, adult persons also may show severe effects. One of the best-known and most dangerous forms in Mexico is *Centruroides suffusus*. At least twenty species occur in the United States, these being found chiefly in the states bordering Mexico and in Florida.

THE CRUSTACEA

The Crustacea are important in medicine only as vectors of human parasites. Representatives of two orders are involved: Copepoda and Decapoda.

Copepods, chiefly of the genus *Cyclops*, are significant as vectors of the nematode *Dracunculus medinensis* and of the cestodes *Diphyllobothrium latum* and *Diphyllobothrium mansoni*. The eggs of these helminths are ingested by *Cyclops*, and larval forms develop in its body cavity. The copepod must then be swallowed by an appropriate vertebrate host for further development to go on. Copepods of the genus *Diaptomus* also are vectors of *Diphyllobothrium latum*. Man serves as a potential host for only the larval stage (plerocercoid) of *Diphyllobothrium mansoni*. He harbors the adult stage of *Diphyllobothrium latum*.

The only significant human parasite carried by decapods is *Paragonimus westermani*. This parasite encysts as a metacercaria in the tissue of the crayfish (*Astacus* sp., *Cambarus* sp.) or crab (*Potamon* sp.), and man is infected by eating such infected tissue. (See Plate XXI, G, facing page 239.)

THE MYRIAPODA

Centipedes (order Chilopoda) have wormlike bodies of many similar segments, each with one pair of legs. There is a distinct head which bears long antennae with many segments. On the first body segment are a pair of fangs, modified from legs. These are connected by a duct with a poison gland. The venom is of exceedingly low potency, and by some is thought to be rather a digestive ferment. Nevertheless, mice can be killed by the bite of some species of centipedes. In man, effects are usually mild, if noted at all. There is often some pain and local edema, at least, following the bite of one species, *Scolopendra heros*. The bite of most forms is harmless. (See Plate XXI, H, facing page 239.)

Millipedes (order Diplopoda) are not venomous. Some forms have been recovered from the human intestine. Certain species are potential intermediate hosts of *Hymenolepis diminuta*.

TABLE 7

ARTHROPODS (EXCLUSIVE OF INSECTS) IMPORTANT
IN MEDICINE

Order	Scientific Name	Common Name	Importance
Acarina	Dermacentor andersoni	spotted-fever tick	vector of rickettsia of Rocky Mountain spotted fever in West
	Dermacentor variabilis	dog tick	vector of rickettsia of Rocky Mountain spotted fever in East
	Amblyomma cajennense		painful bites
	Ornithodorus moubata	human soft tick	vector of relapsing fever in Africa
	Ornithodorus turicata		vector of relapsing fever spirochete in southwest United States
	Sarcoptes scabiei	itch mite	cause of scabies
	Dermanyssus gallinae	chicken mite	cause of dermatitis in man
	Liponyssus bacoti	tropical rat mite	vector of rickettsia of endemic typhus
	Trombicula irritans	North American chigger mite	cause of itching and dermatitis to agricultural workers
	Trombicula akamushi		vector of rickettsia of tsutsugamushi fever
	Pediculoides ventricosus	grain itch mite	cause of dermatitis in grain handlers body
Araneida	Latrodectes mactans	black-widow spider	venom inoculated by bite
Scorpionida	Centruroides suffusus		venom inoculated by sting
Copepoda	Cyclops sp.	Cyclops	vector of *Dracunculus medinensis, Diphyllobothrium latum,* and *Diphyllobothrium mansoni*
Decapoda	Astacus sp. Potamon sp.	crayfish, crab	vector of *Paragonimus westermani*
Chilopoda	Scolopendra heros	centipede	weak venom inoculated by bite

APPENDIX

Appendix

TECHNICAL METHODS

WHENEVER POSSIBLE, parasites are best examined alive. Generally, the living, moving organism reveals much about itself that any preservative will obscure or the most satisfactory dye will fail to show. Yet, in many cases, the parasites are wholly invisible except when fixed and stained, so that special procedures must be resorted to. In the following pages are presented brief summaries of the principal methods used in the preservation and examination of parasitological materials. In preparing materials for present or future examination, the freshness of the specimen is a matter of paramount consideration, since, after the death of either the host or the parasite, significant changes promptly set in.

THE PREPARATION OF ORGANS FOR MUSEUM PURPOSES

Organs may be prepared for museum purposes by preservation by Kaiserling's method or by treatment with alcohol or formalin. The Kaiserling method is definitely best.

KAISERLING METHOD

Two solutions are required for the Kaiserling method of preparing organs. These are:

Solution No. 1:		Solution No. 2:	
Formalin (40% Formaldehyde)	200 cc.	Potassium acetate	200 g.
Potassium nitrite	15 g.	Glycerine	400 cc.
Potassium acetate	30 g.	Water	2000 cc.
Water	1000 cc.	Thymol	1%

Immerse the specimen first in Solution No. 1, being careful that all parts of the specimen are reached by the solution. Solid organs should be injected in several places with from 2 to 5 cc. of the solution by means of a hypodermic syringe. The time required varies with the size and thickness of the specimen, as little as 1 or 2 hours sufficing for a thin bowel, whereas up to

72 hours may be required for a liver or spleen. The organ should be drained, then immersed in alcohol until the original color is restored. It is then placed in Solution No. 2 in a museum jar.

ALCOHOL METHOD

The preservative solution consists of 2 parts of alcohol (95 percent) and 1 part water. Organs can be preserved in this alcohol-water mixture, the fluid being changed daily for the first week. Although this method successfully preserves the organ, the natural color of the organ cannot subsequently be restored. For specimens showing gross pathological changes, it is quite satisfactory.

FORMALIN METHOD

The preservative solution consists of 1 part of formalin (40 percent formaldehyde) and 9 parts of water or physiological saline. This solution is an excellent fixative since it penetrates rapidly, but it spoils the natural colors of the organs. The solution should be changed daily for several days. The specimen can finally be stored in the same fluid.

THE FIXATION AND PRESERVATION OF TISSUES FOR SECTION CUTTING

Tissues and organs prepared for sectioning must first be cut into small pieces not over ¾ inch square by ¼ inch thick. Lengths of intestine or stomach are best pinned out on a flat surface and cut into 1-inch lengths after the whole has been fixed and hardened.

No one fixative satisfies all purposes. One may satisfactorily show the tissue changes but fail to fix the parasites in the tissue. Others preserve the parasites well but are poor for the host tissues. It is, therefore, necessary to discriminate in the choice of fixatives, with regard for the end sought. Several standard fixatives follow:

ZENKER'S SOLUTION

Formula

Potassium bichromate	5 g.
Distilled water	200 cc.
Add, immediately before use:	
Mercuric chloride	5 g.
Formalin	10 cc
Acetic acid (glacial)	10 cc.

Zenker's fixative solution is excellent for all ordinary histopathological purposes in which paraffin blocks will be prepared and is very efficient for tissues containing parasites. It may not penetrate so quickly as other fixatives. Tissues, therefore, are usually left in the solution for from 24 to 48 hours, then placed in running tap water for 24 hours. They may be stored in 70 percent alcohol for an indefinite period thereafter.

BOUIN'S SOLUTION

Formula

Picric acid (saturated solution in distilled water)	75 parts
Formalin (40% formaldehyde)	20 parts
Acetic acid (glacial)	5 parts

Bouin's solution is also an excellent fixative for all general purposes and for most tissues containing parasites. Fix for 24 to 48 hours, renewing the fixative once or twice in the period, then transfer directly to 70 percent alcohol, after draining off the excess Bouin's fluid.

GILSON'S SOLUTION

Formula

Mercuric chloride	5 g.
Nitric acid (80%)	4 cc.
Acetic acid (glacial)	1 cc.
Alcohol (70%)	25 cc.
Distilled water	220 cc.

This is one of the best fixative solutions; it is also especially favorable for trematodes. Tissues may be left in it for 24 hours without injury. After washing in water, specimens are passed through the alcohols to 70 percent to which iodine has been added, then, if desired, stored indefinitely in alcohol of 70 to 85 percent concentration.

SCHAUDINN'S SOLUTION

Formula

Mercuric chloride (saturated solution in water or saline)	2 parts
Absolute alcohol	1 part
Acetic acid (glacial)	3%

This is a good general-purpose fixative solution, especially useful for intestinal protozoa and for cestodes. After fixation for 1 or 2 hours, specimens are transferred successively through the alcohols to 70 percent, in which they can be preserved indefinitely.

THE STAINING OF TISSUE SECTIONS

Tissue sections in paraffin which have been spread upon microscope slides can be stained by the following procedure:

a. Remove paraffin wax *thoroughly* with 3 separate washings with xylol.
b. Rinse off xylol *thoroughly* with 3 separate washings of absolute alcohol, then wash with water.
c. Stain with hematoxylin for 12 minutes, then wash with water.
d. Wash momentarily in 1 percent acid alcohol (6 to 8 seconds); wash with water.
e. Wash in 0.5 percent ammonia water until section turns blue.
f. Stain with eosine (20 to 25 seconds).
g. Dehydrate *thoroughly* with three separate applications of absolute alcohol.

h. Clear with creosote.

i. Remove creosote with xylol.

j. Add Canada balsam and cover with slip.

SPECIAL METHODS FOR BLOOD WORK

CLEANING SLIDES AND COVER SLIPS

It is necessary, particularly in blood work, that the slides and cover slips used be thoroughly clean. Slides may be immersed in 5 percent ammonia water or in hot soapy water, rinsed in water and alcohol, wiped dry with a lint-free towel, and stored away from dust. Cover slips may be cleaned by immersion in 1 percent hydrochloric acid in 95 percent alcohol, rinsed in water, and dried with a handkerchief or other soft cloth prior to use.

MAKING BLOOD FILMS

Thin blood films

a. Place a small drop of fresh blood near one end of a clean slide.

b. Bring a second slide to the edge of the drop and, after the blood has traveled along the line of contact of the slides, spread it to a film.

c. The film may then be stained by the Wright, the Giemsa, or another appropriate stain.

Thick blood films

a. Place four small drops of fresh blood on a clean slide, so as to form corners of a square 1 centimeter on a side.

b. With the edge of a second slide, or with a dissecting needle, cause the drops to flow together to form a very thick film, 1 centimeter square.

c. After the film has dried, the film can be dehemoglobinized in distilled water and stained with a suitable dye.

GENERAL BLOOD STAINS

Wright's stain.—Wright's stain is used principally with thin blood films. The procedure follows:

a. The dry film is covered with Wright's stain for from 1 to 1½ minutes (one volume).

b. Distilled water (2 volumes) is added to the stain on the slide and the mixture is allowed to stand for 5 to 20 minutes.

c. After washing thoroughly in water, the film is allowed to dry and is examined with the oil immersion lens.

Giemsa's stain.—The Giemsa stain may be used with either thin or thick blood films. The procedure for its use follows:

a. Thin films are fixed in methyl alcohol for 5 minutes, then placed in Giemsa stain for 1 hour to overnight. After rinsing in water, they are allowed to dry and are examined with the oil-immersion lens.

b. Thick films are immersed in Giemsa's stain, without being previously de-hemoglobinized, for from 2 hours to overnight, rinsed in water, dried, and examined.

Stained blood films are best not covered, as balsam often gradually destains them. After the films have been examined under the oil-immersion objective lens, the oil may be removed with xylol.

SPECIAL BLOOD STAINS

Eosinophile stain.—The procedure for a special stain for eosinophilic leucocytes follows:

a. Prepare a thin blood film on a clean slide.
b. Fix film in methyl alcohol (1 to 3 minutes).
c. Wash with water.
d. Stain with hematoxylin (7 minutes).
e. Wash with 1 percent acid alcohol (6 to 8 seconds).
f. Wash with ½ percent ammonia water until film turns blue.
g. Stain with eosin (25 seconds).
h. Wash in water 1 minute.
i. Let dry and examine under oil.

Reticulocyte stain.—The procedure for a special stain for reticulocytes follows:

a. Place 1 drop of saturated solution (in absolute alcohol) of brilliant cresyl blue on a perfectly clean slide; let dry.
b. Rub off excess granules by rubbing very lightly with paper.
c. Place a large drop of blood on the film of brilliant cresyl blue.
d. Mix the blood and the stain with a needle.
e. Cover the mixture (to prevent evaporation) and let stand 3 to 4 minutes.
f. Using a second slide, spread out the mixture, following the procedure used with a fresh blood film.
g. Let dry, and examine with oil-immersion objective.
h. (Optional) Counterstain the film with Wright's stain.

PRESERVING AND EXAMINING THE PROTOZOA
A. THE INTESTINAL PROTOZOA

PRESERVATION OF FECES IN BULK

a. Feces containing protozoal cysts can be preserved by adding an abundance of Schaudinn's fluid.
b. After fixation for 24 hours, the supernatant fluid should be decanted off and replaced with 70 percent alcohol.
c. The material should be allowed to settle two or three times and the alcohol changed.
d. Finally the feces should be stored in 70 percent alcohol. (Formalin—10 percent in water or saline—may be substituted for the alcohol, the feces finally being stored in formalin of this same strength.)

CONCENTRATION METHOD FOR PROTOZOAL CYSTS

a. Ten grams of feces should be emulsified in about 200 cc. of distilled water and let stand 30 minutes so that the heavier particles may settle out.
b. The supernatant fluid is then decanted and diluted with distilled water to 1000 cc.
c. After standing in the refrigerator overnight, the supernatant fluid is decanted, and the sediment is washed in water, then precipitated by centrifugation at 2000 revolutions per minute for 2 minutes.
d. The sediment is then examined for protozoal cysts.

FRESH MOUNTS OF INTESTINAL PROTOZOA

Emulsify a small particle of feces in physiological saline or in a water solution of eosine or neutral red. In saline, the chromatoid bar of *Endamoeba histolytica* cysts is brought out clearly. The dyes reveal whether the protozoa are living or dead, only dead cells being stained by them. Nuclei of intestinal protozoan cysts are differentially stained, as are also glycogen granules, if the feces is emulsified in iodine solution. The iodine solution can be made as follows: iodine, 1 g.; potassium iodide, 2 g.; distilled water, 1000 cc.

STAINING INTESTINAL PROTOZOA

The most satisfactory method for staining intestinal protozoa and their cysts is that of Heidenhain by iron-alum hematoxylin. Other simpler staining procedures are also available.

Heidenhain's iron-alum hematoxylin stain.—The procedure is as follows:

a. Fix smears in Schaudinn's fluid.
b. Pass through 70 percent alcohol, 70 percent alcohol plus iodine, 50 percent alcohol, and 30 percent alcohol (5 minutes each).
c. Wash in distilled water for 10 minutes.
d. Leave smear in mordant for 6 hours. (Mordant = 4 percent iron alum.)
e. Wash momentarily in distilled water.
f. Stain with hematoxylin for 6 hours to overnight. (Hematoxylin = 1 g. hematoxylin crystals + 10 cc. 90 percent alcohol + 90 cc. distilled water.)
g. Wash in distilled water. (Smears are now jet black.)
h. Destain in 1 percent iron alum to desired color. (Observe process with scope.)
i. Wash in distilled water.
j. Dehydrate in alcohols to absolute alcohol (5 minutes each).
k. Clear with xylol.
l. Mount in dilute balsam.

Mayer's haemalum stain.—The procedure is as follows:

a. Fix smears in Schaudinn's fluid.
b. Pass smears through 95, 70, 50, and 30 percent alcohol (10 minutes each).
c. Wash in distilled water for 10 minutes.
d. Stain with haematoxylin mixture for 5 to 20 minutes.

Haematoxylin mixture

Haematoxylin	1.0 g.
Sodium iodate	0.2 g.
Potash alum	50.0 g.
Distilled water	1000.0 cc.

e. Wash in running tap water until smear is blue.
f. Dehydrate through alcohol series to absolute alcohol (10 minutes each).
g. Pass through absolute alcohol + xylol (equal parts) for 5 minutes.
h. Clear in xylol.
i. Mount in balsam.

CULTIVATION OF INTESTINAL PROTOZOA

Boeck's and Drbohlav's L.E.S. medium.—Endamoeba histolytica, the non-pathogenic amoebae, *Balantidium coli,* and certain of the intestinal flagellates can be cultivated in the so-called L.E.S. medium described by Boeck and Drbohlav. It consists of a coagulated whole egg slant which is covered to the top of the slant with a fluid made of 1 part inactivated human, horse, or rabbit serum and 6 parts Locke's solution. Cultures must be transplanted every 24 to 48 hours, a generous portion of the sediment being carried over each time with a pipette. The addition of a pinch of rice starch to the culture fluid partially inhibits the bacterial growth. Transfers are best made in a warm room with the culture tube to be inoculated as well as the pipette used for the transfer previously warmed to 37° C.

Craig's medium.—Craig's medium is similar to that of Boeck and Drbohlav but differs in lacking the coagulated egg slant. It consists of 1 part of sterile human, horse, or rabbit serum (freshly inactivated) plus 7 parts of Locke's solution.

Tsuchiya's medium.—Tsuchiya's medium consists of nutrient meat broth (pH 7.0) to which is added a small amount of a mixture of starch and charcoal. It can be used with or without a coagulated egg slant.

Wenyon's medium.—To 9 parts of physiological salt solution add 1 part of 2 percent nutrient agar. After autoclaving, cool to 50° C. and add to each tube containing 10 cc. of the mixture 20 drops of fresh rabbit blood without shaking. After incubation at 37° C. for 24 hours, the medium is ready for use.

B. THE BLOOD PROTOZOA

FRESH PREPARATIONS

Certain of the blood protozoa, e.g., the malarial parasites and the trypanosomes, can be examined in fresh preparations. A drop of fresh blood is placed on a clean slide, covered with a slip, and examined with the high-power objective.

STAINED PREPARATIONS

Thin or thick blood films may be prepared and stained as described above under methods for blood films.

CULTIVATION OF THE BLOOD FLAGELLATES

N.N.N. medium.—Certain of the blood flagellates can be cultivated in a medium prepared as follows:

a. Prepare the following "base" and place 5 cc. in test tubes:

Agar	14 g.
Sodium chloride	6 g.
Distilled water	900 cc.

b. Prior to use, add to the molten base, cooled to 50° C., 2 cc. of fresh defibrinated rabbit blood and let solidify as a slant.
c. After solidification, add 1 cc. of sterile distilled water and incubate 24 hours.
d. Inoculate the fluid in the tube with the flagellates.
e. Push the cotton plug far enough into the tube to permit inserting a cork stopper or covering with foil to prevent evaporation.
f. Incubate at room temperature or at 27° C.

(Bacteriological broth can be substituted for the water.)

FIXING, PRESERVING, AND EXAMINING HELMINTHS

GENERAL DIRECTIONS FOR MOUNTING ISOLATED WORMS

Wash the parasites well in normal saline or, better, in Ringer's solution before fixing, to remove extraneous tissues and mucus. They may be left in Ringer's solution for some time without harmful effects if the solution is changed frequently. Intestinal forms lose the epithelium if left long in saline. Specific directions for subsequent handling of the different groups of helminths follow:

Trematoda

a. Place the parasite in water on a slide and cover with a slip or a second slide, pressing down sufficiently to flatten the worm. If possible without injuring the worm, remove the eggs from the uterus (they are often removed by immersion of the worm in distilled water).
b. Place a drop of Gilson's fixative at one edge of the slip and pull this under by touching a piece of filter paper to the fluid at the opposite side of the slip.
c. After specimen becomes white about the edges, lift the cover several times to bathe all parts of the specimen. Leave in fixative for 2 hours, or longer if possible.
d. Transfer specimen successively through water and 35 and 50 percent alcohol, leaving in each for 2 hours if possible.
e. Wash several times in 70 percent alcohol to which iodine has been added. The worms may be left indefinitely in 70 percent alcohol.
f. Stain in Delafield's hematoxylin in 70 percent alcohol for several hours or overnight. To accelerate staining, place the worm in hematoxylin in a porcelain evaporating dish and heat the stain to steaming (*but not to boiling*) for 5 minutes.
g. Destain in 2 percent acid in alcohol until only a faint pink color remains and the organs are visible.

h. Rinse several times in 70 percent alcohol to which a few drops of ammonia are added until the specimen turns blue.
i. Transfer to 95 percent alcohol, then to absolute alcohol, leaving in each for 2 hours if possible.
j. Clear in creosote, then transfer to xylol.
k. Add Canada balsam drop by drop to the xylol; finally transfer to pure balsam.
l. Mount in balsam.

Cestoda

a. Lift a convenient length of the cestode to a dry glass plate. Flatten it at length upon the glass.
b. Let a film of Schaudinn's fixative solution run the length of the worm. After 15 minutes, immerse the cestode in the fixative.
c. Wash thoroughly in distilled water.
d. Transfer through alcohols to 70 percent + iodine, leaving 2 hours in each dilution. The worms may be left indefinitely in 70 percent alcohol.
e. Stain in Delafield's hematoxylin for 12 hours.
f. Destain with acid 70 percent alcohol until only a rose-red color remains in the organs and until all the red color has left the cortex.
g. Wash in 70 percent alcohol during 2 hours, with frequent changes of fluid.
h. Transfer to 95 percent alcohol for 2 hours, then immerse momentarily in 95 percent alcohol + eosine.
i. Transfer to 100 percent alcohol, to creosote, and to xylol. To the xylol slowly add balsam.
j. Mount in balsam.

Nematoda.—Permanent mounts of nematodes are usually not advised, if other means of preserving the specimens are available. Hot fixing fluids are preferred, since when fixed in cold fluids, nematodes curl into knots. They may be fixed in hot (80° C.) 70 percent alcohol or in hot 5 percent formalin. The worms may be left indefinitely in these solutions, 5 percent glycerin being added to the alcohol solution. Semipermanent mounts in pure glycerin, in glycerin jelly, or in lactophenol may be made of small nematodes. The cover slip of these mounts must be "ringed" first with balsam, then with gold size. Nematodes preserved in formalin can be cleared in 5 to 10 minutes by 88 percent phenol, then examined in temporary mounts in this fluid.

EXAMINING BLOOD FOR HELMINTH LARVAE

Methods similar to those used for the blood protozoa can be employed for helminth larvae of the blood (e.g., microfilariae). Fresh preparations reveal the active living worms. Thick blood films can be stained by Giemsa's stain or by the following method:

O'Connor's stain

a. Fix in alcohol-ether (equal parts) for 5 minutes.
b. Stain in hematoxylin for 8 minutes.
c. Immerse momentarily in acid alcohol.

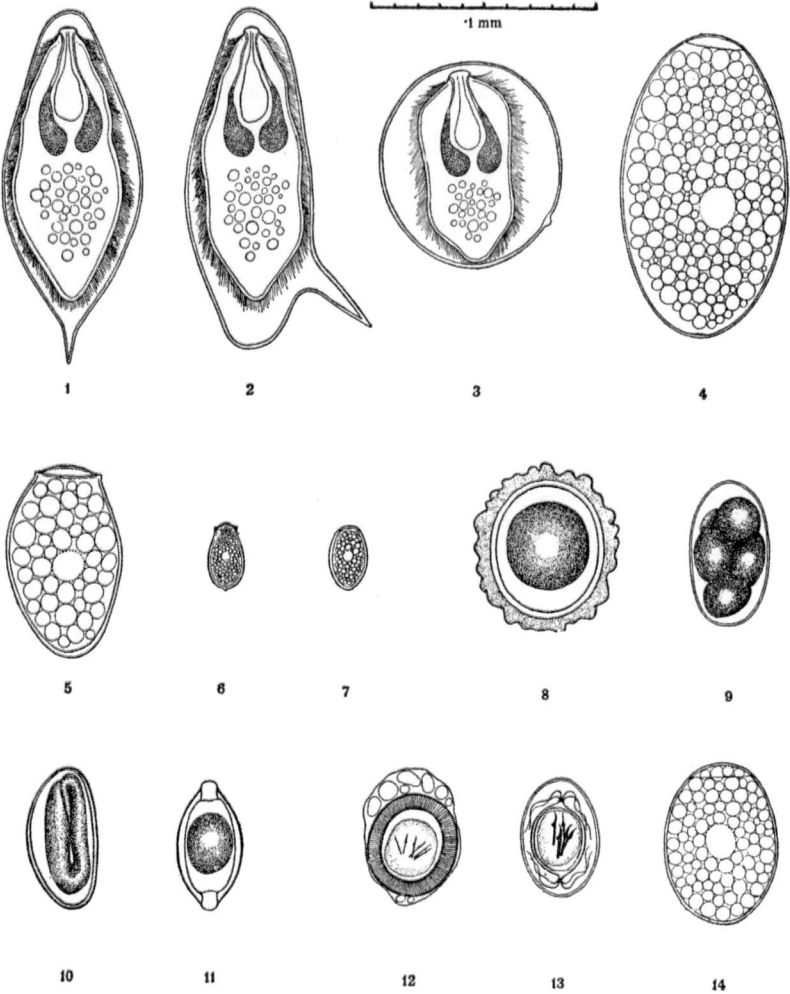

Figure 16. Eggs of medically important helminths: 1, *Schistosoma haematobium*; 2, *Schistosoma mansoni*; 3, *Schistosoma japonicum*; 4, *Fasciolopsis buski*; 5, *Paragonimus westermani*; 6, *Clonorchis sinensis*; 7, *Heterophyes heterophyes*; 8, *Ascaris lumbricoides*; 9, *Necator americanus* or *Ancylostoma duodenale*; 10, *Enterobius vermicularis*; 11, *Trichuris trichiura*; 12, *Taenia* spp.; 13, *Hymenolepis nana*; 14, *Diphyllobothrium latum*.

d. Rinse in ammonia water, then in water.

e. Let dry and examine under the oil-immersion objective.

PRESERVING AND EXAMINING HELMINTH EGGS AND LARVAE IN FECES

a. Mix the feces with an equal volume of 10 percent formalin. This suspension will keep indefinitely.

b. To examine for eggs or larvae, place a drop of the fecal suspension on a slide and cover with a slip. Observe with low then with high power of the microscope. (See Figure 16.)

c. To prepare semipermanent slides, rim the cover slip first with balsam, then with gold size.

CULTIVATION OF HELMINTH EGGS AND LARVAE

Charcoal method.—Mix a known quantity of feces with an equal amount of bone black or sterile soil in a covered vessel and incubate at from 25° to 30° C. After an interval which varies for different species, the appropriate stages will develop. The filariform stage of *Strongyloides stercoralis* generally is found after 36 hours and the same stage of the hookworms after 6 days. The worms may be isolated from the culture by a modification of the Baermann technique, described below.

Filter paper method.—Place a circle of moist filter paper in the lid of a Petri dish. Spread feces in a thin layer over the bottom of the dish. Incubate at 27° C. The larvae will climb the sides of the dish to the blotting paper. For prolonged incubation, seal the dish with plasticine.

Embryonation of helminth eggs.—The eggs of ascarids and some other nematodes must be embryonated before they are infective. This can be done by culture for from 2 to 4 weeks at 27° C. The eggs in a Petri dish are covered to a depth of about 1 centimeter with 0.2 percent formaldehyde water solution to inhibit bacterial growth.

CONCENTRATING HELMINTH EGGS IN FECES

Sedimentation method.—Thoroughly emulsify the feces in water (or, in the case of schistosome eggs, in saline), letting the emulsion stand for 2 hours. Decant the supernatant fluid and discard it. The eggs will be found in the sediment. Repeat this procedure several times.

Flotation method.—Emulsify the feces in 10 to 20 volumes of sugar solution (1 pound of sugar in 12 fluid ounces of water) or in saturated sodium chloride solution, in a vessel filled so that the meniscus is above the top of the container. After from 15 minutes to 1 hour, the floated eggs can be removed from the fluid surface to a slide with the bacteriological loop. As an alternate procedure, a cover slip may be floated on the surface of the solution for the interval (up to 1 hour). The slip will retain many of the eggs which come in contact with it, and these can be observed by lifting the slip, placing it on a slide, and examining with a scope. Hookworm, *Ascaris,* and *Hymenolepis* eggs will rise in the salt solution, and these as well as *Taenia* and *Enterobius* eggs will be floated in the sugar solution. Operculated eggs will not rise in either solution.

Centrifugation method.—Place 4 to 5 grams of feces in a centrifuge tube. Add water and agitate. Fill the tube with water and centrifugalize slowly for 1 minute. Decant the fluid. Completely fill the tube with brine, after thoroughly agitating the sediment. Place a cover slip over the tube and centrifugalize. Eggs will rise and be fastened to the slip. Examine the cover slip by the hanging-drop method.

CONCENTRATING HELMINTH EGGS IN URINE

Let the urine stand for several hours or overnight in a sedimentation cone or else centrifugalize the sample for several minutes at low speed. Transfer the sediment to a slide and examine microscopically. *Schistosoma hematobium* is the only important form whose eggs occur in the urine of man.

COUNTING HELMINTH EGGS IN FECES

Fulleborn's method

    a. Emulsify thoroughly a known weight of feces in brine in a round container.
    b. Float a round cover slip on the surface of the brine for 15 minutes to 1 hour.
    c. With forceps quickly lift off the slip vertically from the fluid surface.
    d. Determine by actual count the number of eggs on the slip.

No. of eggs on slip: Total no. of eggs = Area of cover slip: Area of the container

Stoll's method

    a. Fill a conical flask to the 56 cc. mark with 0.1/N NaOH. Add feces in small pieces to the 60 cc. mark. Add glass beads.
    b. Cork the flask. Shake thoroughly and violently.
    c. Remove 0.15 cc. of fluid to a glass slide. Count all the eggs present under the scope.
    d. Multiply the number of eggs counted by 100 to find the number of eggs per cc. of feces. Accuracy is estimated to be 80 to 90 percent.

ISOLATION OF HELMINTH LARVAE

From cultures or from soil (modification of Baermann technic)

    a. A culture or earth containing larvae is placed in a gauze-lined sieve which is fitted into a funnel. The funnel must be filled to the bottom of the sieve with water at 37° C. and must be closed at the stem end with a clamped length of rubber tube.
    b. After several hours or overnight, the larvae will have migrated down into the stem of the funnel and can be obtained by running out 50 cc. or so of the fluid from the stem.

The method is used chiefly with hookworm larvae.

From muscle

    a. Place the muscle, which has been cut or ground into small pieces, in artificial digestive juice (0.7 percent pepsin in 0.5 percent water solution of hydrochloric acid), using 30 cc. of the juice for each gram of muscle.

b. Keep the mixture in constant agitation and at a temperature of 37° C. for from 3 to 5 hours.

c. At the end of this time, transfer the digest to a large funnel of which the stem is closed with a clamped length of rubber tube.

d. After an interval of 1 to 4 hours, run out a few cc. from the bottom of the funnel into a sedimentation cone.

e. By repeatedly washing the sediment which will contain the larvae, a nearly pure mass of larvae finally can be obtained,

The method is used chiefly with *Trichinella spiralis*.

PRESERVING AND EXAMINING INSECTS

Insects and other arthropods may be preserved (1) dry, (2) in fluid, or (3) in balsam on a slide.

DRY MOUNTS

Such insects as adult mosquitoes and flies are killed with cyanide, chloroform, ether, or tobacco smoke. Large forms are pinned through the thorax with an insect pin and fastened firmly in a cork-bottom box which has been treated with creosote or paradichlorbenzene. Insect eggs as well as small insects may advantageously be fastened to a triangle of paper which is mounted on a pin.

FLUID PRESERVATION

Soft-bodied larvae of flies and mosquitoes, as well as adults and larvae of midges, fleas, and lice, are preserved in 70 to 85 percent alcohol after being killed in hot water and left in 50 percent alcohol for several hours. Heavily chitinized forms may be dropped directly into 85 percent alcohol. The addition of 1 percent glycerin to the final preserving fluid is advantageous.

Other preserving fluids are 10 percent solution of formalin and 5 percent solution of chloral hydrate. Fly larvae may be first fixed in Carnoy's fluid, then preserved in 85 percent alcohol.

Carnoy's fluid	
Chloroform	3 parts
Glacial acetic acid	1 part
Absolute alcohol	6 parts

SLIDE MOUNTS

Entire insects or their appendages (fresh or preserved) may be mounted on slides for study, the following procedure generally being satisfactory.

a. Boil the specimen in 5 to 10 percent caustic potash until it becomes transparent and free of tissue.

b. Soak in water to remove the alkali.

c. Dehydrate by transfer through alcohol to 95 percent alcohol.

d. Stain with acid fuchsin, if necessary.

e. Transfer to absolute alcohol, then to xylol for clearing.

f. To mount, place the specimen on a slide and cover with a drop of balsam.

Leave for 24 hours in order that the specimen may be fastened in position or arrangement on the slide. Then cover with a cover slip.

SELECTED IMMUNOLOGICAL PROCEDURES

Immunological tests are employed chiefly in the diagnosis of parasitic infections of the somatic tissues. They are used for some protozoan diseases but have proved most helpful in the somatic tissue helminthiases such as schistosomiasis, hydatid disease, cysticercosis, trichiniasis, and filariasis.

PREPARATION OF ANTIGEN

Whenever possible, antigen derived from the specific parasite should be used in performing immunological tests. Very often, however, when antigens of the specific parasite cannot be obtained, antigens from a closely related species will serve for the test.

An antigen suitable for most kinds of immunological tests can be prepared from helminth parasites in the following manner: the worm is thoroughly washed and dried, then triturated to a fine powder. One percent of this powder is extracted in Coca's fluid, carbolized saline, or physiological saline for 24 hours at 37° C. The suspension is then centrifugalized, and the supernatant fluid is decanted. This fluid represents a dilution of at least 1 to 100 of the dry substance.

With the protozoans, antigens usually are obtained from culture fluids or by extracting organisms grown in culture.

PRECIPITIN TESTS

Precipitin tests are used routinely by some laboratories for the diagnosis of trichiniasis and hydatid disease. These tests are performed as follows:

    a. With a capillary pipette place 0.1 to 0.25 cc. of the patient's serum in 8 small-bore precipitin tubes.

    b. With a second pipette carefully overlay an equal volume of successive dilutions (in the extractant fluid) of the antigen (from 1–100 to 1–3000) in tubes Nos. 1 to 7. In tube No. 8 place an equal volume of the extractant fluid as a control.

    c. After incubating the tubes for from 40 to 60 minutes, read the tubes for reaction at the interface of the fluids. It is essential also to test a known positive serum and a known negative serum simultaneously with the same antigens. A positive reaction is characterized by the formation of a flocculent precipitate.

COMPLEMENT FIXATION TESTS

The complement fixation test is used for diagnosing such protozoan infections as amoebiasis, malaria, trypanosomiasis, and leishmaniasis. It has had even wider application in the diagnosis of schistosomiasis, hydatid disease, and filariasis. The test is essentially like that of the Wassermann reaction except that the antigens used are derived from the specific parasites. A positive reaction consists in the fixation of complement by the union in vitro of the parasite antigen with specific antibody in the patient's serum. The procedure is so highly specialized that its particulars cannot be included here. The student is referred for details to special books which deal with the reaction.

INTRADERMAL TESTS

The skin of persons who are infected with any of certain kinds of helminths becomes sensitive to the antigens of the parasite. The reaction which follows the intradermal injection of these antigens often aids in identifying the corresponding infections. Usually an immediate response (within 5 to 10 minutes) occurs, although sometimes delayed reactions also are seen. Skin tests are especially helpful in diagnosing schistosomiasis, hydatid disease, trichiniasis, and filariasis. Skin tests have proved unsatisfactory thus far for diagnosing protozoan infections.

In performing the skin test, a small amount (0.1 cc.) of the *sterile* extract is introduced intradermally. An equal amount of the *sterile* extractant is introduced as a control. A positive immediate reaction consists of extension of the initial bleb into a wheal with distinct pseudopodia. An erythematous zone may or may not develop about the site of injection, and is best ignored as a diagnostic sign. It is often well to encircle with pen and ink the initial bleb so that any extension of the wheal can be more easily recognized. In delayed reactions there is local induration which appears in half an hour or so and may persist for from a few hours to a day or more.

BOOKS FOR REFERENCE

GENERAL

Brumpt, E. Précis de parasitologie. 4th ed., Masson, Paris, 1936.

Chandler, A. C. Introduction to Parasitology. 6th ed., Wiley, New York, 1940.

Craig, C. F., and E. C. Faust. Clinical Parasitology. 2d ed., Lea and Febiger, Philadelphia, 1940.

Hegner, R., F. M. Root, D. L. Augustine, and C. G. Huff. Parasitology. Century, New York, 1938.

Manson-Bahr, P. Manson's Tropical Diseases. 11th ed., Cassell, London, 1940.

Stitt, E. R., P. W. Clough, and M. C. Clough. Practical Bacteriology, Hematology, and Animal Parasitology. 9th ed., Blakiston, Philadelphia, 1938.

Strong, R. P. Stitt's Diagnosis, Prevention, and Treatment of Tropical Diseases. 6th ed., Blakiston, Philadelphia, 1942.

PROTOZOA

American Association for the Advancement of Science. A Symposium on Human Malaria, with Special Reference to North America and the Caribbean Region. A.A.A.A., Washington, D.C., 1941.

Becker, E. R. Coccidia and Coccidioses of Domesticated Game, and Laboratory Animals, and Man. Collegiate, Ames (Iowa), 1934.

Boyd, M. F. An Introduction to Malariology. Harvard University, Cambridge (Mass.), 1930.

Calkins, G. N. Protozoa in Biological Research. Columbia University, New York, 1941.

Craig, C. F. Amebiasis and Amebic Dysentery. Thomas, Springfield (Ill.), 1934.

—— Laboratory Diagnosis of Protozoan Diseases. Lea and Febiger, Philadelphia, 1942.

Hegner, R., and W. H. Taliaferro. Human Protozoology. Macmillan, New York, 1924.

Wenyon, C. M. Protozoology. William Wood, New York, 1926.

HELMINTHES

Baylis, H. A. A Manual of Helminthology. 2d ed., London, 1929.

Faust, E. C. Human Helminthology. 2d ed., Lea and Febiger, Philadelphia, 1939.

Lapage, G. Nematodes Parasitic in Animals. Methuen, London, 1937.

Yorke, W., and P. A. Maplestone. The Nematode Parasites of Vertebrates. Blakiston, London, 1926.

ARTHROPODA

Comstock, J. H. An Introduction to Entomology. Rev. ed., Comstock, Ithaca (N.Y.), 1933.

Ewing, H. E. A Manual of External Parasites. Thomas, Springfield (Ill.), 1929.

Fox, C. Insects and Disease of Man. Blakiston, Philadelphia, 1925.

Herms, W. B. Medical Entomology. 3d ed., Macmillan, New York, 1939.

Matheson, R. Medical Entomology. Thomas, Springfield (Ill.), 1932.

Patton, W. S., and A. M. Evans. Insects, Ticks, Mites, and Venomous Animals, Part I, Medical. Croydon (England), 1929.

Riley, W. A., and O. A. Johannsen. Medical Entomology. McGraw-Hill, New York, 1938.

SPECIALIZED TOPICS

Burnet, F. M. Biological Aspects of Disease. Macmillan, New York, 1941.

Culbertson, J. T. Immunity against Animal Parasites. Columbia University, New York, 1941.

Findlay, G. M. Recent Advances in Chemotherapy. 2d ed., Churchill, London, 1939.

Hull, T. G. Diseases Transmitted from Animals to Man. Thomas, Springfield (Ill.), 1930.

Perla, D., and J. Marmorston-Gottesman. Natural Resistance and Clinical Medicine. Little, Brown, Boston, 1941.

Smith, T. Parasitism and Disease. Princeton University, Princeton (N.J.), 1934.

Taliaferro, W. H. The Immunology of Parasitic Infections. Century, New York, 1929.

INDEX